Endovascular Management of Cerebrovascular Disease

Editors

RICARDO A. HANEL
CIARÁN J. POWERS
ERIC SAUVAGEAU

NEUROSURGERY
CLINICS OF NORTH AMERICA

www.neurosurgery.theclinics.com

Consulting Editors

RUSSELL LONSER
ISAAC YANG

July 2014 • Volume 25 • Number 3

ELSEVIER

1600 John F. Kennedy Boulevard • Suite 1800 • Philadelphia, Pennsylvania, 19103-2899

http://www.theclinics.com

NEUROSURGERY CLINICS OF NORTH AMERICA Volume 25, Number 3
July 2014 ISSN 1042-3680, ISBN-13: 978-0-323-31166-3

Editor: Jennifer Flynn-Briggs
Developmental Editor: Yonah Korngold

Neurosurgery Clinics of North America (ISSN 1042-3680) is published quarterly by Elsevier Inc., 360 Park Avenue South, New York, NY 10010-1710. Months of issue are January, April, July, and October. Business and Editorial Offices: 1600 John F. Kennedy Blvd., Suite 1800, Philadelphia, PA 19103-2899. Customer Service Office: 11830 Westline Industrial Drive, St. Louis, MO 63146. Periodicals postage paid at New York, NY, and additional mailing offices. Subscription prices are $380.00 per year (US individuals), $572.00 per year (US institutions), $415.00 per year (Canadian individuals), $711.00 per year (Canadian institutions), $525.00 per year (international individuals), $711.00 per year (international institutions), $185.00 per year (US students), and $255.00 per year (international students). International air speed delivery is included in all *Clinics* subscription prices. All prices are subject to change without notice. **POSTMASTER:** Send address changes to *Neurosurgery Clinics of North America*, Elsevier Periodicals Customer Service, 11830 Westline Industrial Drive, St. Louis, MO 63146. **Customer Service: 1-800-654-2452 (US and Canada). From outside the US and Canada, call: 1-314-453-7041. Fax: 1-314-453-5170. E-mail: JournalsCustomerService-usa@elsevier.com (for print support) and journalsonlinesupport-usa@elsevier.com (for online support).**

Reprints. For copies of 100 or more, of articles in this publication, please contact the Commercial Reprints Department, Elsevier Inc., 360 Park Avenue South, New York, NY 10010-1710. Tel. 212-633-3874; Fax: 212-633-3820; E-mail: reprints@elsevier.com.

Neurosurgery Clinics of North America is covered in *MEDLINE/PubMed (Index Medicus), EMBASE/Excerpta Medica, and Current Contents/Clinical Medicine (CC/CM).*

Contributors

CONSULTING EDITORS

RUSSELL LONSER, MD
Chair, Department of Neurological Surgery, The Ohio State University, Columbus, Ohio

ISAAC YANG, MD
Assistant Professor, Department of Neurosurgery, David Geffen School of Medicine, Jonsson Comprehensive Cancer Center, University of California Los Angeles, Los Angeles, California

EDITORS

RICARDO A. HANEL, MD, PhD
Director of Cerebrovascular and Stroke, Lyerly Neurosurgery, Baptist Health, Jacksonville, Florida

CIARÁN J. POWERS, MD, PhD
Assistant Professor, Department of Neurological Surgery, The Ohio State University Wexner Medical Center, Columbus, Ohio

ERIC SAUVAGEAU, MD
Director of Stroke and Cerebrovascular Surgery, Lyerly Neurosurgery, Baptist Health, Jacksonville, Florida

AUTHORS

BEVERLEY AAGAARD-KIENITZ, MD
Associate Professor of Radiology and Neurological Surgery; Program Director, Neuroendovascular Fellowship: Endovascular Neurosurgery/Neurointerventional Surgery; Co-Director, Neuroendovascular Section, University of Wisconsin Hospital and Clinics, Madison, Wisconsin

TODD ABRUZZO, MD
Chief, Pediatric Interventional Neuroradiology, Department of Radiology; Associate Professor, Department of Neurosurgery, University of Cincinnati College of Medicine; Comprehensive Stroke Center, University of Cincinnati Neuroscience Institute; Mayfield Clinic, Cincinnati, Ohio

AZAM AHMED, MD
Assistant Professor, Departments of Radiology and Neurological Surgery, University of Wisconsin Hospital and Clinics, Madison, Wisconsin

FELIPE C. ALBUQUERQUE, MD
Endovascular Neurosurgeon, Division of Surgery, Barrow Neurological Institute, St Joseph's Hospital and Medical Center, Phoenix, Arizona

MICHAEL J. ALEXANDER, MD
Professor and Vice-Chairman, Department of Neurosurgery, Cedars-Sinai Medical Center, Los Angeles, California

NORBERTO ANDALUZ, MD
Associate Professor of Neurosurgery; Director, Division of Neurotrauma; Medical Director, Neurotrauma Center, Department of Neurosurgery, University of Cincinnati College of Medicine; Comprehensive Stroke Center, University of Cincinnati Neuroscience Institute; Mayfield Clinic, Cincinnati, Ohio

RAMSEY ASHOUR, MD
Chief Resident, Department of Neurological Surgery, Lois Pope LIFE Center, University of Miami Miller School of Medicine, Miami, Florida

KAIZ ASIF, MD
Neurointerventional Fellow, Division of Neurointervention, Department of Neurology, SNN (Stroke, Neurocritical Care, and Neurointerventional) Research Center, Froedtert Hospital, Medical College of Wisconsin, Milwaukee, Wisconsin

ALI AZIZ-SULTAN, MD
Section Chief of Cerebrovascular/ Endovascular, Department of Neurosurgery, Brigham & Women's Hospital, Boston, Massachusetts

CHRISTOPHER D. BAGGOTT, MD
Neurosurgery Resident, Department of Neurological Surgery, University of Wisconsin Hospital and Clinics, Madison, Wisconsin

BERNARD R. BENDOK, MD, MS
Professor of Neurological Surgery, Radiology and Otolaryngology, Northwestern Memorial Hospital, Chicago, Illinois

CARLO BORTOLOTTI, MD
Division of Neurosurgery, Istituto delle Scienze Neurologiche di Bologna, IRCCS Bellaria Hospital, Bologna, Italy

BENJAMIN BROWN, MD
Cerebrovascular Fellow, Department of Neurosurgery, Mayo Clinic, Jacksonville, Florida

ALICIA C. CASTONGUAY, PhD
Assistant Professor of Neurology, Division of Neurointervention, Department of Neurology, Director of the SNN (Stroke, Neurocritical Care, and Neurointerventional) Research Center, Froedtert Hospital, Medical College of Wisconsin, Milwaukee, Wisconsin

NOHRA CHALOUHI, MD
Department of Neurosurgery, Jefferson Hospital for Neuroscience, Thomas Jefferson University, Philadelphia, Pennsylvania

JOHN P. DEVEIKIS, MD
Department of Neurosurgery, University of Alabama at Birmingham, Birmingham, Alabama

PAULA EBOLI, MD
Department of Neurosurgery, Cedars-Sinai Medical Center, Los Angeles, California

TAREK Y. EL AHMADIEH, MD
Post-doctoral Research Fellow, Department of Neurological Surgery, Northwestern Memorial Hospital, Chicago, Illinois

NAJIB E. EL TECLE, MD
Post-doctoral Research Fellow, Department of Neurological Surgery, Northwestern Memorial Hospital, Chicago, Illinois

JORGE L. ELLER, MD
Endovascular Fellow, Department of Neurosurgery, University at Buffalo, State University of New York; Department of Neurosurgery, Gates Vascular Institute, Kaleida Health, Buffalo, New York; Assistant Professor, Cerebrovascular Neurosurgery, PeaceHealth Sacred Heart Medical Center, Springfield, Oregon

PAUL FOREMAN, MD
Department of Neurosurgery, University of Alabama at Birmingham, Birmingham, Alabama

AYMAN GHEITH, MD
Neurointerventional Fellow, Department of Neurology, SNN (Stroke, Neurocritical Care, and Neurointerventional) Research Center, Froedtert Hospital, Medical College of Wisconsin, Milwaukee, Wisconsin

YAIR M. GOZAL, MD, PhD
Department of Neurosurgery, University of Cincinnati College of Medicine, Cincinnati, Ohio

CHRISTOPH J. GRIESSENAUER, MD
Department of Neurosurgery, University of Alabama at Birmingham, Birmingham, Alabama

AARON W. GROSSMAN, MD, PhD
Department of Neurosurgery, University of Cincinnati College of Medicine, Cincinnati, Ohio

YOUSSEF J. HAMADE, MD
Research Assistant, Department of Neurological Surgery, Northwestern Memorial Hospital, Chicago, Illinois

RICARDO A. HANEL, MD, PhD
Director of Cerebrovascular and Stroke, Lyerly Neurosurgery, Baptist Health, Jacksonville, Florida

MARK R. HARRIGAN, MD
Associate Professor, Department of Neurosurgery, University of Alabama at Birmingham, Birmingham, Alabama

DAVID HASAN, MD
Department of Neurosurgery, University of Iowa, Iowa City, Iowa

L. NELSON HOPKINS, MD
Distinguished Professor of Neurosurgery; Professor of Radiology, Departments of Neurosurgery and Radiology, School of Medicine and Biomedical Sciences, University at Buffalo, State University of New York; Toshiba Stroke and Vascular Research Center, School of Medicine and Biomedical Sciences, University at Buffalo, State University of New York; Department of Neurosurgery, Gates Vascular Institute, Kaleida Health; Chief Executive Officer, Jacobs Institute, Buffalo, New York

DANIEL S. IKEDA, MD
Department of Neurological Surgery, The Ohio State University Wexner Medical Center, Columbus, Ohio

PASCAL JABBOUR, MD
Department of Neurosurgery, Jefferson Hospital for Neuroscience, Thomas Jefferson University; Chief, Division of Neurovascular Surgery and Endovascular Neurosurgery; Associate Professor, Department of Neurological Surgery, Thomas Jefferson University Hospital, Philadelphia, Pennsylvania

GIUSEPPE LANZINO, MD
Professor of Neurosurgery, Department of Neurologic Surgery, College of Medicine, Mayo Clinic, Rochester Minnesota

ELAD I. LEVY, MD, MBA, FACS, FAHA
Chairman of the Department of Neurosurgery; Professor, Departments of Neurosurgery and Radiology, School of Medicine and Biomedical Sciences, University at Buffalo, State University of New York; Toshiba Stroke and Vascular Research Center, School of Medicine and Biomedical Sciences, University at Buffalo, State University of New York; Department of Neurosurgery, Gates Vascular Institute, Kaleida Health, Buffalo, New York

JOHN R. LYNCH, MD
Associate Professor of Neurology, Departments of Neurology, Radiology, and Neurosurgery, SNN (Stroke, Neurocritical Care, and Neurointerventional) Research Center, Froedtert Hospital, Medical College of Wisconsin, Milwaukee, Wisconsin

EVAN S. MARLIN, MD
Department of Neurological Surgery, The Ohio State University Wexner Medical Center, Columbus, Ohio

CAMERON G. MCDOUGALL, MD
Chief, Endovascular Neurosurgery, Division of Neurological Surgery, Barrow Neurological Institute, St Joseph's Hospital and Medical Center, Phoenix, Arizona

MAXIM MOKIN, MD, PhD
Endovascular Neurosurgery Fellow, Department of Neurosurgery, School of Medicine and Biomedical Sciences, University at Buffalo, State University of New York; Department of Neurosurgery, Gates Vascular Institute, Kaleida Health, Buffalo, New York

DAVID NIEMANN, MD
Associate Professor, Departments of Radiology and Neurological Surgery, University of Wisconsin Hospital and Clinics, Madison, Wisconsin

MIN S. PARK, MD
Division of Neurological Surgery, Barrow Neurological Institute, St Joseph's Hospital and Medical Center, Phoenix, Arizona

BIRAJ M. PATEL, MD
Clinical Instructor, Departments of Radiology and Neurological Surgery, University of Wisconsin Hospital and Clinics, Madison, Wisconsin

GLEN POLLOCK, MD
Assistant Professor of Neurosurgery, Departments of Neurology and Neurosurgery, SNN (Stroke, Neurocritical Care, and Neurointerventional) Research Center, Froedtert Hospital, Medical College of Wisconsin, Milwaukee, Wisconsin

CIARÁN J. POWERS, MD, PhD
Assistant Professor, Department of Neurological Surgery, The Ohio State University Wexner Medical Center, Columbus, Ohio

STYLIANOS RAMMOS, MD
Arkansas Neuroscience Institute, Little Rock, Arkansas

ANDREW RINGER, MD
Professor of Neurosurgery and Radiology; Director, Division of Cerebrovascular Surgery, Department of Neurosurgery, University of Cincinnati College of Medicine; Comprehensive Stroke Center, University of Cincinnati Neuroscience Institute; Mayfield Clinic, Cincinnati, Ohio

ROBERT H. ROSENWASSER, MD
Department of Neurosurgery, Jefferson Hospital for Neuroscience, Thomas Jefferson University, Philadelphia, Pennsylvania

ROBERT W. RYAN, MD
University Neurosurgery Associates, University of California, San Francisco-Fresno, Fresno, California

MATTHEW R. SANBORN, MD
Division of Neurological Surgery, Barrow Neurological Institute, St Joseph's Hospital and Medical Center, Phoenix, Arizona

ERIC SAUVAGEAU, MD
Director of Stroke and Cerebrovascular Surgery, Lyerly Neurosurgery, Baptist Health, Jacksonville, Florida

JOSEPH C. SERRONE, MD
Department of Neurosurgery, University of Cincinnati College of Medicine, Cincinnati, Ohio

ANDREW SHAW, MD
Department of Neurological Surgery, The Ohio State University Wexner Medical Center, Columbus, Ohio

ADNAN H. SIDDIQUI, MD, PhD
Associate Professor, Departments of Neurosurgery and Radiology, School of Medicine and Biomedical Sciences, University at Buffalo, State University of New York; Toshiba Stroke and Vascular Research Center, School of Medicine and Biomedical Sciences, University at Buffalo, State University of New York; Department of Neurosurgery, Gates Vascular Institute, Kaleida Health; Jacobs Institute, Buffalo, New York

KENNETH V. SNYDER, MD, PhD
Assistant Professor, Departments of Neurosurgery, Neurology, and Radiology, School of Medicine and Biomedical Sciences, University at Buffalo, State University of New York; Toshiba Stroke and Vascular Research Center, School of Medicine and Biomedical Sciences, University at Buffalo, State University of New York; Department of Neurosurgery, Gates Vascular Institute, Kaleida Health, Buffalo, New York

CHRIS SOUTHWOOD, MD
Neurology Resident, Department of Neurology, SNN (Stroke, Neurocritical Care, and Neurointerventional) Research Center, Froedtert Hospital, Medical College of Wisconsin, Milwaukee, Wisconsin

MOHAMED S. TELEB, MD
Neurointerventional Fellow, Division of Neurointervention, Department of Neurology, SNN (Stroke, Neurocritical Care, and Neurointerventional) Research Center, Froedtert Hospital, Medical College of Wisconsin, Milwaukee, Wisconsin

STAVROPAULA I. TJOUMAKARIS, MD
Department of Neurosurgery, Jefferson Hospital for Neuroscience, Thomas Jefferson University, Philadelphia, Pennsylvania

OSAMA O. ZAIDAT, MD, MS
Professor of Neurology, Neurosurgery, and Radiology; Co-Director, Comprehensive Stroke Center; Chief, Neurointerventional Division, Departments of Neurology, Neurosurgery, and Radiology, SNN (Stroke, Neurocritical Care, and Neurointerventional) Research Center, Froedtert Hospital, Medical College of Wisconsin, Milwaukee, Wisconsin

SAMER G. ZAMMAR, MD
Post-doctoral Research Fellow, Department of Neurological Surgery, Northwestern Memorial Hospital, Chicago, Illinois

MARIO ZANATY, MD
Department of Neurosurgery, Jefferson Hospital for Neuroscience, Thomas Jefferson University, Philadelphia, Pennsylvania

MARIO ZUCCARELLO, MD
Frank H. Mayfield Professor & Chairman, Department of Neurosurgery, University of Cincinnati College of Medicine; Director, Neurovascular Division; Co-Medical Director, Comprehensive Stroke Center, University of Cincinnati Neuroscience Institute; Mayfield Clinic, Cincinnati, Ohio

Contents

techniques for those that are ruptured and unruptured. Basilar apex aneurysms are the most common type and are frequently wide-necked, necessitating stent-assisted coiling or balloon remodeling. Other techniques have evolved to forego stenting in acutely ruptured wide-necked aneurysms. The prevention of delayed thromboembolic complications with dual antiplatelet therapy in patients with stents is critical. After treatment, basilar aneurysms require close follow-up to ensure complete occlusion. Basilar apex aneurysms often require delayed re-treatment, especially when previously ruptured.

Cerebral Vasospasm **497**

Christopher D. Baggott and Beverley Aagaard-Kienitz

Cerebral vasospasm causes delayed ischemic neurologic deficits after aneurysmal subarachnoid hemorrhage. This is a well-established clinical entity with significant associated morbidity and mortality. The underlying patholphysiology is highly complex and poorly understood. Large-vessel vasospasm, autoregulatory dysfunction, inflammation, genetic predispositions, microcirculatory failure, and spreading cortical depolarization are aspects of delayed neurologic deterioration that have been described in the literature. This article presents a perspective on cerebral vasospasm, as guided by the literature to date, specifically examining the mechanism, diagnosis, and treatment of cerebral vasospasm.

Endovascular Approaches to Pial Arteriovenous Malformations **529**

Matthew R. Sanborn, Min S. Park, Cameron G. McDougall, and Felipe C. Albuquerque

Endovascular approaches to arteriovenous malformations (AVMs) are often necessary to define and help treat these often complex lesions. Angiography provides important information to help plan surgical or radiosurgical approaches. Modern embolization techniques allow AVMs to be treated with the goals of making surgery safer and easier, eliminating high-risk features in patients with AVMs who are otherwise not candidates for treatment, and even potentially curing the patient of the lesion. Liquid embolic agents have significantly advanced what is possible with endovascular treatment of AVMs.

Endovascular Management of Intracranial Dural Arteriovenous Fistulae **539**

Stylianos Rammos, Carlo Bortolotti, and Giuseppe Lanzino

Endovascular embolization is the primary therapeutic modality for intracranial dural arteriovenous fistulae. Based on access route, endovascular treatment can be schematically divided into transarterial, transvenous, combined, and direct/percutaneous approaches. Choice of access route and technique depends primarily on dural arteriovenous fistulae angioarchitecture, pattern of venous drainage, clinical presentation, and location. Individualized endovascular approaches result in a high degree of cure with a reasonably low complication rate.

Endovascular Treatment of Carotid-Cavernous Fistulas **551**

Mario Zanaty, Nohra Chalouhi, Stavropaula I. Tjoumakaris, David Hasan, Robert H. Rosenwasser, and Pascal Jabbour

Endovascular management has become the treatment of choice for carotid-cavernous fistulas regardless of the fistula type. The endovascular method offers numerous options that render it capable of treating each fistula type by choosing

NEUROSURGERY CLINICS OF NORTH AMERICA

FORTHCOMING ISSUES

October 2014
Pain Management
Andre Machado, Milind S. Deogaonkar, and Ashwini D. Sharan, *Editors*

January 2015
Central Neurocytomas
Dong Gyu Kim and Isaac Yang, *Editors*

RECENT ISSUES

April 2014
Minimally Invasive Spine Surgery
Zachary A. Smith and Richard G. Fessler, *Editors*

January 2014
Advances in Neuromodulation
Kim Won, Antonio De Salles, and Nader Pouratian, *Editors*

October 2013
Intracranial Stereotactic Radiosurgery
Bruce E. Pollock, *Editor*

RELATED INTEREST

Neuroimaging Clinics of North America, November 2013 (Vol. 23, No. 4)
Endovascular Management of Neurovascular Pathology in Adults and Children
Joseph J. Gemmete, and Neeraj Chaudhary, *Editors*
http://www.neuroimaging.theclinics.com/

Preface
Endovascular Management of Cerebrovascular Disease

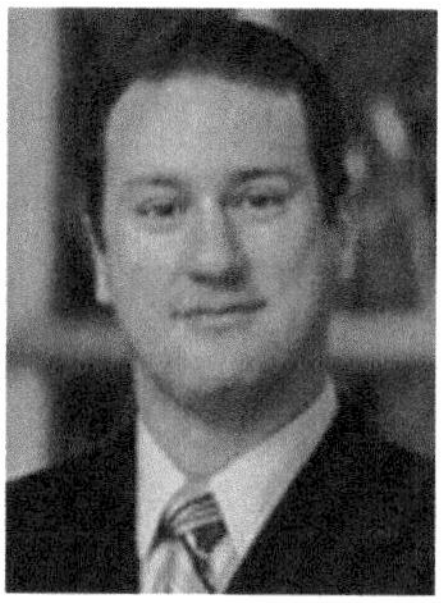
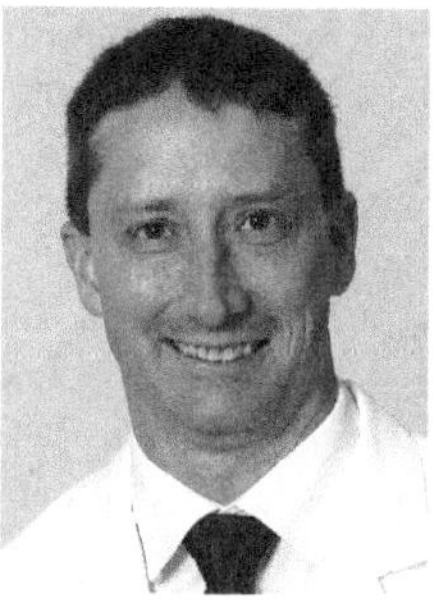
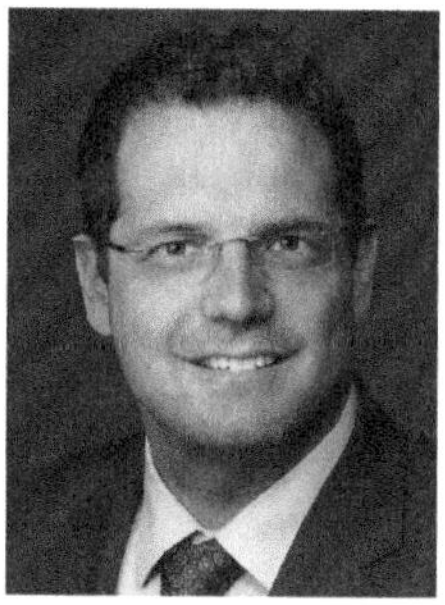

Ricardo A. Hanel, MD, PhD   Ciarán J. Powers, MD, PhD   Eric Sauvageau, MD
Editors

We are fortunate to practice endovascular neurosurgery in an exciting time. Since the concept of endovascular treatment of cerebrovascular disease became a modern reality with the first description of aneurysm coiling in 1991,[1] the field has grown dramatically.

Endovascular treatment of cerebral aneurysms is now a commonplace procedure and has largely superseded the former gold standard of craniotomy for clipping.[2] The primary advantage of endovascular surgery over microsurgery is the minimization of approach-associated morbidity. Even at the hands of the best neurosurgeons, the approach-associated morbidity of a craniotomy is significantly greater than endovascular approach. The liabilities of endovascular treatment, namely, lack of control at the operative site and questionable long-term durability, are increasingly being addressed with incremental innovation in support catheter, balloon technology, and coil/stent technologies. More recently, the advent of flow diverters, a disruptive technology when compared with endosaccular devices, is changing the paradigm of aneurysm treatment and allowing safe treatment of extraordinary lesions with much lower recurrence rates. The immediate future holds the promise for better tools to help us provide the best care for our patients, which should always be at the center of all considerations.

For this reason, we must approach this future with our eyes open and maintain a little skepticism. While the advances of technology in endovascular neurosurgery are impressive, for some pathologic processes, the indications for treatment remain undefined. Nowhere is this more evident than in the treatment of acute ischemic stroke from large vessel occlusion (LVO). With advances in stentriever and suction thrombectomy devices, successful angiographic recanalization rates are now consistently greater than 80%.[3] However, as recent prospective randomized studies have shown, thrombectomy has yet to show a significant improvement in patient outcomes.[4,5] While there are many valid criticisms of these prospective, randomized trials (especially the poor representation of current technology), the key issue is likely patient selection. Simply put, we do not yet know which patients will benefit from thrombectomy for acute LVO. As the practitioners capable of providing these remarkable endovascular treatments, it is incumbent on us to lead the research

Neurosurg Clin N Am 25 (2014) xiii–xiv
http://dx.doi.org/10.1016/j.nec.2014.05.001
1042-3680/14/$ – see front matter

that will determine which patients are the best candidates for therapy.

Arteriovenous malformation also represents an area where patient selection is of the essence to improve patient outcomes. Endovascular therapy definitely represents a valid option or adjunct but the benefit could be nullified by inexperienced hands or if the procedure is directed toward the wrong kind of patient toward the wrong patient.

In summary, it remains primordial to educate present and future generations to be neurovascular specialists and not only mere technological savants. We hope this issue of *Neurosurgery Clinics of North America* will serve as a high-level topic review and keep the readers updated on current and future neurointervention directions.

Ricardo A. Hanel, MD, PhD
Lyerly Neurosurgery
Baptist Health
800 Prudential Drive, Tower B, 11th Floor
Jacksonville, FL 33227, USA

Ciarán J. Powers, MD, PhD
Department of Neurological Surgery
The Ohio State University, Wexner Medical Center
410 West 10th Avenue
Columbus, OH 43210, USA

Eric Sauvageau, MD
Director of Stroke and Cerebrovascular Surgery
Baptist Health, Jacksonville, Florida
Lyerly Neurosurgery
800 Prudential Drive
Tower B 11th Floor
Jacksonville, FL 32207, USA

E-mail addresses:
rhanel@hotmail.com (R.A. Hanel)
Ciaran.Powers@osumc.edu (C.J. Powers)
esauvageau@lyerlyneuro.com (E. Sauvageau)

REFERENCES

1. Guglielmi G, Vinuela F, Dion J, et al. Electrothrombosis of saccular aneurysms via endovascular approach. Part 2: preliminary clinical experience. J Neurosurg 1991;75:8–14.
2. Brinjikji W, Rabinstein A, Nasr DM, et al. Better outcomes with treatment by coiling relative to clipping of unruptured intracranial aneurysms in the United States, 2001-2008. AJNR Am J Neuroradiol 2011;32:1071–5.
3. Nogueira RG, Lutsep HL, Gupta R, et al. Trevo versus Merci retrievers for thrombectomy revascularisation of large vessel occlusions in acute ischaemic stroke (TREVO 2): a randomised trial. Lancet 2012;380:1231–40.
4. Broderick JP, Palesch YY, Demchuk AM, et al. Endovascular therapy after intravenous t-PA versus t-PA alone for stroke. N Engl J Med 2013;368:893–903.
5. Ciccone A, Valvassori L, Nichelatti M, et al. Endovascular treatment for acute ischemic stroke. N Engl J Med 2013;368:904–13.

Endovascular Tools Available for the Treatment of Cerebrovascular Disease

Christoph J. Griessenauer, MD, Paul Foreman, MD, John P. Deveikis, MD, Mark R. Harrigan, MD*

KEYWORDS

• Endovascular • Neurointervention • Angiography

KEY POINTS

- A guide catheter is a catheter that is typically placed in the internal carotid artery or vertebral artery and accommodates microcatheters and other devices.
- Since the introduction of the detachable coil by Guglielmi (GDC coils) in 1991, coiling has become the mainstay of endovascular treatment of aneurysms.
- Flow diversion functions by placing a wire mesh stent within the parent vessel, across the aneurysm, leading to thrombosis of the aneurysm with preservation of flow through the parent vessel and its branches.
- Balloons have found a variety of neurointerventional applications, including extracranial and intracranial balloon angioplasty, balloon-assisted thrombectomy and thrombolysis, balloon-assisted coiling, balloon test occlusion, and balloon-expandable stent placement.
- Currently, several self-expanding stents are available for carotid angioplasty and stenting. Stents used for this indication are either tapered or straight and manufactured with open- or closed-cell design.

CATHETERS AND WIRES

Diagnostic Catheters and Wires

Several catheters are suitable for diagnostic cerebral and spinal angiography (**Fig. 1**). Angled taper and vertebral catheters are both excellent all-purpose diagnostic catheters. Simmons 1 through 3 catheters are preferred for spinal angiography, left common carotid artery access, and a tortuous or bovine-configured aortic arch. The CK-1, or HN-5, facilitates left common carotid artery or right vertebral artery access, while the H1, or Headhunter, is preferred for right subclavian and right vertebral artery access. The Newton catheter is another alternative for tortuous anatomy on older patients. Hydrophilic wires of variable diameter (eg, angled Glidewire [Terumo Medical, Somerset, NJ, USA]) are used for catheter navigation.

Guide Catheters

A guide catheter is a catheter that is typically placed in the internal carotid artery or vertebral artery and accommodates microcatheters and other devices. Preferably it is 6 French in caliber to allow for guide catheter angiograms with microcatheters or other devices in place and is available with straight or angled tips. A straight catheter, as the name would imply, is useful in relatively straight vessels but usually requires a wire exchange, while angled catheters are easier to navigate and advantageous when the final position of the catheter tip

Disclosures: None.
Department of Neurosurgery, University of Alabama at Birmingham, Birmingham, AL, USA
* Corresponding author. Faculty Office Tower 1005, 510 20th Street South, Birmingham, AL 35294.
E-mail address: mharrigan@uabmc.edu

Neurosurg Clin N Am 25 (2014) 387–394
http://dx.doi.org/10.1016/j.nec.2014.04.001
1042-3680/14/$ – see front matter

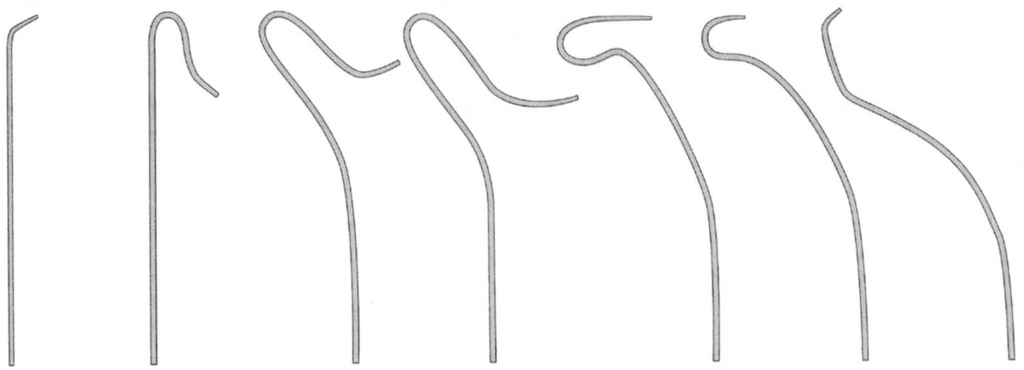

Fig. 1. Recommended diagnostic catheter tips.

is in the curve of a vessel. Commonly used guide catheters include the Neuron system (Penumbra, San Leandro, CA, USA), Guider Softip XF (Stryker Neurovascular, Fremont, CA, USA), Envoy (Codman, Raynham, MA, USA), Cook Shuttle and Northstar Lumax (Cook, Bloomington, IN, USA), Merci Balloon Guide (Concentric Medical, Mountain View, CA, USA), ReFlex (Reverse Medical, Irvine, CA, USA), Berenstein (Boston Scientific, Natick, MA, USA), and Pinnacle Destination (Terumo Medical, Somerset, NJ, USA). The 6F 0.053 in Neuron is soft and flexible, allowing for positioning in the distal internal carotid or vertebral artery but less stable than other catheters. The Guider Softip XF has a soft, atraumatic tip that minimizes risk of vasospasm and dissection in narrow, tortuous vessels but is prone to fall into the aortic arch. The Envoy is relatively rigid and provides a good platform in tortuous vessels with large internal lumen but has a stiff, sharp-edged tip, thus increasing the risk of vessel damage. The Cook Shuttle is another catheter that provides a very large, stable platform.

Balloon Guide Catheters

The Merci Balloon Guide catheter is capable of temporarily occluding flow in the carotid or vertebral artery during thrombectomy but is prone to fall into the aortic arch. The Berenstein and Cello (eV3 Neurovascular, Irvine, CA, USA) balloon guides allow for control of proximal flow to prevent distal migration of embolic agents.

Microcatheters

A microcatheter provides access for treatment of a vascular lesion and is available in various sizes and shapes. Preshaped microcatheters are preferred for accessing aneurysms that arise from the parent vessel at an acute angle. When appropriately preshaped devices are unavailable, steam shaping is an option. Catheters have hydrophilic coating to reduce thrombogenicity.[1] Smaller microcatheters permit better guide catheter angiograms, while larger and stiffer microcatheters provide stability when catheter access is tenuous because of the vascular anatomy. Single-tip and two-tipped microcatheters are available, and two-tipped microcatheters are necessary for aneurysm coiling. The two tips in microcatheters used for aneurysm coiling are always 3 cm apart and can be used for measurements or calibration. Commonly used microcatheters include the Excelsior SL-10 and Excelsior 1018 (Stryker Neurovascular, Fremont, CA, USA), Echelon 10, Ultraflow, and Marksman (all ev3, Irvine, CA, USA), Magic microcatheter (AIT-Balt, Miami, FA, USA), and Prowler Select Plus (Codman, Raynham, MA, USA). The Excelsior SL-10 can be used for 10- and 18-system coils. The Echelon 10 and Ultraflow are compatible for onyx and N-butyl cyanoacrylate (NBCA) embolization. The Marksman is fairly robust and useful for Neuroform EZ (Stryker Neurovascular, Fremont, CA, USA) stent deployment. The Excelsior 1018 accommodates 10- and 18-system coils and is suitable for polyvinyl alcohol (PVA) embolization. Use of the Prowler Select Plus is preferred with the Enterprise Vascular Reconstruction System (Codman, Raynham, MA, USA).

Microwires

Various microwires are available that differ in size, degree of stiffness, visibility on fluoroscopy, and the ability to shape, steer, track, and torque. Commonly used microwires include the Synchro-14, Transend EX Floppy tip, or Platinum (all Stryker Neurovascular, Fremont, CA, USA); the Neuroscout 14 Steerable Guidewire (Codman, Raynham, MA, USA); and Headliner J-tip (Terumo Medical,

Somerset, NJ, USA). The Synchro-14 is flexible, suitable for navigation through complex anatomy and into small aneurysms. The Neuroscout 14 Steerable Guidewire maintains shape, permitting exceptional torque control. The Headliner J-tip is good for uncomplicated anatomy, as the J-tip is atraumatic and tends to follow the straightest vessel.

Intermediate Catheters

Intermediate catheters (eg, Distal Access Catheter [Stryker Neurovascular, Fremont, CA, USA], Revive Intermediate Catheter [Codman, Raynham, MA, USA], and Fargo and FargoMAX [Balt Extrusion, Montmorency, France]) are sized between a guide catheter and a microcatheter and provide stable access by functioning as a bridge between the 2 catheters in triaxial arrangement (microwire and microcatheter, intermediate catheter, and guide catheter). First developed to stabilize the Merci devices (Stryker Neurovascular, Fremont, CA, USA), intermediate catheters have been found to be helpful with tortuous cerebrovascular anatomy, need for remote access, and thrombectomy by reducing the laxity and bend of the microcatheter, therefore facilitating navigation.[2,3]

COILS

Since the introduction of the detachable coil by Guglielmi (GDC coils) in 1991, coiling has become the mainstay of endovascular treatment of aneurysms.[4] The next 20 years witnessed an evolution in coiling technology, allowing for the endovascular treatment of numerous cerebrovascular conditions.

Platinum Coils

Various platinum coils, differing in size, shape, design, stiffness, and detachment system are available; despite the abundance of coiling options, no particular coil has proven superior for the treatment of aneurysms. Coils consist of a fine platinum thread looped around a thicker platinum core that is connected to a pusher wire, where the detachment mechanism is located. There are 3 basic coil shapes (**Fig. 2**). Framing coils assume a 3-dimensional configuration designed to give the aneurysm a spherical shape through gentle radial force. Ideally, they extend across the neck to reduce the effective neck area. Examples include the Micrusphere (Micrus, Mountainview, CA, USA), Target 360 (Stryker Neurovascular, Fremont, CA, USA), and Orbit Galaxy (Codman, Raynham, MA, USA) complex coils. Filling coils are helical and are intended to occupy space within the aneurysms. Examples include Helipaq (Micrus, Mountainview, CA, USA), Target 360 soft (Stryker Neurovascular, Fremont, CA, USA), and Orbit Galaxy (Codman, Raynham, MA, USA) fill coils. Finishing coils are the softest coils and are designed for final packing of the aneurysm. Examples include Deltapaq (Micrus, Mountainview, CA, USA), Deltaplush (Micrus, Mountainview, CA, USA), Target Ultra (Stryker Neurovascular, Fremont, CA, USA), Orbit Galaxy Xtrasoft (Codman, Raynham, MA, USA), and Microplex HyperSoft (Terumo Medical, Somerset, NJ, USA) coils.

Coil sizes have been traditionally categorized into 10-system and 18-system, a nomenclature that originated with the introduction of the first

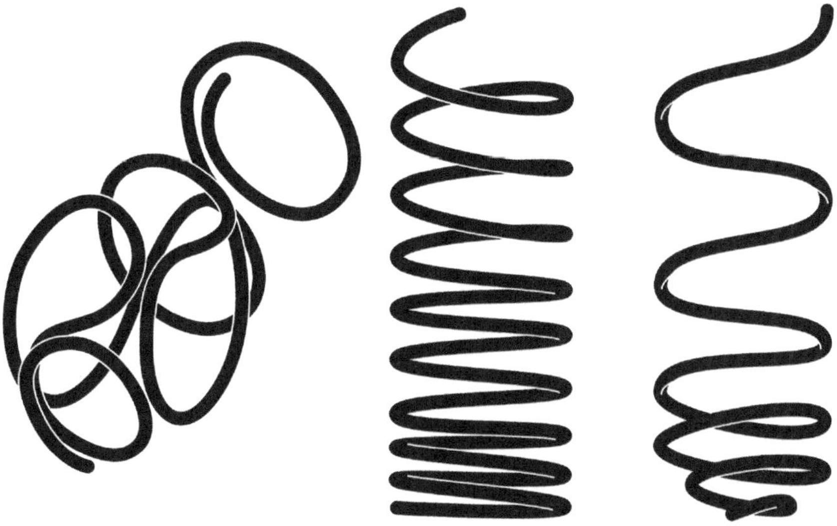

Fig. 2. Basic coil shapes. Three-dimensional framing coil (*left*), Helical filling coil (*middle*), 2-diameter finishing coil (*right*).

microcatheters used to deploy GDC coils, the Tracker-10 and Tracker-18 (formerly Target Therapeutics, now Stryker Neurovascular, Fremont, CA, USA). The actual diameter of 10- and 18-system coils is 0.008 and 0.016 in, respectively. Although the 10-system is adequate for most aneurysms, 18-system coils are preferred for framing of larger, unruptured aneurysms. Today there are several coils on the market that have a larger diameter (Orbit Galaxy [Codman, Raynham, MA, USA], Cashmere [Micrus, Mountainview, CA, USA], and Penumbra Coil 400 [Penumbra, San Leandro, CA, USA]) while maintaining the softness of the 10-system.

Augmented Coils

Augmentation of platinum coils with bioactive materials (Polyglycolic polylactic acid [PGLA], hydrogel) to decrease the rate of aneurysm recanalization has shown variable efficacy. Two prospective, randomized trials (Cerecyte and Matrix And Platinum Science [MAPS]) failed to show benefit with PGLA-augmented coils over bare platinum coils.[5,6] Hydrogel, on the other hand, appears to decrease recanalization rates, at least in the short term.[7] Examples include Matrix2 (Stryker Neurovascular, Fremont, CA, USA), Cerecyte (Codman, Raynham, MA, USA), Nexus (ev3 Neurovascular, Irvine, CA, USA), HydroCoil (Terumo Medical, Somerset, NJ, USA). Several alternative coil designs have been developed to increase packing density in an effort to reduce recanalization rates.

Pushable Coils

Pushable coils including platinum coils with thrombogenic fibers (eg, Trufill [Codman, Raynham, MA, USA], Hilal and Tornado Micorcoils [Cook, Bloomington, IN, USA], and Fibered Platinum and Vortx [Boston Scientific, Natick, MA, USA]), or short straight or helical coils are impelled through the microcatheter into the vessel using rapid saline injection for embolization of vessels of medium size. Detachable coils alone are rarely used for extracranial embolization as they are slower to deploy, more expensive, and less thrombogenic. There are, however, detachable fibered coils available (eg, Sapphire NXT [ev3 Neurovascular, Irvine, CA, USA]).

FLOW DIVERSION

Flow diversion functions by placing a wire mesh stent within the parent vessel, across the aneurysm, leading to thrombosis of the aneurysm with preservation of flow through the parent vessel and its branches. Currently the Pipeline Embolization Device (PED, ev3 Neurovascular, Irvine, CA, USA) is the only US Food and Drug Administration (FDA)-approved flow diverter, with approval granted in 2011 (**Fig. 3**). Flow PED's surface area coverage of approximately 30% is considerably greater than that provided by other stents.[8] The device is available in variable diameters and lengths, with a maximum diameter and length of 5 and 35 mm, respectively. Device diameter is chosen to approximate the parent vessel diameter. The length should be at least 6 mm greater than the aneurysm neck. If there is a difference in parent vessel diameter proximal and distal to the aneurysm, the stent is either sized to the larger diameter, or multiple stents, sized to fit the proximal and distal arteries, are selected.

Despite the early experience with flow diverters, data suggest that treatment of aneurysms utilizing this technology is effective and results high rates of occlusion rates. The associated morbidity and mortality, however, are not negligible.[9]

BALLOONS

Balloons have found a variety of neurointerventional applications including extracranial and intracranial balloon angioplasty, balloon-assisted thrombectomy and thrombolysis, balloon-assisted coiling, balloon test occlusion, and balloon-expandable stent placement.

Extracranial Balloon Angioplasty

Balloon angioplasty is a component of carotid angioplasty and stenting and is performed to dilate the stenotic region to accommodate the stent. Smaller angioplasty balloons, typically 2.0 to 2.5 mm in diameter and long enough to cover the extent of stenosis, are favored as they are associated with improved results.[10] Stents currently used for carotid angioplasty and stenting are self-expanding and do not rely on a balloon.

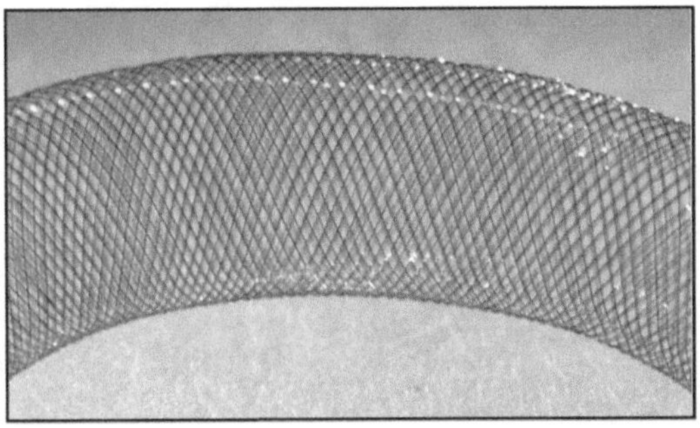

Fig. 3. Photograph of the Pipeline embolization device (ev3 Neurovascular, Irvine, CA, USA).

Balloon-mounted coronary drug-eluding stents are reserved for carotid or vertebral artery origin stenosis.[11]

Intracranial Balloon Angioplasty

Both compliant and noncompliant balloons are used for intracranial balloon angioplasty. Examples of the former and latter include Hyperglide and Hyperform (ev3 Neurovascular, Irvine, CA, USA); Maverick2 Monorail Balloon Catheter and NC Ranger Balloon Catheter (Boston Scientific, Natick, MA, USA); and NC Raptor (Cordis, Miami, FL, USA), respectively. Compliant balloons are generally softer and easier to navigate in small and tortuous vessels. They can be inflated repeatedly to gently dilate the vessel through multiple low-pressure inflations. The diameter, however, greatly varies with the amount of inflation, and overdilation and vessel rupture have been observed. Noncompliant balloons are rigid and more suitable for proximal, higher-caliber vessels. They are less likely to overinflate, as they stop inflating as they reach their nominal size. Noncompliant balloons can only be inflated a single time.

Both balloon types have shown comparable results for treatment of cerebral vasospasm after aneurysmal subarachnoid hemorrhage.[12] Small noncompliant balloons (eg, Maverick2 Monorail Balloon Catheter [Boston Scientific, Natick, MA, USA]) are also used for balloon angioplasty to augment thrombolysis superimposed on atherosclerotic lesions. Rescue angioplasty has shown favorable results for recanalization of occluded vessels that prove refractory to other methods of thrombolysis, but it carries a risk of subarachnoid hemorrhage.[13]

Balloon-Assisted Coiling

Balloon-assisted coiling is an alternative strategy for the treatment of wide neck aneurysms. The concept relies on placement of a framing coil that shapes the aneurysm to provide a stable structure suitable for coiling while a balloon is inflated in the parent vessel. Both Hyperglide and Hyperform, both single-lumen over-the-wire balloons, can be used for this purpose. The balloon will inflate after an appropriately sized wire is advanced past the catheter tip, which seals the catheter. The Ascent (Codman, Raynham, MA, USA) has a double lumen that allows for coiling through a central lumen while the balloon is inflated.

Balloon Test Occlusion

Several balloons can be used for the purpose of test occlusion. A double-lumen balloon catheter with 1 lumen for inflation of the balloon and an additional lumen is soft to avoid vessel trauma. Over-the-wire balloons (eg, Hyperglide and Hyperform) are the most commonly used balloons for test occlusions, because they are soft and easy to navigate. Although they cannot be used for pressure measurements because of their single-lumen design, they have the benefit of being rapidly deflated by simply withdrawing the wire. The GuardWire (Medtronic, Santa Rosa, CA, USA) is an inflatable balloon mounted on a small-diameter wire with an inner lumen for inflation. It does not allow pressure measurements, deflates slowly, and is stiffer than the balloons mentioned previously and thus should not be used in the intracranial circulation.

STENTS

Extracranial Stents

Currently, several self-expanding stents are available for carotid angioplasty and stenting. Stents used for this indication are either tapered or straight and manufactured with open- or closed-cell design. Open-cell stents have connecting and nonconnecting struts that extend into the lumen and can interfere with embolic protection device (EPD) passage. Closed-cell stents have overlapping or fully connecting struts that do not extend into the lumen. They do not, however, conform to curved vessels as well. The stent selected should have a diameter 1 to 2 mm wider than the normal vessel at full expansion to exert radial force and enhance apposition to the vessel wall; it should cover the entire lesion in length. In 2004, the FDA approved the Acculink stent (Abbott Laboratories, Santa Clara, CA, USA), an open-cell stent, for carotid angioplasty and stenting for patients at high risk for adverse events from carotid endarterectomy (**Fig.** 4A). In 2011, after review of the Carotid Revascularization Endarterectomy versus Stenting Trial (CREST)[14] results, the approval was expanded for use in patients at standard risk for adverse events from carotid endarterectomy. Other examples of open-and closed-cell stents approved for patients considered to be at high risk for carotid endarterectomy include Precise (Cordis, Miami Lakes, FL, USA), NexStent (Boston Scientific, Natick, MA, USA), Protege (ev3 Neurovascular, Irvine, CA, USA) and Xact (Abbott Laboratories, Santa Clara, CA, USA), and Wallstent (Boston Scientific, Natick, MA, USA) (see **Fig.** 4B) respectively.

Intracranial Stents

Several devices are available for intracranial angioplasty and stenting designed primarily for

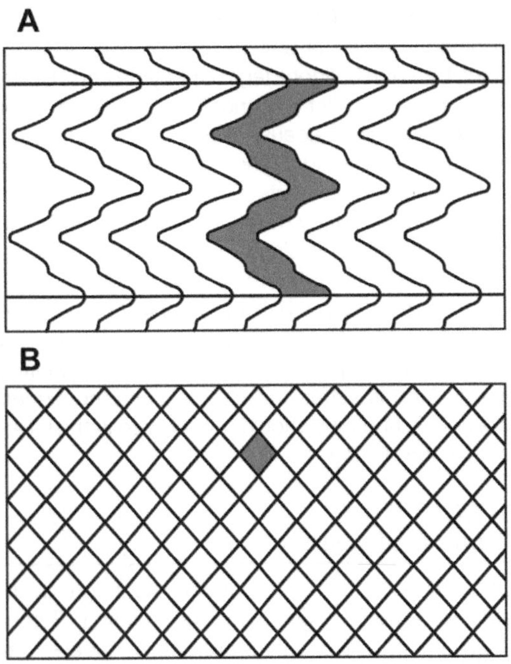

Fig. 4. Schematic drawings of open cell (Acculink stent (Abbott Laboratories, Santa Clara, CA, USA) [*A*]) and closed cell (Wallstent (Boston Scientific, Natick, MA, USA) [*B*]) stent design.

indications of symptomatic atherosclerotic stenosis. Other systems are used for treatment of intracranial aneurysms.

Balloon-Expandable Stents

The PHAROS Vitesse (Codman, Raynham, MA, USA) and balloon-mounted coronary stents are examples of balloon-expandable stents designed for atherosclerotic stenosis. In acute ischemic stroke, they may help to prevent rethrombosis after successful recanalization. Prior to the development of cerebrovascular-specific devices, balloon-mounted coronary stents were used for intracranial arterial disease and were associated with high complication rates due to rigidity and difficulty navigating the tortuous intracranial anatomy.[10]

Self-Expanding Stents

The Wingspan Stent System is a self-expanding stent available under a Humanitarian Device Exemption and is specifically designed for intracranial atherosclerotic stenosis. The Neuroform3 (Stryker Neurovascular, Fremont, CA, USA) and the Enterprise Vascular Reconstruction Device and Delivery System (Codman, Raynham, MA, USA) are examples of self-expanding stents currently used for stent-assisted coiling of wide neck intracranial aneurysms, and they have been used to prevent rethrombosis after successful recanalization in acute ischemic stroke. These self-expanding stents are made of nitinol, a metal alloy of nickel and titanium, and self-expand after deployment in the parent vessel across the neck of the aneurysm. Neuroform has been available under the humanitarian device exemption since 2002 and is more established than Enterprise. Enterprise, however, is more flexible, easier to navigate, and can be repositioned during deployment as long no more than 80% of the stent is placed outside the microcatheter. In contrast to Enterprise, which has a closed-cell design and is prone to kinking in a tight curve, Neuroform has an open-cell design more suitable for placement in sharp curves. The size selection is also more limited for the Enterprise, and it cannot be used in vessels smaller than 2.5 mm diameter.

Two self-expanding, closed-cell stent-like devices used in the treatment of acute ischemic stroke are the Solitaire device (ev3 Neurovascular, Irvine, CA, USA) and Trevo device (Stryker Neurovascular, Fremont, CA, USA). Both utilize a similar concept, which involves retrievable stent deployment into the thrombus to capture and withdraw the thrombus. The Solitaire differs from the Trevo in its open-ended design. It is also available as a detachable version in Europe for stent-assisted coiling.

EMBOLIC PROTECTION DEVICE

Embolic protection devices (EPDs) are placed to avoid embolization of debris during carotid angioplasty and stenting and have been routinely used since 2000. The first EPD was introduced in 1990 and consisted of a catheter with a latex balloon mounted to the end that was inflated to arrest flow in the carotid artery during stent placement and allow for aspiration of debris after stent deployment.[15] There are several conceptually similar balloon occlusion devices currently on the market in North America (Guardwire Temporary Occlusion and Aspiration System [Medtronic, Santa Rosa, California] and MO.MA [Invatec, Roncadelle, Italy]). Flow-reversal devices (Parodi Anti-Emboli System) (W.L. Gore & Associates, Flagstaff, Arizona) involve inflation of balloons in the External carotid artery (ECA) and common carotid artery (CCA) to reverse flow in the internal carotid artery (ICA) and prevent embolization.[16] Filters are the most commonly used EPD and preserve ICA flow during stent placement. Examples include Accunet and Emboshield (both Abbott Laboratories, Santa Clara, CA, USA), FilterWire EZ (Boston Scientific, Natick, MA, USA), Angioguard (Cordis, Miami Lakes, CA, USA), SpiderFX (ev3 Neurovascular, Irvine, CA, USA), Interceptor PLUS (Medtronic, Santa Rosa, CA, USA), and Rubicon (Rubicon Medical, Salt Lake City, Utah).

THROMBECTOMY AND THROMBOLYSIS

Various devices for mechanical thombectomy in acute ischemic stroke are currently available.

Microsnares

Microsnares (eg, Amplatz Goose Neck microsnare [ev3 Neurovascular, Irvine, CA, USA]) can be used for thrombus retrieval and maceration and are preferentially used in combination with thrombolytic drugs.[17] They may be most useful in the treatment of basilar artery occlusion.[18]

Alligator Retriever Device

This Alligator Retriever device (ev3 Neurovascular, Irvine, CA, USA) has microforceps in the shape of claws that can be advanced through a microcatheter and used for thrombus retrieval. The size selected should match the size of the vessel in which the thrombus is located.

Merci Retriever

The Merci Retrieval system (Stryker Neurovascular, Fremont, CA, USA), approved in 2004 following the MERCI trial, was the first FDA-approved neurointerventional device for acute ischemic stroke.[19] It relies on a nitinol wire that assumes helical shape once it emerges from the microcatheter distal to the thrombus and is used with the Merci balloon catheter to temporarily arrest blood flow during the retrieval process.

Penumbra System

The Penumbra System (Penumbra, San Leandro, CA, USA), the second FDA-approved device for acute ischemic stroke, uses a microcatheter attached to an electrical aspiration pump for thrombus aspiration. A soft wire, the Separator, is inserted into the microcatheter to physically break up the thrombus and prevent clogging of the microcatheter. Unlike the Merci Retriever, this device works proximal to the thrombus, eliminating the need to navigate distal to the thrombus.

Stentrievers for Thrombectomy

As discussed previously, stent-like devices including Solitaire (ev3 Neurovascular, Irvine, CA, USA) and Trevo (Stryker Neurovascular, Fremont, CA, USA) are used to retrieve thrombus and have revolutionized the field. These stentrievers are much more effective in rapidly reducing flow compared with earlier systems.

Additional Devices for Mechanical Thrombectomy

Several other devices are available or are actively being evaluated in clinical trials for the treatment of acute ischemic stroke in the United States. The EKOS system (EKOS, Bothell, Washington) consists of a microcatheter with a piezoelectric ultrasound element at its tip allowing for deeper penetration of tPA into the thrombus. The EN Snare (Merit Medical, South Jordan, Utah) is designed with 3 interlaced loops to retrieve foreign bodies. Angiojet (Possis Medical, Minneapolis, Minnesota) is a 2-lumen device that combines local suction and mechanical disruption of a thrombus by creating a localized low-pressure zone with multiple high-velocity, high-pressure saline jets (Bernoulli principle).[20]

NeuroFlo

The NeuroFlo system (CoAxia, Maple Grove, Minnesota) improves cerebral blood flow by partially and temporarily obstructing flow in the abdominal aorta, thus diverting blood flow to the brain. The device was FDA-approved under the Humanitarian Device Exemption in 2005 for cerebral vasospasm after aneurysmal hemorrhage[21] and may also be beneficial in a subset of patients with acute ischemic stroke.[22]

CLOSURE DEVICES

Closure devices are used for closure of the percutaneous femoral artery puncture site. They allow the earlier patient ambulation and may be particularly useful in patients on antithrombotic medications. However, they carry a slightly increased risk of complication over mechanical compression.[23] Currently there are 3 commonly used devices on the market, all using different mechanisms. Perclose Pro-GlideTM (Abbott Vascular, Abbott Park, Illinois) utilizes a closure stitch, while Angio-Seal (St. Jude Medical, St. Paul, Minnesota) anchors a collagen sponge to the arteriotomy site. Mynx Cadence (AccessClosure, Mountain View, CA, USA) places an expanding glycolic sealant over the arteriotomy. No 1 device has proven superior to the others, and the choice remains an operator preference.

REFERENCES

1. Kallmes DF, McGraw JK, Evans AJ, et al. Thrombogenicity of hydrophilic and nonhydrophilic microcatheters and guiding catheters. AJNR Am J Neuroradiol 1997;18(7):1243–51.
2. Spiotta AM, Hussain MS, Sivapatham T, et al. The versatile distal access catheter: the Cleveland Clinic experience. Neurosurgery 2011;68(6):1677–86.

3. Binning MJ, Yashar P, Orion D, et al. Use of the Outreach Distal Access Catheter for microcatheter stabilization during intracranial arteriovenous malformation embolization. AJNR Am J Neuroradiol 2012; 33(9):E117–9.
4. Dovey Z, Misra M, Thornton J, et al. Guglielmi detachable coiling for intracranial aneurysms: the story so far. Arch Neurol 2001;58(4):559–64.
5. Molyneux AJ, Clarke A, Sneade M, et al. Cerecyte coil trial: angiographic outcomes of a prospective randomized trial comparing endovascular coiling of cerebral aneurysms with either cerecyte or bare platinum coils. Stroke 2012;43(10):2544–50.
6. Harrigan MR, Deveikis JP. Intracranial aneurysm treatment. In: Harrigan MR, Deveikis JP, editors. Handbook of cerebrovascular disease and neurointerventional technique. 2nd edition. New York: Humana Press; 2013. p. 196.
7. White PM, Lewis SC, Gholkar A, et al. Hydrogel-coated coils versus bare platinum coils for the endovascular treatment of intracranial aneurysms (HELPS): a randomised controlled trial. Lancet 2011;377(9778):1655–62.
8. Kallmes DF, Ding YH, Dai D, et al. A new endoluminal, flow-disrupting device for treatment of saccular aneurysms. Stroke 2007;38(8):2346–52.
9. Brinjikji W, Murad MH, Lanzino G, et al. Endovascular treatment of intracranial aneurysms with flow diverters: a meta-analysis. Stroke 2013;44(2):442–7.
10. Kessler IM, Mounayer C, Piotin M, et al. The use of balloon-expandable stents in the management of intracranial arterial diseases: a 5-year single-center experience. AJNR Am J Neuroradiol 2005;26(9): 2342–8.
11. Stayman AN, Nogueira RG, Gupta R. A systematic review of stenting and angioplasty of symptomatic extracranial vertebral artery stenosis. Stroke 2011; 42(8):2212–6.
12. Terry A, Zipfel G, Milner E, et al. Safety and technical efficacy of over-the-wire balloons for the treatment of subarachnoid hemorrhage-induced cerebral vasospasm. Neurosurg Focus 2006;21(3):E14.
13. Ringer AJ, Qureshi AI, Fessler RD, et al. Angioplasty of intracranial occlusion resistant to thrombolysis in acute ischemic stroke. Neurosurgery 2001;48(6): 1282–8 [discussion: 1288–90].
14. Brott TG, Hobson RW 2nd, Howard G, et al. Stenting versus endarterectomy for treatment of carotid-artery stenosis. N Engl J Med 2010;363(1):11–23.
15. Theron J, Courtheoux P, Alachkar F, et al. New triple coaxial catheter system for carotid angioplasty with cerebral protection. AJNR Am J Neuroradiol 1990; 11(5):869–74 [discussion: 875–7].
16. Parodi JC, Schonholz C, Ferreira LM, et al. "Seat belt and air bag" technique for cerebral protection during carotid stenting. J Endovasc Ther 2002;9(1):20–4.
17. Harrigan MR, Deveikis JP. Treatment of acute ischaemic stroke. In: Harrigan MR, Deveikis JP, editors. Handbook of cerebrovascular disease and neurointerventional technique. 2nd edition. New York: Humana Press; 2013. p. 196.
18. Nesbit GM, Luh G, Tien R, et al. New and future endovascular treatment strategies for acute ischemic stroke. J Vasc Interv Radiol 2004;15(1 Pt 2): S103–10.
19. Smith WS, Sung G, Starkman S, et al. Safety and efficacy of mechanical embolectomy in acute ischemic stroke: results of the MERCI trial. Stroke 2005;36(7):1432–8.
20. Lee MS, Singh V, Wilentz JR, et al. AngioJet thrombectomy. J Invasive Cardiol 2004;16(10):587–91.
21. Lylyk P, Vila JF, Miranda C, et al. Partial aortic obstruction improves cerebral perfusion and clinical symptoms in patients with symptomatic vasospasm. Neurol Res 2005;27(Suppl 1):S129–35.
22. Shuaib A, Bornstein NM, Diener HC, et al. Partial aortic occlusion for cerebral perfusion augmentation: safety and efficacy of NeuroFlo in Acute Ischemic Stroke trial. Stroke 2011;42(6):1680–90.
23. Nikolsky E, Mehran R, Halkin A, et al. Vascular complications associated with arteriotomy closure devices in patients undergoing percutaneous coronary procedures: a meta-analysis. J Am Coll Cardiol 2004;44(6):1200–9.

General Technical Considerations for the Endovascular Management of Cerebral Aneurysms

Paula Eboli, MD[a], Robert W. Ryan, MD[b],
Michael J. Alexander, MD[a,*]

KEYWORDS

• Cerebral aneurysms • Endovascular techniques • Coil embolization • Stent assistance
• Flow diversion

KEY POINTS

- Direct endosaccular coil embolization is usually possible in aneurysms with a dome/neck ratio of 1.6 or higher.
- Aneurysms with wide necks are more likely to need adjunctive technology with balloon or stent assistance.
- The degree of initial aneurysm occlusion is highly predictive of a durable aneurysm occlusion on delayed imaging.
- Flow-diverting devices have been developed for large aneurysms with a wide neck and have superior long-term occlusion rates to coil embolization in large and giant aneurysms.
- Patients with ruptured aneurysms may be better treated surgically if there is a significant intracerebral hematoma with mass effect or in wide-necked aneurysms in which antiplatelet therapy is thought to be too risky to the patient.

INTRODUCTION: NATURE OF THE PROBLEM

Cerebral aneurysms pose a threat to patients because of their risk of rupture causing subarachnoid hemorrhage (SAH), and the goal of treatment is the exclusion of the aneurysm from the circulation to prevent bleeding (in the case of unruptured aneurysms) or rebleeding (in the case of ruptured aneurysms). Although there are different types and sizes of aneurysms, occurring at many locations within the cerebral vasculature and in patients of all ages, the general approach to the endovascular management of these lesions requires the same basic steps: (1) diagnosing the aneurysm and determining its suitability for endovascular treatment; (2) gaining endovascular access to the aneurysm; (3) excluding the aneurysm from the circulation; (4) avoiding complications during treatment; and (5) following up to monitor the durability of the treatment. This article explores these general technical considerations for the endovascular management of intracranial aneurysms.

RELEVANT ANATOMY AND PATHOPHYSIOLOGY

Endovascular Access

In contrast with open surgical treatment of aneurysms, in which the focus is on the regional

[a] Department of Neurosurgery, Cedars-Sinai Medical Center, 127 South San Vicente Boulevard, ASHP Building, Suite A6303, Los Angeles, CA 90048, USA; [b] University Neurosurgery Associates, 2335 E. Kashian Lane, Suite 301, UCSF-Fresno, Fresno, CA, USA
* Corresponding author.
E-mail address: michael.alexander@cshs.org

Neurosurg Clin N Am 25 (2014) 395–404
http://dx.doi.org/10.1016/j.nec.2014.04.016

neurosurgery.theclinics.com

intracranial vascular anatomy, during endovascular treatment of aneurysms consideration must also be given to peripheral vascular anatomy, aortic arch, and great vessel anatomy in addition to the intracranial vascular anatomy. Gaining endovascular access to the arteries of the brain requires first accessing the peripheral vascular system, usually by a transfemoral route (although transbrachial or transradial routes may be used),[1] navigating the aortic arch, and selecting the desired carotid or vertebral artery. Increased tortuosity of the great vessels, which is common with increasing age, or aberrant branching patterns from the arch can make it difficult to pass a catheter or can decrease its stability during the treatment.

Consideration must also be given to the course, orientation, and disease state of the cervical portion of the carotid and vertebral arteries. A high-grade cervical stenosis, or excessive tortuosity, may limit the ability to access intracranial lesions or may increase the risk of complications from the endovascular procedure, and strategies for treating or navigating these obstacles should be planned ahead of time, based on preoperative imaging studies. The final step of endovascular access is navigation of the intracranial vessels, and, again, review of preoperative imaging is important, because individual variability is high. The use of biplane angiography and biplane roadmapping is the standard of care in the endovascular treatment of cerebral aneurysms. Having 2 separate views of the regional arterial anatomy and the aneurysm increases the safety of the procedure by reducing the risk of parent artery or aneurysm perforation during aneurysm access and coil delivery.

In general, aneurysm treatment is performed by the most direct route available, usually via the ipsilateral carotid or vertebral artery. However, it is important to assess the patency of the circle of Willis, and give consideration to alternate access routes, based on the shape and orientation of the aneurysm, and in case of emergency, such as loss of access from the ipsilateral side during treatment.

Aneurysm and Parent Artery Anatomy

As described by Rhoton,[2] aneurysms tend to occur at branch points of the parent artery, usually where the vessel takes a curve, and point in the direction blood would have flowed if the branch or curve did not occur. Almost 80% of aneurysms occur in the anterior circulation, with the remaining 20% in the posterior circulation. The location and direction of the aneurysm with respect to the parent artery has important implications for the strategy used to access the inside of the lesion. For example, aneurysms arising at major bifurcations, such as the carotid T or basilar Y are usually entered with a straight or 45° angled microcatheter, whereas those occurring at smaller branch bifurcations, such as the posterior communicating or ophthalmic artery, may require a 90° or J-shaped microcatheter for access. For aneurysms of the anterior circulation, attention should be paid to whether the carotid siphon has an open or closed configuration, because the increased tortuosity of the latter can make catheter tracking more difficult.

For the most common type of intracranial aneurysm, the saccular aneurysm, numerous morphologic and geometric descriptors have been used. The most basic anatomic assessment is size, measured as the maximum diameter dimension of the aneurysm dome, and is important because increasing size is correlated with an increased risk of rupture according to data from the International Study of Unruptured Intracranial Aneurysms (ISUIA).[3] The shape of the aneurysm is also important, because the presence of irregularities or a daughter sac was associated with increased risk of rupture in the Japanese Unruptured Cerebral Aneurysm Study (UCAS).[4] Other geometric assessments based on ratios, such as the aspect ratio (dome height to neck width) and size ratio (aneurysm size to parent artery size) have also been positively associated with rupture risk.[5,6]

With regard to the suitability of aneurysms for endovascular treatment, alone or with adjuvants, the determination of the aneurysm as wide necked is important. The traditional definition of a wide-necked aneurysm is a neck width greater than 4 mm[7] or a dome to neck ratio of less than 2,[8] and was based on the likelihood of successful coiling in the early era of endovascular treatment. With the advent of coils with complex or three-dimensional (3D) shapes, it was suggested that aneurysms with dome to neck ratios down to 1.5 could be routinely treated with coiling alone.[9] In the modern era of adjunctive endovascular techniques, especially balloon remodeling and stent assistance, the assessment of morphology can help determined which aneurysms will require an adjunct. A retrospective review found that aneurysms with a dome to neck ratio of greater than 1.6, and an aspect ratio greater than 1.6, rarely required adjuncts for coiling, whereas those with dome to neck and aspect ratios of less than 1.2 almost always required an adjunctive technique. Aneurysms in the middle range, from 1.2 to 1.6, were equally divided between needing adjunctive techniques and not.[10] A recent large national registry study from Japan found that adjunctive techniques were applied in 54.8% of procedures for the endovascular treatment of unruptured aneurysms, highlighting their common use for managing lesions that would previously not have been able to be treated by endovascular therapy.[11]

Another important anatomic consideration is the presence of branch arteries in proximity to the aneurysm. Some of the most common branch vessels to consider include the ophthalmic, posterior communicating, anterior choroidal, posterior inferior cerebellar, large lenticulostriate perforators, and the recurrent artery of Heubner. The precise origin of these small vessels can be difficult to appreciate using conventional imaging techniques, but 3D rotational angiography can provide exquisite detail of their relation to the aneurysm neck. If the vessels arise from the parent artery, treatment of the aneurysm with conventional techniques and adjuncts is usually safe. If the branch arises from the base of the neck of the aneurysm, coiling may still be possible, although great care must be taken to preserve the origin of the vessel, and a neck remnant may be left to achieve this end. If the branch arises from higher up the neck or from the dome, coiling may present too high a risk for vessel occlusion with ischemic complication, or may leave too large a remnant for effective treatment of the aneurysm.

CLINICAL PRESENTATION AND DIAGNOSIS

Cerebral aneurysms present in one of 2 general categories: ruptured and unruptured. Because the morbidity and mortality from aneurysmal rupture are high, early and accurate diagnosis is important. The classic presentation of a ruptured aneurysm is the sudden onset of the worst headache of the patient's life, and strongly suggests that aneurysm rupture with SAH has occurred. However, not all patients have classic presentations, and a recent decision-making tool has been described to identify those requiring further investigation in the emergency department. It included patients that were alert, had a Glasgow Coma Scale (GCS) score of 15, with nontraumatic headache with onset less than 1 hour, and any of these 6 variables: age more than 40 years, neck pain or stiffness, witnessed loss of consciousness, onset during exertion, thunderclap or instant onset, and limited neck range of motion on examination.[12] Using this algorithm had a sensitivity of 100% and specificity of 15%, capturing all patients with SAH in the study and restricting unnecessary investigations. For patients with GCS less than 15, new neurologic deficits, or prior history of aneurysm or SAH, follow-up tests were always ordered.

The first test for SAH is nonenhanced computed tomography (CT) of the brain, because modern scanners have sensitivity nearing 100% for detecting aneurysmal SAH when performed within 3 days of the onset of symptoms.[13] After this time, as blood may clear from the cerebrospinal fluid (CSF) spaces, patients with no SAH visualized on CT but a suggestive clinical history should undergo lumbar puncture and examination of the CSF for xanthochromia; if positive, dedicated vascular imaging is needed.[14] CT angiogram (CTA) is the preferred initial cerebral vascular study in patients with SAH, because it provides sufficient anatomic information about aneurysm morphology, location, presence of branch vessels, and parent vessel anatomy to determine whether endovascular coiling or open clipping is the preferred treatment, and it also limits the risks associated with an invasive diagnostic angiogram. The addition of a CTA of the neck and arch vessels can help predict any challenges for endovascular access, and allows the operator to be prepared with appropriate catheter selection.

In contrast with ruptured aneurysms, unruptured aneurysms are rarely symptomatic, and are usually discovered incidentally on cerebral imaging performed for other indications, or as part of familial screening. Enlarging or changing aneurysms may cause a focal neurologic deficit from compression of an adjacent neural structure, such as a third nerve palsy from a posterior communicating artery aneurysm, or diplopia from a basilar artery aneurysm, and warrant prompt investigation and management. Magnetic resonance angiography (MRA) is a favored imaging modality for unruptured aneurysms, because it avoids the risks of radiation exposure and thromboembolic complications associated with CTA and digital subtraction arteriography, respectively, and in many cases can supply sufficient anatomic information to allow treatment planning, especially if it includes images of the neck and arch. As with ruptured aneurysms, the important technical considerations during assessment of diagnostic imaging are the routes of access (femoral/arch/cervical/intracranial) and the likelihood for needing adjunctive devices for aneurysm embolization based on lesion morphology.

ENDOVASCULAR CONSIDERATIONS

Background and Historical Perspectives

Although endovascular neurosurgery is a young discipline, advances in imaging technology and materials science have produced rapid progression, and recognition of new challenges continues to lead to new innovations. Neurointerventional suites have developed from single-arm, cathode ray tube–coupled image intensifiers, to biplane, flat-panel detectors with enhanced resolution and magnification, and the capability 3D rotational angiograms, 3D roadmap capability, aneurysm metric analysis, and virtual stenting ability (**Fig. 1**). Linked to modern image analysis software, the anatomic detail of the cerebral vasculature that can be obtained allows expanded application of endovascular techniques. The earliest intra-arterial treatments of aneurysms are attributed to Serbinenko,[15] who used detachable balloons to occlude aneurysm lumens. The development of detachable platinum coils by Guglielmi and colleagues[16] revolutionized endovascular treatment, and has created an industry of coil design based on different sizes, shapes, and materials.

Vascular access in the past was limited by the stiffness of guides and microcatheters, and by the thrombogenic properties of many wires. Advances in materials sciences have seen the introduction of highly flexible guide catheters that can be navigated more distally, or used in tandem with smaller catheters, providing a triaxial system of support consisting of a long flexible sheath, an intermediate distal access catheter, and a microcatheter. Hydrophilic coatings on wires reduce thrombus formation, and modern construction can produce soft but supportive and navigable devices. The desire to treat more complex intracranial lesions by endovascular means saw the introduction of numerous adjuncts to assist in coil embolization, most notably balloon and stent remodeling of aneurysm necks. The first stents were borrowed from interventional cardiology and were very stiff, often balloon mounted, and difficult to use in intracranial vessels. The advent of flexible, self-expanding nitinol stents that could be easily tracked through brain arteries permitted the treatment of wide-necked aneurysms that could not otherwise have been coiled,[17] and provided the impetus for the design of other stents both to support coiling and for stand-alone aneurysm treatment by flow diversion.

Available Techniques

The endovascular management paradigms for aneurysms can be broadly divided into deconstructive strategies (parent artery occlusion) with or without revascularization, and reconstructive strategies (aneurysm occlusion with parent artery preservation). Reconstructive strategies include coil embolization alone or with balloon or stent assistance, intrasaccular liquid polymer embolization, low-porosity flow-diverting intraluminal stents, and endosaccular flow-diverting devices.

Deconstructive techniques produce aneurysm occlusion by directly stopping inflow through parent artery occlusion at the origin of the aneurysm; by inducing thrombosis through a type of hunterian ligation, with occlusion of the parent artery proximal to the aneurysm origin; or by trapping the aneurysm with parent artery occlusion both proximal and distal to the aneurysm origin. The original method for parent artery occlusion, still available in many countries, is inflation and deployment of detachable balloons, which has the advantage of rapid occlusion of the parent artery at the site of delivery but can be difficult to

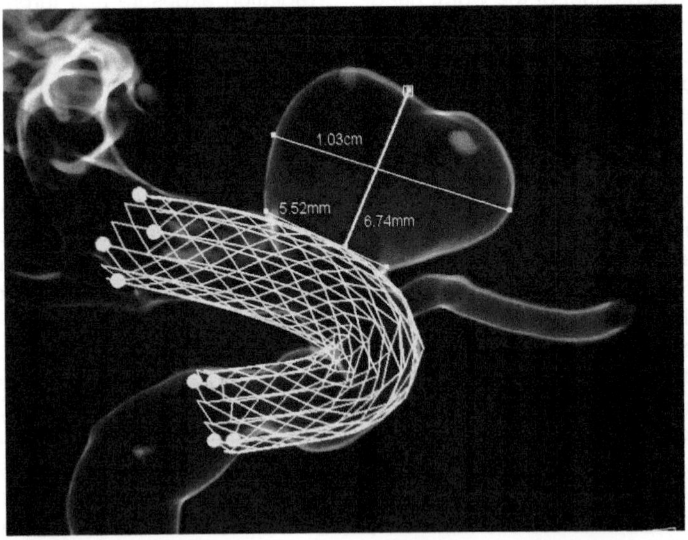

Fig. 1. Three-dimensional rotational angiogram reconstruction with virtual stenting of wide-necked aneurysm and morphologic analysis measurements.

navigate and has a risk of premature detachment. The other endovascular technique for parent artery occlusion (and the only technique currently available in the United States) is delivery of detachable coils into the lumen. An advantage of this method is that coils may be placed over a shorter segment of the vessel than a balloon, reducing the risk to perforating arteries, but a drawback is increased time for delivery and usually more devices are needed compared with balloons. The most important consideration before parent artery occlusion is the status of collateral circulation, which should be assessed both anatomically by presence of communicating arteries, and functionally, such as with balloon test occlusion, to minimize the risk of ischemic complications with vessel sacrifice. As reconstructive treatments continue to expand and improve, deconstructive techniques are being used less commonly, but may still be used for cases such as dissecting aneurysms, progressively enlarging fusiform aneurysms such as those of the vertebrobasilar system, and giant cavernous segment aneurysms.

Reconstructive strategies are intended to exclude aneurysms from the circulation and preserve normal vessels. Primary coiling with detachable coils is the first choice in reconstructive techniques in most cases. Selection of an appropriate size and shape for the first coil based on aneurysm morphology creates a stable frame, allowing subsequent coils to be delivered inside for progressive aneurysm occlusion. Most coil manufacturers provide a range of sizes, shapes, and stiffness levels, designed for different types of aneurysms and different stages of the procedure. The initial framing coil is usually selected to have a complex 3D shape and to be stiffer, to provide stability for the coil mass and to keep it within the aneurysm. Subsequent filling coils are generally softer, smaller, and may have complex or helical shapes to fill the remaining space within the aneurysm and promote thrombosis. Despite advances in coil shape technology, aneurysms with unfavorable morphology (wide necks, low dome to neck and aspect ratios) present a risk for coil herniation into the parent artery, and operators tend to be less aggressive about achieving high packing densities, leading to lower rates of complete occlusion, increased neck remnants, and more recurrences over time. To address these concerns, the adjunctive techniques of balloon and stent remodeling have been developed.

The first technique developed to assist in coil delivery for wide-necked aneurysms was balloon remodeling with temporarily inflatable, nondetachable balloons.[18,19] By this method, a microcatheter capable of delivering coils is positioned inside the aneurysm, and a balloon is then inflated in the parent artery across the neck of the aneurysm, stabilizing the catheter and allowing coil delivery without herniation into the parent artery. The balloon is usually then deflated, and if the coil remains in place it is detached; recently, some investigators have advocated delivering and detaching several coils during 1 balloon inflation to increase the complexity and stability of the coil mass.[20] The benefits of balloon-assisted coiling are the ability to treat wide-necked lesions and achieve higher packing densities without the need for implanted devices or antiplatelet therapy; this latter point is especially important for reducing hemorrhagic complications with ruptured aneurysms. Some risks of using a balloon include arterial injury or rupture during inflation, or rupture of the aneurysm. Thrombotic and embolic complications are higher with balloon use, but can be mitigated with judicious periprocedural anticoagulation. Balloon inflation causes temporary cessation of blood flow and risk of ischemia if collateral circulation is limited; slow coil detachment systems can increase the time at risk, whereas more rapid detachments facilitate shorter inflation times. In addition, with balloon deflation, there is a small risk of prolapse or frank herniation and migration of the coil mass, especially if several coils have been detached together.[21]

Stent-assisted coiling is another reconstructive technique to allow the endovascular treatment of wide-necked aneurysms. The 2 most common stents currently used for supporting aneurysm coiling are the open-cell Neuroform stent (Stryker Neurovascular, Fremont, CA) and the closed-cell Enterprise stent (Codman and Shurtleff, Raynham, MA), although several other stents designed to support coiling are available in other countries and are currently in clinical trials in the United States. In the closed-cell design, all of the stent tynes are connected and the stent moves as single piece, with the pores fixed and closed; in the open-cell design, about half of the tynes are not connected, allowing some of the pores to be open. These properties may affect the stent apposition to the wall of the artery and the support provided by the device, and open-cell stents are often used in more tortuous artery segments.

The goal of stent delivery is to cover the neck of the aneurysm, providing a structural support to keep coils inside. The stent may also provide a hemodynamic benefit, redirecting flow inside the normal vessel lumen (although to a significantly lesser degree than a flow-diverter device), and may also serve as a scaffold for endothelialization. There are numerous methods by which stent-assisted coiling can be performed. The stent may be delivered followed by reaccessing the aneurysm by passing the microcatheter through the stent cells for coiling, requiring the use of only a single microcatheter. Alternatively, 2 microcatheters may be used, with the first positioned inside the aneurysm, then the second used to deliver the stent, jailing the first in a stable configuration for coiling and removing the need for passing through the stent (**Fig. 2**). For aneurysms occurring near the origin of small branch vessels, such as the ophthalmic or posterior communicating artery, typically only a single stent is required, and care must be taken to preserve the branch during coiling. For bifurcation aneurysms, such as at the basilar apex, carotid terminus, or middle cerebral artery, a Y-stent technique may be used, with stents placed in both branches to fully protect the parent arteries during coiling.[22]

For Y stenting, the first device is preferably an open-cell design so that the second device, which may be open or closed cell, can fit through without becoming narrowed. The first stent is deployed in the branch that is the most challenging to access, because the interstices of the stent can make subsequent selection of the contralateral branch more difficult, so it is better to access the more favorable vessel at this point. With both branches protected, the aneurysm is then reaccessed through the struts of the stent and coils are deployed, or, alternatively, the microcatheter jailing technique may also be used. In order to prevent thromboembolic complications and thrombosis of the stent, patients are started on dual antiplatelet therapy before the procedure. Several investigators have advocated the preprocedural assessment of antiplatelet medication therapeutic effect and correction if necessary.[23]

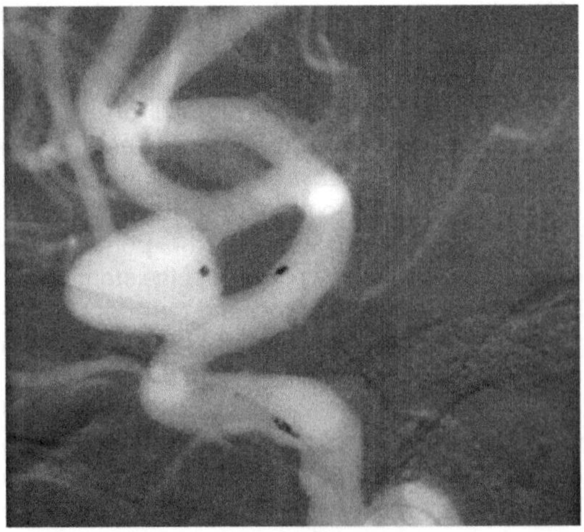

Fig. 2. Roadmap lateral angiogram view showing the microcatheter jailing technique. The tip of the first microcatheter is located in the aneurysm dome. A second microcatheter crosses the neck of the aneurysm with a stent ready to be deployed.

Although subtherapeutic values may increase the risk for thromboembolic complications, supratherapeutic values may increase the risk for hemorrhagic complications. The risk of hemorrhagic complications from these medications is typically very low for unruptured cases, but it increases dramatically for ruptured aneurysms, especially with respect to other neurosurgical procedures such as ventriculostomy and ventriculoperitoneal shunting. A recent review found roughly double the number of complications in stent-assisted coiling of ruptured versus unruptured aneurysms (13% vs 6%–7%).[24] Another potential concern with the use of stents is occlusion of perforators or small branch arteries. Although the porosity of the commonly used stents is high, with a small amount of metal compared to the size of the interstices, it is still possible that a strut may cover the ostium of a perforator and acutely occlude it, or that occlusion may occur gradually as the stent heals into the parent vessel wall and is covered by endothelium. In addition, as noted in coronary and other vessels in the body, intracranial stents are at risk of developing in-stent stenosis, which can be more problematic in small vessels and, although rarely symptomatic, warrants judicious follow-up, although this seems to occur less frequently with aneurysm stents compared with stents placed for the treatment of atherosclerotic disease.

Another available reconstructive technique for endovascular treatment of aneurysms is the use of stand-alone flow-diverting stents. Flow-diverting stents differ from other intracranial stents by having lower porosity, favoring intraluminal blood flow, and leading to stagnation and thrombosis within a covered aneurysm, but permitting ongoing demand-based flow into covered branches and perforating arteries (**Fig. 3**). The 2 devices with the most clinical experience are the Pipeline embolization device (Covidien, Irvine, CA), currently approved by the US Food and Drug Administration for anterior circulation aneurysms larger than 10 mm and proximal to the superior hypophyseal artery, and the Silk stent (Balt Extrusion, Montmorency, France), available in Europe. The Pipeline for the Intracranial Treatment of Aneurysms (PITA) trial[25] evaluated 31 patients who had placement of the Pipeline flow diverter for treatment of unruptured cerebral aneurysms. Delayed follow-up angiography showed a 93% complete aneurysm occlusion rate. The Pipeline for Uncoilable or Failed aneurysm Study (PUFS) trial[26] evaluated 107 patients with large or giant aneurysms with a wide neck and found a delayed complete

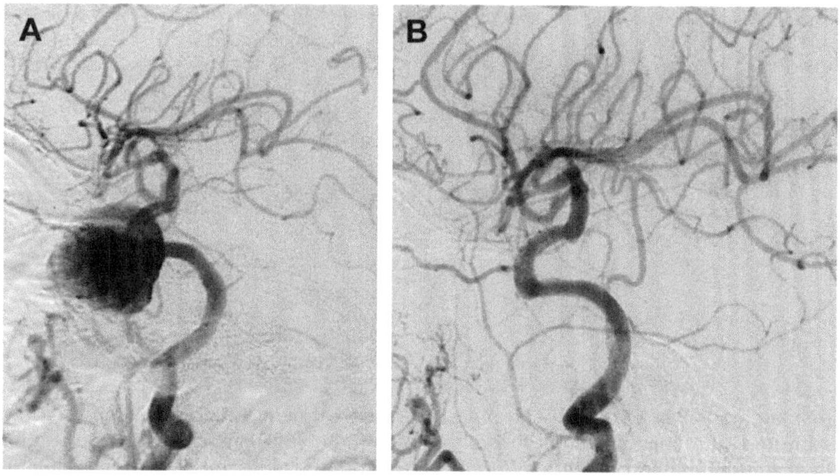

Fig. 3. (*A*) Lateral angiographic view of symptomatic giant cavernous internal carotid artery aneurysm with a wide neck. (*B*) Delayed follow-up lateral angiogram 12 months following the placement of a single Pipeline flow-diverter device and no endosaccular coils showing complete obliteration of the aneurysm and preservation of the ophthalmic artery.

aneurysm occlusion rate of 74%. Use of flow diverters also requires dual antiplatelet medications, with the attendant risks described earlier.

Indications and Contraindications

Patients with ruptured aneurysms require treatment to prevent rebleeding, and based on current evidence the most recent guidelines on the management of aneurysmal SAH suggested that for aneurysms amenable to either endovascular or surgical treatment, endovascular therapy should be considered first.[27] Although there may be considerable variation based on operator experience and comfort level in determining which aneurysms are amenable to either treatment, the modern endovascular toolbox allows a coil-first policy to be reasonable in many cases. Some contraindications to endovascular therapy include the presence of life-threatening intracerebral hematoma, requiring surgical evacuation, and, if feasible, clipping the aneurysm may be performed at the same time. Other anatomic features are contraindications to coiling, such as the presence of important branch arteries arising from the body of the aneurysm, or proximal vessel tortuosity that preclude endovascular access. In addition, wide-necked ruptured aneurysms that would require stent-assisted coiling and the use of dual antiplatelet agents, and especially those with ventriculostomy, may be better treated with surgery, because they are at higher risk of hemorrhagic complications from endovascular therapy. This clinical decision is based on the treating team's level of expertise and the patient's clinical condition.

For patients with unruptured aneurysms, the indications for treatment are based on size, shape, location, and patient factors. A review of the national inpatient sample from 2001 to 2008 identified patients undergoing coiling as having lower morbidity and mortality compared with those treated by surgical clipping, and there was a trend toward a higher percentage of coil embolization treatments over time, from 20% in 2001 to 63% in 2008.[28] Again, modern endovascular techniques and adjuncts, including the safer use of dual antiplatelets in this population, make it reasonable to approach patients who do not have a contraindication using an endovascular first policy. Some contraindications include important branch vessels arising from the aneurysm that could not be preserved with endovascular treatment, and restrictions of endovascular access. Other factors that some investigators have suggested to favor surgical clipping include young patient age (because clipping durability is argued to be higher) and middle cerebral artery (MCA) location, although both of these have been debated in the literature. A recently published endovascular series by Alexander and colleagues[29] of 184 MCA aneurysms reported that 38% of the MCA aneurysms that were embolized required stent assistance, with an overall periprocedural complication rate of 3.8%, suggesting that MCA location by itself is not a contraindication to embolization (**Fig. 4**).

Pearls and Pitfalls

Clinical outcomes

For patients with ruptured aneurysms, outcome is often related to presenting grade, as well as numerous other patient and clinical factors; however, overall, the results from 2 large randomized

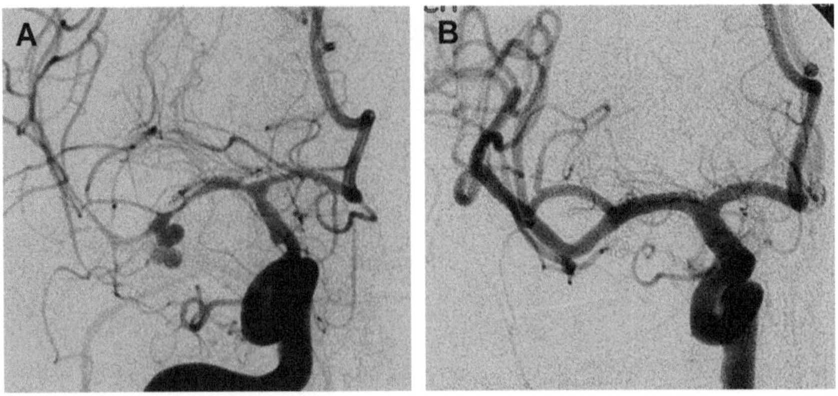

Fig. 4. (*A*) Initial angiogram of a patient who presented for treatment 6 days following subarachnoid hemorrhage with a ruptured MCA aneurysm and concomitant vasospasm. (*B*) Six-month follow-up angiogram showing complete MCA aneurysm obliteration with a durable angiographic result and resolution of the previously seen vasospasm.

trials showed that the number of patients who were dead or disabled at 1 year after SAH was 23% for those treated with endovascular coiling compared with 30% to 33% in the clipping group.[30,31] For unruptured aneurysms, assessment of the national inpatient sample from 2001 to 2008 showed that 4.9% of patients treated with coiling were discharged to long-term facilities, suggesting disability, with a 0.6% mortality, compared with 14% and 1.2% respectively for clipped patients.[28]

Another outcome that is important to assess for aneurysms treated by endovascular coiling is the degree of occlusion at the end of the procedure, because incompletely treated lesions have increased risk for recurrence, regrowth, and rupture. A commonly used classification for degree of aneurysm occlusion is the Raymond scale, a 3-point classification that grades treatment as class1 if completely occluded, class 2 if a neck remnant is present, and class 3 if there is residual filling of the aneurysm.[32] Based on angiographic follow-up, none of the aneurysms initially graded as class 1 showed progression to class 3 or required retreatment, whereas 12% of the class 2 aneurysms progressed to class 3.

Another assessment of the degree of aneurysm occlusion is based on a calculated packing density, in which the volume of the aneurysm is assessed by its angiographic dimensions, and the percent volume filled is determined by the length and caliber of the coils deposited, yielding a percent packing density. Some studies have suggested a relationship between higher packing densities and lower rates of recurrence on follow-up angiography, but the optimum packing density for any given aneurysm is not precisely known, and other hemodynamic factors such as inflow at the neck may be equally important.[33,34] In general, Raymond class 1 occlusion and packing densities more than 20% are generally considered desirable to reduce the risk of recurrence.

Follow-up considerations

Most large series show that, for coil embolization, larger aneurysms have a higher chance of delayed aneurysm recurrence by coil compaction or interval aneurysm growth. It is therefore considered the standard of care to obtain delayed intracranial vascular imaging to assess for aneurysm occlusion stability. The modality for imaging follow-up has been controversial, with some investigators advocating diagnostic catheter angiography and others recommending high-resolution MRA imaging. Recommendations for the initial follow-up imaging have been at 3 or 6 months following embolization, and again at 1 or 2 years following treatment, with longer follow-up recommended by some investigators.

SUMMARY

The safety of the endovascular treatment of cerebral aneurysms is contingent on appropriate preprocedural planning and the stepwise sequential analysis and management based on the aneurysm size, shape, neck, proximal arterial anatomy, and clinical factors. With a comprehensive toolbox of coils, stents, liquid polymers, flow-diverting devices, and advanced imaging, these procedures can be effective in a wide range of ruptured and nonruptured cerebral aneurysms with equivalent or superior outcomes to traditional open surgical therapy, as shown by multiple randomized clinical trials and national clinical outcomes database assessment. This field continues to develop with additional innovative devices soon to be available.

REFERENCES

1. Zaidat OO, Szeder V, Alexander MJ. Transbrachial stent-assisted coil embolization of right posterior inferior cerebellar artery aneurysm: technical case report. J Neuroimaging 2007;17(4):344–7.
2. Rhoton AL Jr. Aneurysms. Neurosurgery 2002; 51(Suppl 4):S121–58.
3. Wiebers DO, Whisnant JP, Huston J 3rd, et al, International Study of Unruptured Intracranial Aneurysms Investigators. Unruptured intracranial aneurysms: natural history, clinical outcome, and risks of surgical and endovascular treatment. Lancet 2003; 362(9378):103–10.
4. UCAS Japan Investigators, Morita A, Kirino T, et al. The natural course of unruptured cerebral aneurysms in a Japanese cohort. N Engl J Med 2012; 366(26):2474–82.
5. Weir B, Amidei C, Kongable G, et al. The aspect ratio (dome/neck) of ruptured and unruptured aneurysms. J Neurosurg 2003;99(3):447–51.
6. Rahman M, Smietana J, Hauck E, et al. Size ratio correlates with intracranial aneurysm rupture status: a prospective study. Stroke 2010;41(5): 916–20.
7. Guglielmi G, Vinuela F, Duckwiler G, et al. Endovascular treatment of posterior circulation aneurysms by electrothrombosis using electrically detachable coils. J Neurosurg 1992;77(4):515–24.
8. Debrun GM, Aletich VA, Kehrli P, et al. Selection of cerebral aneurysms for treatment using Guglielmi detachable coils: the preliminary University of Illinois at Chicago experience. Neurosurgery 1998;43(6): 1281–95.
9. Cloft HJ, Joseph GJ, Tong FC, et al. Use of three-dimensional Guglielmi coils in the treatment of wide-necked cerebral aneurysms. AJNR Am J Neuroradiol 2000;21(7):1312–4.
10. Brinjikji W, Cloft HJ, Kallmes DF. Difficult aneurysms for endovascular treatment: overwide or undertall? AJNR Am J Neuroradiol 2009;30(8):1513–7.
11. Shigematsu T, Fujinaka T, Yoshimine T, et al, JR-NET Investigators. Endovascular therapy for asymptomatic unruptured intracranial aneurysms: JR-NET and JR-NET2 findings. Stroke 2013;44(10):2735–42.
12. Perry JJ, Stiell IG, Sivilotti ML, et al. Clinical decision rules to rule out subarachnoid hemorrhage for acute headache. JAMA 2013;310(12):1248–55.
13. Cortnum S, Sorensen P, Jorgensen J. Determining the sensitivity of computed tomography scanning in early detection of subarachnoid hemorrhage. Neurosurgery 2010;66(5):900–2.
14. Horstman P, Linn FH, Voorbij HA, et al. Chance of aneurysm in patients suspected of SAH who have a "negative" CT scan but a "positive" lumbar puncture. J Neurol 2012;259(4):649–52.
15. Serbinenko FA. Balloon catheterization and occlusion of major cerebral vessels. J Neurosurg 1974; 41(2):125–45.
16. Guglielmi G, Vinuela F, Sepetka I, et al. Electrothrombosis of saccular aneurysms via endovascular approach. Part 1: electrochemical basis, technique, and experimental results. J Neurosurg 1991;75(1): 1–7.
17. Wanke I, Doerfler A, Schoch B, et al. Treatment of wide-necked intracranial aneurysms with a self-expanding stent system: initial clinical experience. AJNR Am J Neuroradiol 2003;24(6):1192–9.
18. Moret J, Cognard C, Weill A, et al. The "remodeling technique" in the treatment of wide neck intracranial aneurysms. Angiographic results and clinical follow up in 56 cases. Interv Neuroradiol 1997;3(1):21–35.
19. Lefkowitz MA, Gobin YP, Akiba Y, et al. Balloon-assisted Guglielmi detachable coiling of wide-necked aneurysms: part II – clinical results. Neurosurgery 1999;45(3):531–7.
20. Fiorella D, Woo HH. Balloon assisted treatment of intracranial aneurysms: the conglomerate coil mass technique. J Neurointerv Surg 2009;1(2):121–31.
21. Fiorella D, Kelly ME, Moskowitz S, et al. Delayed symptomatic coil migration after initially successful balloon-assisted aneurysm coiling: technical case report. Neurosurgery 2009;64(2):E391–2.
22. Chow MM, Woo HH, Masaryk TJ, et al. A novel endovascular treatment of a wide-necked basilar apex aneurysm by using a Y-configuration, double stent technique. AJNR Am J Neuroradiol 2004;25(3): 509–12.
23. Drazin D, Choulakian A, Nuno M, et al. Body weight: a risk factor for subtherapeutic antithrombotic therapy in neurovascular stenting. J Neurointerv Surg 2011;3(2):177–81.
24. Bodily KD, Cloft HJ, Lanzino G, et al. Stent-assisted coiling in acutely ruptured intracranial aneurysms: a qualitative, systematic review of the literature. AJNR Am J Neuroradiol 2011;32(7):1232–6.
25. Nelson PK, Lylyk P, Szikora I, et al. The pipeline embolization device for the intracranial treatment of aneurysms trial. AJNR Am J Neuroradiol 2011; 32(1):34–40.
26. Becske T, Kallmes DF, Saatci I, et al. Pipeline for uncoilable or failed aneurysms: results from a multicenter clinical trial. Radiology 2013;267(3):858–68.
27. Connolly ES Jr, Rabinstein AA, Carhuapoma JR, et al. Guidelines for the management of aneurysmal subarachnoid hemorrhage: a guideline for healthcare professionals from the American Heart Association/American Stroke Association. Stroke 2012; 43(6):1711–37.
28. Brinjikji W, Rabinstein AA, Nasr DM, et al. Better outcomes with treatment by coiling relative to clipping

of unruptured intracranial aneurysms in the United States, 2001-2008. AJNR Am J Neuroradiol 2011; 32(6):1071–5.
29. Eboli P, Ryan RW, Alexander JE, et al. Evolving role of endovascular treatment for MCA bifurcation aneurysms: case series of 184 aneurysms and review of the literature. Neurol Res 2014;36(4):332–8.
30. Molyneux AJ, Kerr RS, Yu LM, et al, International Subarachnoid Aneurysm Trial (ISAT) Collaborative Group. International Subarachnoid Aneurysm Trial (ISAT) of neurosurgical clipping versus endovascular coiling in 2143 patients with ruptured intracranial aneurysms: a randomised comparison of effects on survival, dependency, seizures, rebleeding, subgroups, and aneurysm occlusion. Lancet 2005;366(9488):809–17.
31. Spetzler RF, McDougall CG, Albuquerque FC, et al. The barrow ruptured aneurysm trial: 3-year results. J Neurosurg 2013;119(1):146–57.
32. Roy D, Milot G, Raymond J. Endovascular treatment of unruptured aneurysms. Stroke 2001;32(9): 1998–2004.
33. Kawanabe Y, Sadato A, Taki W, et al. Endovascular occlusion of intracranial aneurysms with Guglielmi detachable coils: correlation between coil packing density and coil compaction. Acta Neurochir (Wien) 2001;143(5):451–5.
34. Sluzewski M, van Rooij WJ, Slob MJ, et al. Relation between aneurysm volume, packing, and compaction in 145 cerebral aneurysms treated with coils. Radiology 2004;231(3):653–8.

Pitfalls and Complications Management in the Endovascular Treatment of Aneurysms

Samer G. Zammar, MD, Youssef J. Hamade, MD, Tarek Y. El Ahmadieh, MD, Najib E. El Tecle, MD, Bernard R. Bendok, MD, MS*

KEYWORDS

• Intracranial aneurysms • Endovascular • Complications • Outcomes assessment

KEY POINTS

- It is crucial to recognize and understand the potential complications associated with endovascular treatment of intracranial aneurysms.
- Understanding the complications associated with endovascular treatment of intracranial aneurysms allows the health care provider to account for several measurements that could potentially avoid the complications and provide more efficiency in their treatment.
- Improved patient selection for endovascular treatment, meticulous planning and preparation of the procedure, anticipating potential complications and preparing for management, building databases that include patients' outcomes assessment, and allowing peer rating and feedback on operative skill can all help to avoid complications.
- The importance of the operator's expertise cannot be overemphasized in the prevention and successful management of these complications.
- Current advancements in simulation, 3-dimensional printing, and holography can potentially play a crucial role in training the novices in endovascular management of intracranial aneurysms and increasing the level of proficiency of the graduating physicians, thus decreasing the incidence of complications.

INTRODUCTION

Complications associated with the endovascular management of intracranial aneurysms can be devastating.[1–4] Successful patient management requires vigilant avoidance, recognition, and management of complications. Both neurologic and nonneurologic complications can occur. Several patient-related and procedure-related parameters can increase the incidence of complications. Reduction of complication rates can be achieved by careful patient selection, meticulous planning and preparation for the procedure, anticipating potential complications, and preparing for their management. Tracking outcomes and a robust case conference for discussion of cases and

Disclosures: None.
Department of Neurological Surgery, Northwestern Memorial Hospital, 676 North St. Clair, Suite 2210, Chicago, IL 60611, USA
* Corresponding author.
E-mail address: bbendok@nmff.org

Neurosurg Clin N Am 25 (2014) 405–413
http://dx.doi.org/10.1016/j.nec.2014.04.002

complications can further enhance outcomes. Education of the care team and a collaborative environment can foster greater focus on complication avoidance. This article reviews complications associated with the endovascular management of intracranial aneurysms, focusing on risk factors, avoidance, recognition, and management.

RISK FACTORS

Patient-Related Risk Factors

Age

Using the National Inpatient Sample (NIS) database, Lawson and colleagues[5] retrieved data on 14,050 patient admissions and concluded that endovascular procedures may confer greater risks than aneurysmal rupture in patients older than 80 years. On the other hand, patients younger than 70 years may have greater benefits from endovascular coiling. Similarly, Brinjikji and colleagues[6] collected data from the NIS on patients undergoing clipping or coiling of unruptured intracranial aneurysms in the United States between 2001 and 2008 to assess the effect of age on clinical outcome. Their analysis showed that for both treatment groups, morbidity and mortality rates increased with age yet were more pronounced in the surgical group. Furthermore, the biggest difference in outcome was seen in the age group of 80 years and older, whereby morbidity reached 33.5% for clipping versus 9.8% for coiling ($P<.0001$) and mortality reached 21.4% for clipping versus 2.4% for coiling ($P<.0001$).[6] On a more specific level, rising trends of morbidity and mortality with age were also seen in patients undergoing endovascular coiling, starting respectively from 3.5% and 0.6% in the age group younger than 50 years, to 0.5% and 4.0% in patients aged 50 to 64 years, to 0.8% and 6.9% in patients aged 65 to 79 years, and reaching 2.4% and 9.8% in those older than 80 years.[6] Fifi and colleagues[7] conducted a retrospective study to assess clinical predictors of complications in 3636 diagnostic catheter cerebral angiograms at a single center. Among predictors including patient age, sex, inpatient versus outpatient status, and indications for angiography, only age older than 65 years was significantly associated with development of complications. Patients in this age group were 4 times more likely (95% confidence interval 1.268–13.859) than younger patients to develop procedural complications.[7] Similar findings were reported by Willinsky and colleagues,[8] who evaluated prospectively a total of 2899 cerebral digital subtraction angiograms to determine risk factors for neurologic complications related to cerebral angiography. Patients aged 55 years and older were found to be significantly more prone than their younger counterparts to develop neurologic complications (1.8% vs 0.9%, respectively; $P<.035$). Although age seems an important risk factor to take into consideration, it may be difficult to determine a specific cutoff beyond which risks of endovascular procedures would significantly increase, as cutoff ages have been shown to vary among studies.

Cerebrovascular risk factors

Cerebrovascular risk factors have been implicated in increasing the risk of neurologic complications following cerebral angiography.[2,8–16] Of these, stroke and transient ischemic attacks (TIAs) have been shown to increase the rate of complications the most.[13] Cloft and colleagues[17] conducted a meta-analysis to assess patients who presented with subarachnoid hemorrhage, cerebral arteriovenous malformation, and aneurysms. The risk of transient and permanent neurologic complications was found to be greater in the presence of TIAs and strokes (3.7%) than in patients with subarachnoid hemorrhage (1.8%) or aneurysms/arteriovenous malformations (0.3%).

Cardiovascular risk factors

The presence of cardiovascular risk factors such as elevated blood pressure, diabetes, and heart failure also has an impact on the risk of procedural complications. A systolic blood pressure of more than 160 mm Hg appears to be significantly associated with the risk of complications.[8,11] In their prospective study, Earnest and colleagues[11] found an increased risk of local (small hematomas) and neurologic complications with the presence of systolic blood pressure greater than 160 mm Hg. Similar findings were also reported by Willinsky and colleagues,[8] who noted a 2.3% risk of complications in patients with a history of cardiovascular disease. Diabetes was found to increase the risk of neurologic complications between 24 and 72 hours following cerebral angiography procedures.[2]

Renal and hydration status

Although contrast-induced nephropathy (CIN) is a well-known complication of angiography with severe consequences, its incidence has decreased remarkably since the advent of nonionic contrast media. In the absence of other causes of renal damage, CIN can be defined as a decline in renal function with more than 25% increase in serum creatinine levels within 24 hours following exposure to contrast agents.[18–21] The risk of CIN tends to increase with the presence of comorbidities such as diabetes and heart failure, in addition to a state of hydration before endovascular procedures.[5,19] Earnest and colleagues[11] found that elevated serum creatinine levels and overall poor preprocedural renal status were associated with a higher risk of neurologic complications. With a significant amount of information on CIN now available in the cardiac literature with a reported average complication risk of 14% in patients undergoing diagnostic procedures for coronary intervention,[5,19] there is wide consensus that patient hydration is an effective way to prevent the development of CIN. However, there is controversy regarding adjuvant empiric steps such as the use of *N*-acetylcysteine (NAC) or sodium bicarbonate. Some studies of coronary angiography reported benefit with the administration of NAC even after the use of moderate and high doses of contrast agent.[19,22] By contrast, other studies reported no benefit from the use of NAC compared with normal saline alone.[23–25] This finding has also been confirmed recently by the Acetylcysteine for Contrast-Induced Nephropathy Trial (ACT), which showed no advantage of NAC in preventing CIN in patients undergoing vascular or coronary angiography.[26] As for sodium bicarbonate, there exists even more controversy regarding its usefulness as a renoprotective agent. In a retrospective study conducted at the Mayo Clinic involving 7977 patients, findings show that administration of sodium bicarbonate may have harmful effects in comparison with saline.[22]

Procedural-Related Risk Factors

Type of contrast agent

Several studies have compared ionic and nonionic contrasts in endovascular interventions, with varying results in relation to the rate of complications. In a prospectively reviewed series of 230 arch and carotid arteriograms that used ionic contrast agents in 98 patients and nonionic contrast agents in 132 patients, McIvor and colleagues[23] found no significant difference in neurologic outcome. On the other hand, Skalpe[24] evaluated neurologic complications of 1509 cerebral angiograms that used ionic contrast agent in a comparison with 1000 angiograms that used nonionic contrast. He found higher complication rates with ionic agents (2%) than with nonionic agents (1.3%). Whereas some studies have linked the use of ionic agents in angiography to an increased risk of renal damage and cerebrovascular complications, with respect to nonionic contrast agents the evidence may be controversial.[2,23–25]

Volume of injected contrast agent

The volume of injected contrast agent appears to be related to an increased risk of procedural complications. Dion and colleagues[2] found that using high volumes of contrast agent increased the risk of neurologic events in the first 24 hours (P = .03) and between 24 and 72 hours (P = .001) following cerebral angiography procedures. There was also an increased risk of nonneurologic events, especially wound hematomas of less than 5 cm in diameter (P<.00001).[2]

Time of the procedure

An increase in procedural time has been associated with an increased risk of complications and overall patient clinical outcome in a wide range of surgical specialties. Mani and Eisenberg[27] assessed the procedural time of 4795 consecutive cerebral angiograms and reported a high complication rate when the time of procedure surpassed 80 minutes (P<.01). Similar conclusions were also drawn by Heiserman and colleagues,[9] who analyzed 1000 cerebral angiograms. Nevertheless, many investigators consider fluoroscopy time to be an important measure of procedural difficulty. In their study, Willinsky and colleagues[8] found that the rate of neurologic complications increased significantly after 10 minutes of fluoroscopy time.

Catheter exchange

Frequent catheter exchange and manipulation during endovascular procedures may reflect the difficulty of the case at hand (tortuous vasculature) or even the inexperience of the operator, and several studies have reported higher rates of neurologic complications with increased number of catheters used.[2,11,28] Dion and colleagues[2] noted an increasing trend of neurologic complications in the first 24 hours following cerebral angiography when 3 or more catheters were used (P = .08). Nonneurologic complications, especially small wound hematomas, also increased significantly in relation to the number of catheters used (P<.00001). Even more than 24 hours following the procedure, frequent catheter use was associated with higher rates of neurologic complications and was found to be a prognostic indicator for patients' neurologic outcome, irrespective of their diagnosis or complexity of the lesions.[11]

Operator experience

Whereas some studies did not show an association between operator experience and the rate of neurologic complications,[9] many others have demonstrated higher complication rates with inexperienced hands.[8,13,23,25,29] Mani and colleagues[25] retrospectively analyzed 5000 cerebral angiograms and found an increased rate of procedural complications in training hospitals in comparison with nontraining hospitals (3.9% vs 0.9%), but the rate of permanent complications was similar in both groups (0.1%). On the other hand, Willinsky and colleagues[8] compared procedures done by faculty members and those by fellows alone but did not find a difference in the rate of neurologic complications, although this rate seemed to increase when the procedures were jointly performed by faculty members and fellows. However, in many of these instances the patient had been older with a worse disease history.

Technique

A complete review of aneurysm coiling techniques is beyond the scope of this article, but it is worth mentioning some nuances of aneurysm coiling as they relate to complication avoidance.[30] Femoral-access complications can be minimized by careful attention to anatomic landmarks and thoughtful use of fluoroscopy to avoid traumatic placement of a sheath. Radial access should be considered in selected cases if femoral access is not feasible or is considered high risk.[31] Guide-catheter placement in the target cervical vessel should be done carefully to avoid complications. Newer guide catheters[32] have dramatically enhanced the stability and safety of such catheters. Three-dimensional angiography has proved to be a useful tool to optimize working views and the understanding of what can be highly complex anatomy. Microcatheter placement in the target aneurysm should be approached with caution and high-magnification road-map fluoroscopy. Sizing of the coils and their choice should be methodical, and the placement of every loop should be carefully monitored. It is important to avoid placing very small coils at the neck, which are not interwoven into the coil matrix, to avoid distal embolization. When a stent is needed the authors typically jail the catheter in the aneurysm first. Though not necessary, the authors have found that this technique avoids the need to traverse a newly paced stent, which can be difficult occasionally. Knowing when to stop adding coils is as much art as it is individual. Although complete aneurysm occlusion is ideal, leaving a neck remnant may be a good tradeoff in favor of safety. Staging may be needed in complex scenarios. Final angiography should carefully rule out dissections and thromboembolic complications. Closure of the access site should be meticulous to avoid hemorrhagic and ischemic complications. Because of the potential for aneurysm recurrence after coiling, a clear follow-up plan must be in place and carefully explained to the patient.

COMPLICATIONS

Thromboembolic

Despite their low risk of occurrence, clinically relevant ischemic events associated with endovascular treatments of intracranial abnormalities can be serious.[1,2,33] In diagnostic cerebral angiography, the rate of permanent neurologic deficits is estimated to be 0.14% to 0.50%.[5] Moreover, with the emergence of diffusion-weighted magnetic resonance imaging (DW-MRI) techniques, clinically silent ischemic events appear to be associated with cerebral angiographic procedures in 10% to 40% of cases.[5,8,9,33–35] In a study that included 72 patients who underwent DW-MRI before and after cerebral angiographic procedures, Park and colleagues[33] reported 1 to 23 lesions in 37 patients. Most of these lesions were smaller than 5 mm and lacunar in nature. Interestingly these lesions occurred in vessels that were not directly related to the endovascular treatment, and were lodged mostly in the cerebral cortical border zone area and the cerebellar hemispheres rather than deep perforating arterial territories. Although clinically silent, these "soft"[36] infarcts have the potential to cause neurocognitive impairments.[36,37] The microemboli occurring during endovascular treatment of aneurysms can be either gaseous or thrombotic. Air emboli can appear when drawing the syringe quickly after contrast injection, during catheter flushing, and when exchanging guide wires.[35,38,39] Thrombotic emboli can be dislodged from intravascular plaques while manipulating the catheter, or can propagate from a thrombus originating at the catheter tip. In an attempt to decrease the incidence of thromboembolic complications, Bendszus and colleagues[35] conducted a prospective study in which they performed 150 cerebral angiography procedures randomized to 50 procedures using either a conventional angiographic technique, systemic heparin treatment throughout the procedure, or air filters between the catheter and both the contrast-medium syringe and catheter flushing. DW-MRI performed before and after the procedure revealed 18 lesions in 11 patients in the control group, and 4 lesions in 3 patients in each of the heparin and air-filter groups. The study concluded that air filters and heparin reduce the incidence of silent strokes ($P = .002$) and have the potential to lower clinically overt ischemic events.

Thromboembolic Complications Associated with Treatment of Endovascular Aneurysms

Thromboembolic events resulting from endovascular coiling of cerebral aneurysms is estimated to be 8.2%.[28,40] There are several potential mechanisms: coil migration into the vessel lumen and distal migration, dislodgment of a preexisting intra-aneurysmal thrombus, thrombus formation in the aneurysmal remnant after incomplete obliteration of the aneurysm, and endothelial injury.[28,40] Most of these events occur preoperatively; therefore, although heparin is not routinely administered in diagnostic cerebral angiography, it is recommended to administer early anticoagulation during endovascular coiling of unruptured intracranial aneurysms. Several studies have advocated the additional use of heparin postoperatively in unruptured aneurysms to further decrease the incidence of thromboembolic events, although this can be challenging for ruptured aneurysms.[28,40–43] In a meta-analysis, Qureshi and colleagues[28] advocated that the postoperative administration of heparin is beneficial only in cases of coil migration and the presence of cerebral ischemia. Exact guidelines for ruptured aneurysm coiling are lacking. An option could be to administer half the dose of heparin at the beginning of the procedure and the other half after the first coil is secured in the aneurysm.[30,44]

There is evidence from coronary angiography and coronary endovascular interventions that antiplatelet therapy before intervention has the potential to decrease the risk of thromboembolic complications.[45] Aspirin and/or clopidogrel administration may therefore form an integral component for prevention of thromboembolic complications in endovascular management of intracranial aneurysms.[46] The general trend is to administer aspirin and clopidogrel simultaneously in aneurysmal coiling, especially when a stent might be needed.[47] In a retrospective study, Hwang and colleagues[47] reviewed 328 aneurysms treated with elective coil embolization by microcatheter technique. The investigators compared 3 groups of patients: group 1 (95 cases) received no antiplatelet therapy, group 2 (61 cases) received either aspirin or clopidogrel, and group 3 (172 cases) received both aspirin and clopidogrel. There was no significant difference in the thromboembolic rate in the group that received antiplatelet therapy compared with the group that did not receive antiplatelet therapy (1.8% without antiplatelet, 2.2% with antiplatelet; P = 1.00) in the cases where the aneurysms were simple and noncomplex. However, in the cases of complex aneurysm configuration that necessitated the use of multiple catheters, there was a significant reduction in the rate of thromboembolic events in patients who received antiplatelet therapy compared with those who did not (12.8% no antiplatelet vs 2.1% with antiplatelet; P = .023). Overall, there was an 85.2% reduction in thromboembolic events. Furthermore, there was no increase in hemorrhagic complications in unruptured aneurysms with antiplatelet therapy (P = .171). The investigators concluded that complex aneurysmal configuration should prompt the use of antiplatelets (aspirin 100 mg/d and clopidogrel 75 mg/d for at least 5 days before coiling) to reduce the risk of thromboembolic events. The results of this study are in accord with those of other studies[48,49] that demonstrated the importance of antiplatelet administration before endovascular coiling of intracranial aneurysms to decrease the risk of procedure-related thromboembolic events. Heparin administration after endovascular access at the beginning of a case to achieve activated coagulation time of 250 to 300 seconds is common practice. In general it is likely preferable to avoid antiplatelets in most patients presenting with ruptured intracranial aneurysms, as they can increase the risk of hemorrhage.

Intraoperative Rupture or Rerupture

Intraoperative aneurysmal rupture or rerupture can be devastating complications in the endovascular treatment of intracranial aneurysms. Aneurysmal rupture and rerupture can manifest with either frank extravasation of the contrast from the aneurysmal dome or sluggishness of flow, and should be suspected whenever there is abrupt change in vital signs and/or an increase in intracranial pressure (ICP). Pierot and colleagues[4] conducted a prospective study involving 739 unruptured intracranial aneurysms treated selectively by coils alone (50.4%), balloon remodeling (37.3%), or stenting (7.8%). The investigators reported an intraprocedural risk of aneurysmal rupture in 2.6% of the cases, with 27.8% permanent clinical consequences and a 16.7% mortality rate. Intraoperative aneurysmal rerupture occurs in 3% to 5% of ruptured cases, and is associated with very high mortality rate ranging from 30% to 100%.[5] The presence of intraprocedural aneurysmal rupture or rerupture should prompt immediate management and control. Inflating a balloon at or proximal to the neck can allow control while further packing of the aneurysm is achieved. Placement of an external ventricular drain should be considered once the aneurysm bleeding has been controlled.[50,51] Under select circumstances, the patient may need to be taken to the operating room to undergo an emergent craniotomy to evacuate a hematoma and clip the ruptured aneurysm.[50,51] Craniotomy may be needed to manage ICP.

Vascular Dissections

Iatrogenic vascular dissections are uncommon complications of neuroendovascular procedures with a mostly benign course, occurring at rates ranging from 0.14% to 0.4%.[17,52,53] The clinical manifestation of an arterial dissection varies based on the vessel involved and the occlusive nature of the dissection. Most of the nonocclusive dissections can undergo resolution, especially when a patient's initial manifestations do not involve ischemic symptoms.[17,54] Several studies have reported that iatrogenic arterial dissection can occur more frequently during interventional procedures in comparison with diagnostic cerebral angiography alone.[7,39,52,53,55] However, Cloft and colleagues[17] reviewed 2437 diagnostic cerebral angiography cases and 675 endovascular interventional procedures, and reported 12 cases of arterial dissection (focal, <3 cm) in total, divided into 0.3% in the diagnostic cerebral angiograms and 0.7% in the neurointerventional procedures, with no statistical significance in the difference between the 2 groups ($P>.1$). The investigators reported that none of the patients who had dissections developed ischemic symptoms, although one was noted later to have a small asymptomatic infarction in the region fed by the dissecting artery. Nine of these patients showed improvement of arterial lumen compromise on follow-up angiography after medical treatment, and the remaining 3 had conditions that remained unchanged. Two patients developed pseudoaneurysms that remained asymptomatic after a 9-month follow-up period. It was noted that most dissections occurred at the time of contrast-material injections, which can damage the arterial lumen when the jet flowing from the catheter tip hits the arterial wall. Furthermore, arterial luminal damage can occur during the manipulation of the catheter and guide wire. The investigators concluded that arterial dissections may be prevented by paying particular attention to the angiogram during test injections.[17] Moreover, the operator can minimally retract the catheter after the tip is in position to dissipate the remaining tension and avoid its erosion over the intima. The authors recommend treatment with systemic heparinization followed by bridging to warfarin or switching to antiplatelet therapy. Surgery and other interventional procedures should be used as a last resort when medical therapy fails and ischemic symptoms progress.[17,54]

Puncture-Site Hematoma

Puncture-site hematomas are common complications of neuroendovascular procedures.[2,3,7,25,27] Their occurrence is not linked to the arterial-site puncture and can follow radial, brachial, or femoral access.[1,2] Kaufmann and colleagues[3] reviewed retrospectively 19,826 patients who underwent diagnostic cerebral angiography and reported arterial site hematoma as the most common complication, occurring with an overall rate of 4.2%. In a prospective study on 1002 cerebral angiographic procedures, Dion and colleagues[2] reported that hematoma was the most common complication, occurring in 6.9% of cases. Advanced age was a risk factor for hematoma formation, as 50% of patients with hematoma were older than 60 years. One-third of those patients who were older than 70 years necessitated fluid replacement or surgical repair of the hematoma. Other risk factors included contrast volume, the number of guide wires used, the use of 3 or more catheters, catheters with a caliber higher than 6.5F, hypertension, procedural duration of more than 60 minutes, and the presence of TIAs at presentation. In a prospective study of more than 1500 cerebral angiograms, Earnest and colleagues[11] reported a 4.4% rate of hematoma formation that was associated with advanced age. Another study by Fifi and colleagues[7] reviewed 3636 cerebral angiograms, and reported that access-site hematoma accounted for 50% of the complications and was noted in 0.15% of the cases.

Arterial closure devices (ACDs) can efficiently seal the arteriotomy site, and have been proved to be safe and effective even in patients on antiplatelet or anticoagulation therapy.[56–58] In their multicenter study comparing 1162 patients who received ACDs with 1162 patients managed by manual compression, Allen and colleagues[59] reported that major bleeding significantly decreased in patients treated with ACDs (2.4% vs 5.2%, $P<.001$). Furthermore, the use of ACDs significantly reduced both the formation of pseudoaneurysms (0.3% vs 1.1%, $P = .028$) and the duration of hospitalization (1.9 ± 1.9 vs 2.3 ± 5.3 days, $P = .007$). Despite many studies proving the efficacy of ACDs,[56–59] a meta-analysis conducted by Das and colleagues,[60] which included 24 studies and more than 3600 patients, demonstrated no statistically significant difference in complications when comparing ACDs with manual compressions but marginally fewer complications with the use of ACDs were noted (odds ratio 0.87, 95% confidence interval 0.52–1.58; $P = .13$). The investigators reported that many of the included studies had poor methodology, and emphasized the need for randomized controlled studies to further evaluate the usefulness of ACDs.

Pearls to prevent complications

A thoughtful approach to patient care and technique can help reduce complications. There are 5 areas worth emphasizing: (1) patient selection, (2) meticulous planning and preparation, (3) anticipation of potential complications, (4) careful and meticulous technique, and (5) careful review of results.

1. A complete knowledge and understanding of the natural history of intracranial aneurysms and their treatment options, a careful assessment of the patient's risk factors, and a thorough evaluation of the patient in his or her bio-psycho-social background are the most important steps in preventing complications. Other alternatives should be carefully considered in each case (eg, open surgical treatment vs observation). Wide aneurysm neck size, poor dome to neck ratio, and difficult access can all increase risk.[61]
2. When the decision for endovascular treatment of the aneurysm is made, the patient's medical condition should be reviewed and optimized.
3. The physician should be aware and prepared for the worst-case scenario. Anticipating complications is one way to minimize them.
4. Although not reviewed in this article, case volume and high-quality training have an impact on results and avoidance of complications. Meticulous attention to detail in the procedure is clearly important. Balancing efficiency with caution is an art that should be respected and embraced.
5. Careful assessment of results can help minimize complications. Birkmeyer and colleagues[62] conducted a study involving 20 bariatric surgeons who submitted videotapes of themselves while performing a laparoscopic gastric bypass. These videotapes were used by peer surgeons to evaluate the technical skills of the performing physicians on a scale of 1 to 5 (higher number indicating higher performance). Across the 20 bariatric surgeons, the scores ranged from 2.6 to 4.8, and in comparison with the top quartile the bottom quartile was shown to have higher complication rates (14.5% vs 5.2%, $P<.001$), higher mortality (0.26% vs 0.05%, $P = .01$), longer operations (137 minutes vs 98 minutes, $P<.001$), higher rates of reoperation (3.4% vs 1.6%, $P = .01$) and higher readmission rates (6.3% vs 2.7%, $P<.001$).[62]

SUMMARY

It is crucial to recognize and understand the complications that might arise from the endovascular treatment of intracranial aneurysms. Such knowledge allows the health care provider to adopt several measures that could potentially avoid the complications and provide more efficient treatment. Improved patient selection for endovascular treatment, meticulous planning and preparation of the procedure, anticipating potential complications and preparing for management, building databases that include patients' outcome assessment, and allowing peer rating and feedback on operative skill can all help to avoid complications. The importance of the operator's expertise cannot be overemphasized in the prevention and successful management of these complications. Current advancements in simulation, 3-dimensional printing, and holography can potentially all play a crucial role in training novices in endovascular management of intracranial aneurysms and in increasing the level of proficiency of the graduating physicians, thus decreasing the incidence of complications.

REFERENCES

1. Dion J, Gates P, Fox AJ, et al. Clinical events following neuroangiography. A prospective study. Acta Radiol Suppl 1986;369:29–33.
2. Dion JE, Gates PC, Fox AJ, et al. Clinical events following neuroangiography: a prospective study. Stroke 1987;18(6):997–1004.
3. Kaufmann TJ, Huston J 3rd, Mandrekar JN, et al. Complications of diagnostic cerebral angiography: evaluation of 19,826 consecutive patients. Radiology 2007;243(3):812–9.
4. Pierot L, Spelle L, Vitry F, et al. Immediate clinical outcome of patients harboring unruptured intracranial aneurysms treated by endovascular approach: results of the ATENA study. Stroke 2008;39(9): 2497–504.
5. Lawson MF, Velat GJ, Fargen KM, et al. Interventional neurovascular disease: avoidance and management of complications and review of the current literature. J Neurosurg Sci 2011;55(3):233–42.
6. Brinjikji W, Rabinstein AA, Lanzino G, et al. Effect of age on outcomes of treatment of unruptured cerebral aneurysms: a study of the National Inpatient Sample 2001-2008. Stroke 2011;42(5):1320–4.
7. Fifi JT, Meyers PM, Lavine SD, et al. Complications of modern diagnostic cerebral angiography in an academic medical center. J Vasc Interv Radiol 2009;20(4):442–7.
8. Willinsky RA, Taylor SM, TerBrugge K, et al. Neurologic complications of cerebral angiography: prospective analysis of 2,899 procedures and review of the literature. Radiology 2003;227(2): 522–8.

9. Heiserman JE, Dean BL, Hodak JA, et al. Neurologic complications of cerebral angiography. AJNR Am J Neuroradiol 1994;15(8):1401–7 [discussion: 1408–11].
10. Theodotou BC, Whaley R, Mahaley MS. Complications following transfemoral cerebral angiography for cerebral ischemia. Report of 159 angiograms and correlation with surgical risk. Surg Neurol 1987;28(2):90–2.
11. Earnest FT, Forbes G, Sandok BA, et al. Complications of cerebral angiography: prospective assessment of risk. AJR Am J Roentgenol 1984;142(2): 247–53.
12. Eisenberg RL, Bank WO, Hedgcock MW. Neurologic complications of angiography in patients with critical stenosis of the carotid artery. Neurology 1980;30(8):892–5.
13. Faught E, Trader SD, Hanna GR. Cerebral complications of angiography for transient ischemia and stroke: prediction of risk. Neurology 1979;29(1): 4–15.
14. Komiyama M, Yamanaka K, Nishikawa M, et al. Prospective analysis of complications of catheter cerebral angiography in the digital subtraction angiography and magnetic resonance era. Neurol Med Chir 1998;38(9):534–9 [discussion: 539–40].
15. Leffers AM, Wagner A. Neurologic complications of cerebral angiography. A retrospective study of complication rate and patient risk factors. Acta Radiol 2000;41(3):204–10.
16. Leow K, Murie JA. Cerebral angiography for cerebrovascular disease: the risks. Br J Surg 1988; 75(5):428–30.
17. Cloft HJ, Jensen ME, Kallmes DF, et al. Arterial dissections complicating cerebral angiography and cerebrovascular interventions. AJNR Am J Neuroradiol 2000;21(3):541–5.
18. Kay J, Chow WH, Chan TM, et al. Acetylcysteine for prevention of acute deterioration of renal function following elective coronary angiography and intervention: a randomized controlled trial. JAMA 2003;289(5):553–8.
19. McCullough PA, Wolyn R, Rocher LL, et al. Acute renal failure after coronary intervention: incidence, risk factors, and relationship to mortality. Am J Med 1997;103(5):368–75.
20. Weisberg LS, Kurnik PB, Kurnik BR. Risk of radiocontrast nephropathy in patients with and without diabetes mellitus. Kidney Int 1994;45(1):259–65.
21. Porter GA. Contrast medium-associated nephropathy. Recognition and management. Invest Radiol 1993;28(Suppl 4):S11–8.
22. From AM, Bartholmai BJ, Williams AW, et al. Sodium bicarbonate is associated with an increased incidence of contrast nephropathy: a retrospective cohort study of 7977 patients at mayo clinic. Clin J Am Soc Nephrol 2008;3(1):10–8.
23. McIvor J, Steiner TJ, Perkin GD, et al. Neurological morbidity of arch and carotid arteriography in cerebrovascular disease. The influence of contrast medium and radiologist. Br J Radiol 1987;60(710): 117–22.
24. Skalpe IO. Complications in cerebral angiography with iohexol (Omnipaque) and meglumine metrizoate (Isopaque cerebral). Neuroradiology 1988; 30(1):69–72.
25. Mani RL, Eisenberg RL, McDonald EJ Jr, et al. Complications of catheter cerebral arteriography: analysis of 5,000 procedures. I. Criteria and incidence. AJR Am J Roentgenol 1978;131(5):861–5.
26. ACT Investigators. Acetylcysteine for prevention of renal outcomes in patients undergoing coronary and peripheral vascular angiography: main results from the randomized Acetylcysteine for Contrast-induced nephropathy Trial (ACT). Circulation 2011;124(11):1250–9.
27. Mani RL, Eisenberg RL. Complications of catheter cerebral arteriography: analysis of 5,000 procedures. III. Assessment of arteries injected, contrast medium used, duration of procedure, and age of patient. AJR Am J Roentgenol 1978;131(5):871–4.
28. Qureshi AI, Luft AR, Sharma M, et al. Prevention and treatment of thromboembolic and ischemic complications associated with endovascular procedures: part II–clinical aspects and recommendations. Neurosurgery 2000;46(6):1360–75 [discussion: 1375–6].
29. Davies KN, Humphrey PR. Complications of cerebral angiography in patients with symptomatic carotid territory ischaemia screened by carotid ultrasound. J Neurol Neurosurg Psychiatry 1993; 56(9):967–72.
30. Bendok BR, Hanel RA, Hopkins LN. Coil embolization of intracranial aneurysms. Neurosurgery 2003; 52(5):1125–30 [discussion: 1130].
31. Levy EI, Boulos AS, Fessler RD, et al. Transradial cerebral angiography: an alternative route. Neurosurgery 2002;51(2):335–40 [discussion: 340–2].
32. Hurley MC, Sherma AK, Surdell D, et al. A novel guide catheter enabling intracranial placement. Catheter Cardiovasc Interv 2009;74(6):920–4.
33. Park KY, Chung PW, Kim YB, et al. Post-interventional microembolism: cortical border zone is a preferential site for ischemia. Cerebrovasc Dis 2011;32(3):269–75.
34. Waugh JR, Sacharias N. Arteriographic complications in the DSA era. Radiology 1992;182(1):243–6.
35. Bendszus M, Koltzenburg M, Bartsch AJ, et al. Heparin and air filters reduce embolic events caused by intra-arterial cerebral angiography: a prospective, randomized trial. Circulation 2004; 110(15):2210–5.
36. Pugsley W, Klinger L, Paschalis C, et al. The impact of microemboli during cardiopulmonary bypass on

neuropsychological functioning. Stroke 1994;25(7):1393–9.
37. Braekken SK, Reinvang I, Russell D, et al. Association between intraoperative cerebral microembolic signals and postoperative neuropsychological deficit: comparison between patients with cardiac valve replacement and patients with coronary artery bypass grafting. J Neurol Neurosurg Psychiatry 1998;65(4):573–6.
38. Mamourian AC, Weglarz M, Dunn J, et al. Injection of air bubbles during flushing of angiocatheters: an in vitro trial of conventional hardware and techniques. AJNR Am J Neuroradiol 2001;22(4):709–12.
39. Omran H, Schmidt H, Hackenbroch M, et al. Silent and apparent cerebral embolism after retrograde catheterisation of the aortic valve in valvular stenosis: a prospective, randomised study. Lancet 2003;361(9365):1241–6.
40. Qureshi AI, Luft AR, Sharma M, et al. Prevention and treatment of thromboembolic and ischemic complications associated with endovascular procedures: part I–pathophysiological and pharmacological features. Neurosurgery 2000;46(6):1344–59.
41. Rowe JG, Molyneux AJ, Byrne JV, et al. Endovascular treatment of intracranial aneurysms: a minimally invasive approach with advantages for elderly patients. Age Ageing 1996;25(5):372–6.
42. Tournade A, Courtheoux P, Sengel C, et al. Saccular intracranial aneurysms: endovascular treatment with mechanical detachable spiral coils. Radiology 1997;202(2):481–6.
43. Vinuela F, Duckwiler G, Mawad M. Guglielmi detachable coil embolization of acute intracranial aneurysm: perioperative anatomical and clinical outcome in 403 patients. J Neurosurg 1997;86(3):475–82.
44. Rahme RJ, Zammar SG, El Ahmadieh TY, et al. The role of antiplatelet therapy in aneurysm coiling. Neurol Res 2014;36(4):383–8.
45. Willard JE, Lange RA, Hillis LD. The use of aspirin in ischemic heart disease. N Engl J Med 1992;327(3):175–81.
46. Fiehler J, Ries T. Prevention and treatment of thromboembolism during endovascular aneurysm therapy. Klin Neuroradiol 2009;19(1):73–81.
47. Hwang G, Jung C, Park SQ, et al. Thromboembolic complications of elective coil embolization of unruptured aneurysms: the effect of oral antiplatelet preparation on periprocedural thromboembolic complication. Neurosurgery 2010;67(3):743–8 [discussion: 748].
48. Ries T, Buhk JH, Kucinski T, et al. Intravenous administration of acetylsalicylic acid during endovascular treatment of cerebral aneurysms reduces the rate of thromboembolic events. Stroke 2006;37(7):1816–21.
49. Yamada NK, Cross DT 3rd, Pilgram TK, et al. Effect of antiplatelet therapy on thromboembolic complications of elective coil embolization of cerebral aneurysms. AJNR Am J Neuroradiol 2007;28(9):1778–82.
50. Vlak MH, Algra A, Brandenburg R, et al. Prevalence of unruptured intracranial aneurysms, with emphasis on sex, age, comorbidity, country, and time period: a systematic review and meta-analysis. Lancet Neurol 2011;10(7):626–36.
51. Piche SL, Haw CS, Redekop GJ, et al. Rare intracanalicular ophthalmic aneurysm: endovascular treatment and review of the literature. AJNR Am J Neuroradiol 2005;26(8):1929–31.
52. Lang EK. A survey of the complications of percutaneous retrograde arteriography: Seldinger technic. Radiology 1963;81:257–63.
53. Gilbert GJ, Melnick GS. Pathophysiology of subintimal hematoma formation during retrograde arteriography. Radiology 1965;85:306–19.
54. Anson J, Crowell RM. Cervicocranial arterial dissection. Neurosurgery 1991;29(1):89–96.
55. Pham MH, Rahme RJ, Arnaout O, et al. Endovascular stenting of extracranial carotid and vertebral artery dissections: a systematic review of the literature. Neurosurgery 2011;68(4):856–66 [discussion: 866].
56. Fargen KM, Hoh BL, Mocco J. A prospective randomized single-blind trial of patient comfort following vessel closure: extravascular synthetic sealant closure provides less pain than a self-tightening suture vascular compression device. J Neurointerv Surg 2011;3(3):219–23.
57. Fields JD, Liu KC, Lee DS, et al. Femoral artery complications associated with the Mynx closure device. AJNR Am J Neuroradiol 2010;31(9):1737–40.
58. Kim HY, Choo SW, Roh HG, et al. Efficacy of femoral vascular closure devices in patients treated with anticoagulant, abciximab or thrombolytics during percutaneous endovascular procedures. Korean J Radiol 2006;7(1):35–40.
59. Allen DS, Marso SP, Lindsey JB, et al. Comparison of bleeding complications using arterial closure device versus manual compression by propensity matching in patients undergoing percutaneous coronary intervention. Am J Cardiol 2011;107(11):1619–23.
60. Das R, Ahmed K, Athanasiou T, et al. Arterial closure devices versus manual compression for femoral haemostasis in interventional radiological procedures: a systematic review and meta-analysis. Cardiovasc Intervent Radiol 2011;34(4):723–38.
61. Zammar SG, El Ahmadieh TY, El Tecle NE, et al. Thoughtful selection of low risk aneurysms for observation does not eliminate rupture risk. Neurosurgery 2013;73(6):N18–9.
62. Birkmeyer JD, Finks JF, O'Reilly A, et al. Surgical skill and complication rates after bariatric surgery. N Engl J Med 2013;369(15):1434–42.

Endovascular Management of Cavernous and Paraclinoid Aneurysms

Benjamin Brown, MD[a], Ricardo A. Hanel, MD, PhD[b,*]

KEYWORDS

• Endovascular • Cavernous • Paraclinoid • Aneurysms • Flow diversion • Coil • Stent

KEY POINTS

- Cavernous and paraclinoid aneurysms are among the most challenging microsurgical lesions due to location and complex anatomy.
- Endovascular methods have evolved over the last 2 decades with coiling, liquid embolic agents, stent-assisted coiling, and flow diverters being developed and used over time.
- The concept of flow diversion is based on placing a stent across the neck of an intracranial aneurysm, which then results in flow away from the aneurysm, inducing thrombosis and occlusion of the aneurysm over time.
- The stent itself experiences neointimal coverage, thus resulting in a remodeling of the parent vessel. As the use and application of flow diverters become more widespread, some important questions remain relating to the effective treatment of dual antiplatelet therapy, the occurrence of delayed aneurysm ruptures and intraparenchymal hemorrhages, and long-term patency rates.

INTRODUCTION

In this article the endovascular treatment of aneurysms arising from the internal carotid artery between its exit from the foramen lacerum and the takeoff of the posterior communicating artery is considered. These aneurysms often present a challenge for microsurgery because of the complex anatomy of the internal carotid artery in the region of the cavernous sinus and anterior clinoid process. Microsurgery of paraclinoid aneurysms frequently requires extensive bone removal for exposure of the neck and to achieve proximal control. Delicate dissection and manipulation of the optic nerve may be required for obtaining a surgical corridor. Aneurysms located more proximally in the cavernous sinus are often inoperable and require internal carotid artery sacrifice with or without bypass. These challenges have encouraged clinicians to develop alternative solutions to reduce morbidity and have ushered in an age of minimally invasive techniques.

In the modern era, endovascular treatment began with the use of balloons, when in 1974, Serbinenko reported 82 patients treated by occlusion of the carotid siphon with latex detachable balloons. In 1991, Guglielmi detachable coils became available and revolutionized the way neurosurgeons thought about cerebral aneurysms and their treatment.[1,2] Since this time, endovascular techniques have evolved into stent- and balloon-assisted coiling and most recently the concept of

[a] Department of Neurosurgery, Mayo Clinic, Jacksonville, FL, USA; [b] Lyerly Neurosurgery, Baptist Health, 800 Prudential Drive Tower B 11th Floor, Jacksonville, FL 33227, USA
* Corresponding author.
E-mail address: rhanel@lyerlyneuro.com

Neurosurg Clin N Am 25 (2014) 415–424
http://dx.doi.org/10.1016/j.nec.2014.04.017
1042-3680/14/$ – see front matter

flow diversion. In this article these techniques as well as the pertinent anatomy, clinical findings, and complications that arise when treating aneurysms of the cavernous and paraclinoid internal carotid artery are reviewed.

RELEVANT ANATOMY AND PATHOPHYSIOLOGY

For the purposes of this article, it is concerned with aneurysms arising from the internal carotid artery from the entrance into the cavernous sinus until just before the takeoff of the posterior communicating artery, which contains segments C4 through C6 in the classification of Bouthillier and colleagues.[3]

Cavernous Aneurysms

Cavernous aneurysms arise from segments C4 and C5. Segment C4, or the cavernous segment, extends from the petrolingual ligament to the proximal dural ring. Within this segment, the carotid is intimately associated with the cavernous sinus, which transmits cranial nerves III, IV, VI, V1, and V2. Therefore, aneurysms of this segment can present with any of the above cranial neuropathies. The postganglionic sympathetic fibers running with the internal carotid artery enter the cavernous sinus here, raising the possibility of Horner syndrome as well.[4]

The carotid then proceeds to segment C5, or the clinoidal segment. This segment is defined by the proximal and distal dural ring. The distal dural ring completely surrounds the carotid, making hemorrhage proximal to this point unlikely to result in subarachnoid hemorrhage.

Paraclinoid Aneurysms

Paraclinoid aneurysms are defined as those aneurysms occurring in segment C6, or the ophthalmic segment. This segment begins at the distal dural ring and continues until just before the takeoff of the posterior communicating artery. The ophthalmic segment contains 2 main arterial branches, the ophthalmic artery originating dorsomedially, followed by the superior hypophyseal artery arising from the ventromedial surface. Aneurysms of the ophthalmic artery generally project in a superomedial direction, whereas those of the superior hypophyseal artery generally project medially.[3,5] Various classification schemes exist for these aneurysms, but they can be broadly grouped into 3 categories:

- Carotid ophthalmic—these aneurysms arise at the base of the ophthalmic artery or just distal to this on the dorsal side of the internal carotid artery
- Ventral paraclinoid—aneurysms arising from the ventral C6 segment and not associated with any particular branch of the internal carotid artery
- Superior hypophyseal—those aneurysms arising from the medial aspect of the C6 segment and associated with the superior hypophyseal artery.[6]

Approximately 33% to 59% of paraclinoid aneurysms are associated with the ophthlamic artery; 27% to 47% are associated with the superior hypophyseal artery, and 14% to 20% are not associated with any arterial branch.[7,8]

CLINICAL PRESENTATION AND DIAGNOSIS

Presentation

Cavernous aneurysms

True cavernous aneurysms are located proximal to the proximal dural ring and account for about 4% of all intracranial aneurysms. There is a strong female preponderance and average age at presentation is 60. They almost never present with subarachnoid hemorrhage because of their extradural location.[9–13] Most commonly, they are found incidentally during evaluation for an unrelated problem, or in investigating cranial neuropathy of those nerves traveling within the cavernous sinus (III, IV, VI, V1, and V2). In cases of rupture, the patient typically presents with signs and symptoms of carotid-cavernous fistula rather than subarachnoid hemorrhage. Carotid cavernous fistula was the presenting symptoms in 9% of cases in a series of 87 cavernous aneurysm patients by Higashida and colleagues.[1]

Diplopia is the presenting symptom in approximately 65% of cases, whereas retro-orbital pain or headache is the presenting symptom in approximately 59% of cases. A relatively high percentage (18%–20%) present asymptomatically. Decreased visual acuity affects approximately 16% of patients presenting with cavernous segment aneurysm.[12,14] With regards to visual symptoms, a variety of constellations may present (**Table 1**).[12] Epistaxis has also been reported rarely.[12,14]

Subarachnoid hemorrhage has been reported as a presenting symptom of cavernous aneurysms in 0% to 5% of cases.[2,12,14–16] The varying rates are likely due to variations in classification scheme and whether the aneurysm was truly of the cavernous segment and therefore completely intradural. The annual risk of rupture is estimated to be between 0% and 1.6%.[2,17]

Table 1
Neuro-ophthalmologic findings at presentation in 206 cavernous carotid aneurysms

Clinical Finding	Treated Patients (n = 74)	Untreated Patients (n = 132)
Third, fourth, sixth pareses (8 with trigemninal involvement)	26	12
Third and sixth pareses (2 with V1)	12	9
Third and fourth nerve pareses (4 with V1)	3	4
Isolated third nerve paresis	11	14
Fourth nerve paresis alone	0	0
Sixth nerve paresis alone	16	18
Reduced or absent corneal reflex	15	1
V dysesthesia	11	5
Horner pupil	3	0
Compressive optic neuropathy	8	7

Adapted from Stiebel-Kalish H, Kalish Y, Bar-On RH, et al. Presentation, natural history, and management of carotid cavernous aneurysms. Neurosurgery 2005;57(5):850–7. [discussion: 850–7].

It is important to determine whether an aneurysm is truly from the cavernous segment to stratify for risk of subarachnoid hemorrhage. On imaging, the optic strut can be used as a useful landmark to approximate the location of the distal dural ring. Computed tomographic angiography (CTA) can show this relationship well to define whether the aneurysm is intradural or extradural.[18] In larger aneurysms, the bony anatomy may be distorted, which may make this more difficult. An alternative method is to identify a "waist" on cerebral angiography. Waist is an indentation on the dorsomedial aspect of the aneurysm where the aneurysm is compressed by the distal dural ring. The portion of aneurysm distal to this waist can be considered in the subarachnoid space.[11]

Paraclinoid aneurysms

Paraclinoid aneurysms are defined above as those aneurysms arising from the distal dural ring to the origin of the posterior communicating artery. They present in bilateral fashion as much as 31% of the time.[7] They present at a mean age of 53 to 55 with a female preponderance of 87% to 92%.[6,7] Paraclinoid aneurysms can present with subarachnoid hemorrhage, headache, and visual symptoms, or incidentally. In unruptured aneurysms, approximately 80% present incidentally, whereas 10% present with headache, and 10% present with visual symptoms.[6,7] The visual symptoms are due to mass effect from the aneurysm on the optic nerve and may result in visual field cut or reduced visual acuity. Risk of rupture is relatively rare. Ruptured paraclinoid aneurysms are thought to comprise between 1.4% and 9.1% of all ruptured aneurysms.[19,20]

Diagnosis

The diagnosis of cerebral aneurysms is most often made by CTA or digital subtraction angiography (DSA). Although CTA has improved in resolution, DSA remains the gold standard for obtaining the greatest detail as well as dynamic data, such as flow stasis and inflow and outflow zones. In the case of ruptured cerebral aneurysms, CT scan defines the typical pattern of diffuse subarachnoid hemorrhage within the basal cisterns. In the event of a negative CT scan, subarachnoid hemorrhage can be confirmed or ruled out using lumbar puncture and testing for xanthocromia.

ENDOVASCULAR CONSIDERATIONS

Historically, the risk of open surgical treatment of cavernous and paraclinoid aneurysms is higher than other anterior circulation aneurysms given the complex anatomy of the cavernous sinus and skull base and the difficulty associated with establishing proximal control,[21–26] which has led to an explosion of endovascular techniques. Indications and the techniques common to both locations of aneurysms are discussed, followed by technical nuances suited to each location.

Indications for Treatment

In determining the need for treatment, cavernous and paraclinoid aneurysms can be categorized as ruptured or unruptured. Ruptured aneurysms producing either subarachnoid hemorrhage or a carotid cavernous fistula should be treated to prevent rerupture in the former and to preserve cranial nerve function and decrease intraocular pressure and possible cortical venous drainage in the latter. The unruptured aneurysms can be further subdivided into symptomatic or asymptomatic.

The unruptured, asymptomatic aneurysm

For unruptured, asymptomatic lesions, the largest study regarding the natural history of these lesions comes from the International Study of Unruptured

Intracranial Aneurysms (ISUIA). All told, this study involved 4060 patients from the United States, Europe, and Canada. With regard to the natural history, these patients were followed for a mean of 4.1 years. They were grouped into 2 categories, those patients without history of prior subarachnoid hemorrhage (group 1) and those with a prior history of subarachnoid hemorrhage (group 2). Aneurysms were then stratified for risk of rupture based on size. For all sizes, group 1 and group 2 had no statistically significant difference in rupture rates except for those aneurysms less than 7 mm. The data for ISUIA are summarized in **Tables 2** and **3**.[17]

Although these data are very helpful, each patient should be evaluated on an individual basis, taking into consideration factors such as age, smoking status, comorbidities, growth on serial imaging, and the risk of the proposed procedure. In practical terms, it is not recommended treatment for asymptomatic intracavernous lesions less than 13 mm. For lesions larger than 13 mm and asymptomatic, the decision is made on a case-by-case basis.

For transitional aneurysms and paraophthalmic lesions, practice of individualized medicine is exercised. ISUIA and other large natural history series serve as guideline for management discussion, with the decision made on an individual basis, taking into consideration each individual and lesion characteristics.

Last, as mentioned previously in this article, it is very important to differentiate truly intracavernous lesions from transitional lesions. ISUIA demonstrated that intracavernous lesions less than 13 mm presented no risk for hemorrhage, whereas transitional lesions behave like other internal carotid artery aneurysms (an exception is made to posterior communicating segment ones). The authors typically use CTA or DSA with dual volume reconstruction to define the relationship between aneurysm and the optic strut and consider intracavernous lesions, aneurysms below the strut level, with transitional lesions expanding beyond the level of the optic strut.

Table 2
Raymond classification for aneurysm embolization

Classification	Description
Class 1	Complete occlusion
Class 2	Residual neck
Class 3	Residual aneurysm

Adapted from Raymond J, Guilbert F, Weill A, et al. Long-term angiographic recurrences after selective endovascular treatment of aneurysms with detachable coils. Stroke 2003;34(6):1398–403.

The unruptured, symptomatic aneurysm

The natural history of cranial neuropathy associated with cavernous and paraclinoid aneurysms is also not well defined and can have a variable course.[13,27] Over time, however, the neuropathy is likely to worsen, and generally, these aneurysms warrant treatment to halt and, it is hoped, to reverse the progression of neuropathy. Given the intradural location of aneurysms of the cavernous sinus, and the relatively benign natural history, any treatment of aneurysms in the cavernous sinus should be very well tolerated. Open surgical repair of these lesions has been discussed historically, but no longer is used due to high morbidity and mortality, with the exception of carotid ligation.[28–30]

Techniques, Results, and Outcomes

The endovascular techniques available for the treatment of cavernous and paraclinoid aneurysms are similar. Where appropriate, differences in techniques or special considerations for the respective locations are highlighted within subsections.

Detachable balloon therapy for cavernous aneurysms

Historically, balloons have been placed within cavernous aneurysms to preserve the parent vessel in aneurysms with an appropriate neck. In this technique, the aneurysm dome is accessed and a silicone detachable balloon (**Figs. 1–3**) is inflated within the aneurysm using a liquid polymerizing material.[1] Detachable balloons are no longer available in the United States.

Occlusion of the internal carotid

It was Barney Brooks in 1930 who pioneered the intravascular approach to treating cerebral pathologic abnormality when he embolized a carotid cavernous fistula by inserting a piece of muscle into the internal carotid artery. By 1974, Serbinenko published a series of 82 patients treated with detachable balloon therapy to occlude the carotid artery.[31] Occlusion of the carotid has survived into the modern era as a durable and viable solution to treating aneurysms of the cavernous segment. Typically, carotid occlusion is performed with partial coiling of the aneurysm and full-thickness coiling of the carotid.[32] Internal carotid artery occlusion results in complete thrombosis of the aneurysm in nearly 100% of the aneurysms.[1,2,33] Symptomatic improvement of

Table 3
ISUIA data for cavernous and paraclinoid aneurysms 5-year risk

	<7 mm	7–12 mm	13–24 mm	>24 mm
Cavernous segment	0	0	3	6.4
Paraclinoid segment	0/1.5[a]	2.6	14.5	40

[a] If history of previous subarachnoid hemorrhage.

presenting cranial nerve deficits has been reported as high as 100%.[1] Reports of permanent neurologic deficit following internal carotid occlusion rage from 2% to 4.4%.[1,2,33]

Endovascular occlusion of the internal carotid artery does have some drawbacks. As mentioned earlier, cavernous and paraclinoid aneurysms are often not found in isolation. Sacrificing an internal carotid artery may limit options in treating a contralateral lesion. There are also case reports of de novo remote aneurysm formation following carotid sacrifice, which may be due to changes in flow patterns.[34–36]

In this strategy, it is advisable to perform a balloon test occlusion of the parent internal carotid artery before sacrifice. If the patient does not pass, it is advisable to perform a high-flow extracranial to intracranial (EC-IC) bypass before internal carotid artery sacrifice. These additional procedures may add additional resources and morbidity.[37]

Balloon test occlusion

Balloon test occlusion is carried out by placing a balloon in the carotid in question and occluding the circulation while performing cerebral angiography from the contralateral internal carotid artery or from the vertebral artery. The balloon is maintained for 30 minutes and serial neurologic examinations are performed. In addition, a 10-minute period of imposed hypotension may be used as an extra level of safety. The patient is considered to "fail" the balloon test occlusion if they become in any way symptomatic from a neurologic standpoint, or if the venous phase is delayed by more than 0.5 seconds in the hemisphere being tested.[38]

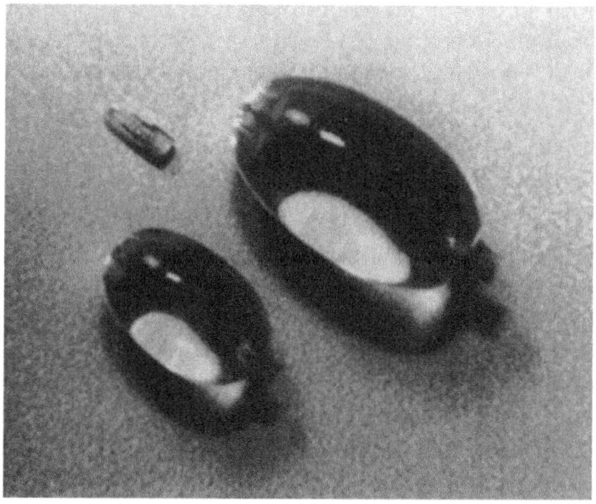

Fig. 1. Detachable silicone balloon previously used in aneurysm embolization and carotid sacrifice. (*From* Higashida RT, Halbach VV, Dowd C, et al. Endovascular detachable balloon embolization therapy of cavernous carotid artery aneurysms: results in 87 cases. J Neurosurg 2009;72(6):857–63; with permission. Available at: http://thejns.org/doi/abs/10.3171/jns.1990.72.22.0857. Accessed December 10, 2013.)

Coil embolization

In 1995, the Guglielmi detachable coil was approved by the US Food and Drug Administration (FDA) for use in the United States. Since that time, the use of coils has dramatically increased in the treatment of cerebral aneurysms. Coil embolization has the benefit over vessel sacrifice of preserving the anatomy of the parent vessel while excluding the aneurysm from the circulation.

Coiling is performed through the insertion of a microcatheter into the dome of the aneurysm and placing coils into the aneurysm dome. Historically, coiling was reserved for those aneurysms with a favorable dome-to-neck ratio; however, over time, techniques have evolved to expand treatment to aneurysms with less favorable anatomy, including the use of balloons and stents. In addition, dual microcatheter technique has been introduced[39] to facilitate coiling of wider necked aneurysms without the use of a stent. Degree of occlusion is generally represented by the Raymond classification (see **Table 2**).[40] Raymond class 1 (complete occlusion) is achieved between 19% and 66% with coil embolization.[40–43] Overall, coil embolization is well tolerated with an approximate 5% rate of procedural morbidity and mortality.[44]

Cavernous aneurysms Because the risk of subarachnoid hemorrhage is very low in cavernous aneurysms, the indications for treatment of cavernous sinus aneurysms are largely based on symptomatology. Common indications for treatment are bone erosion, head, eye, or face pain attributable to the aneurysm, diplopia, visual

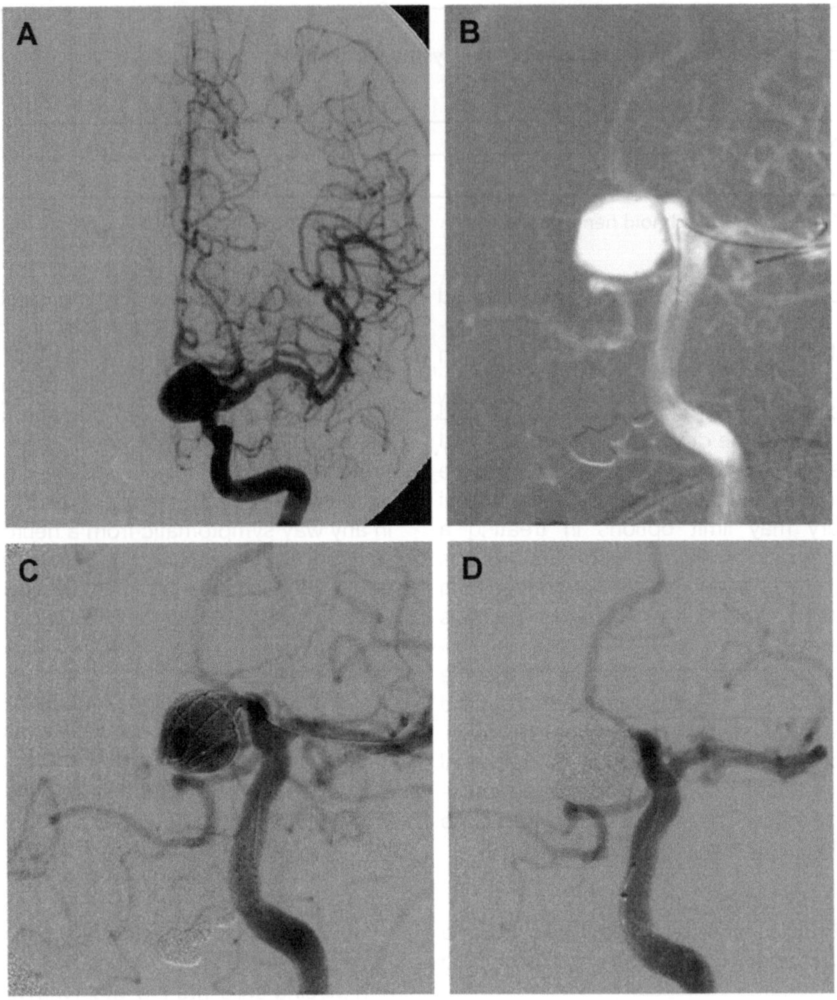

Fig. 2. Case illustration. A 40-year-old woman presented with subarachnoid hemorrhage. Cerebral angiogram demonstrated large superior hypophyseal aneurysm (*A*); roadmap imaging obtained (*B*); treatment perform with primary coiling—initial coil in place (*C*); final result (*D*) demonstrated complete aneurysm occlusion.

loss, carotid-cavernous fistula, or cerebral infarction due to embolus from aneurysm thrombus.[12]

Generally coil embolization of cavernous segment aneurysms is very well tolerated. van Rooij[33] reported no complications in a series of 31 coiled cavernous aneurysms. Occlusion rates after coiling were complete in 32%, near complete in 55%, and incomplete in 13%. Incomplete treatment and recurrence, as demonstrated by this and many other authors, were very high for cavernous aneurysms, because of a high incidence of wide-necked lesions at this region.

Paraclinoid aneurysms The degree of occlusion varies widely between series for paraclinoid aneurysms. Raymond classification of 1 is established in 40% to 72% of paraclinoid aneurysms, whereas near complete occlusion is achieved in 8.2% to 39%, and partial occlusion is achieved in 5% to 19.2% of paraclinoid aneurysms. Higher rates of occlusion are obtained with stent-assisted coiling and in smaller aneurysms.[6,7,43,45]

The overall rate of permanent morbidity and mortality is between 0%–8.3% and 0%–2.2%, respectively, in coiling of paraclinoid aneurysms, and 4% to 7% of patients experience early thromboembolic complications, which often result in only transient morbidity.[6,7,45–47] Recurrences occur in between 14% and 17% of those aneurysms treated with coil embolization.[7,46] There is a trend toward less recurrence of aneurysms with stent-assisted coiling.[7,43]

Flow diversion

Flow diversion for the treatment of aneurysm was introduced in the United States with FDA approval

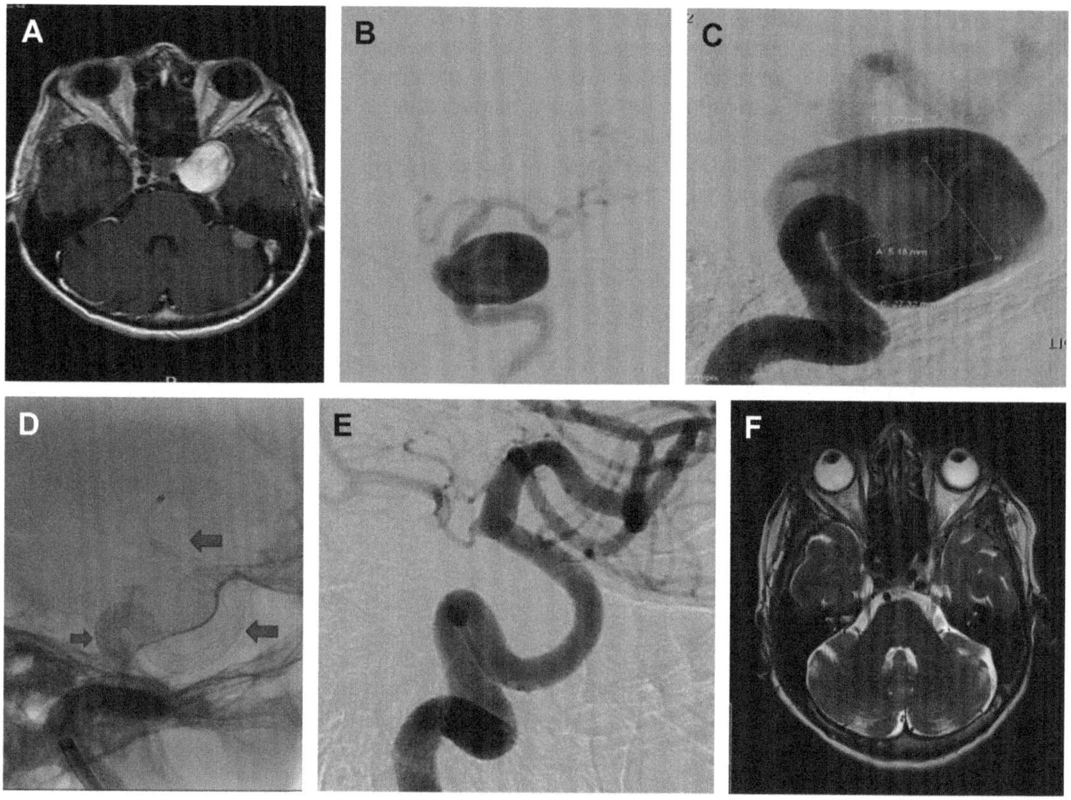

Fig. 3. Case illustration. Sexagenarian woman presented with ophthalmoplegia. Magnetic resonance imaging (MRI) Head with contrast demonstrated left internal carotid artery aneurysm (*A*); cerebral angiogram confirmed presence of wide neck, giant, cavernous segment aneurysm (*B*, AP; *C*, lateral); treatment performed with single flow diverter (*arrows*) (*D*); 6-month follow-up angiography demonstrated complete aneurysm occlusion (*E*); 12-month follow-up MRI demonstrated complete involution of cavernous mass (*F*).

of the Pipeline embolization device (PED) in April of 2011 (Chestnut Medical Technologies, Menlo Park, CA, USA). Flow diverters work by decreasing the flow of blood within the aneurysm, thereby decreasing laminar flow and increasing the tendency to clot. As clot forms within the aneurysm, the device acts as a scaffold over which endothelium can grow, eventually excluding the aneurysm from circulation.

The occlusion rate seen with flow diversion is approximately 69% to 94% at 6 months and 86.8% to 95% at 1 year.[48–53] The risk of morbidity and mortality following flow diversion has been reported between 0% and 19%[48–51,53,54]; however, reports vary widely on types of aneurysms treated and morbidity criteria. There are several theoretical advantages to flow diversion over traditional coil embolization. First, one is not required to directly catheterize the aneurysm, thus reducing the risk of an intraoperative rupture. Second, a flow diverter treats the entire diseased segment of a parent artery by facilitating neointimal growth along the segment, including across the aneurysm neck, resulting in a more anatomically sound treatment. Last, because nothing is left within the aneurysm sac, over time the dome may atrophy, potentially relieving any mass effect it may be applying.

Pipeline for uncoilable or failed aneurysms The Pipeline for Uncoilable or Failed Aneurysms trial is a multicenter, prospective, interventional, single-arm trial of the PED for the treatment of uncoilable or failed aneurysms of the internal carotid artery. It consisted of 108 patients with recently discovered unruptured large and giant wide-necked aneurysms. The primary treatment endpoint was angiographic evaluation that demonstrated complete aneurysm occlusion and absence of major stenosis at 6 months. The primary safety endpoint was the occurrence of a major ipsilateral stroke or neurologic death at 180 days.

There were a total of 106 aneurysms eligible for evaluation of the primary treatment endpoint. The median number of pipeline devices placed was 3 with a range of 1 to 15. Of the 106 aneurysms, 73.6% met the treatment endpoint of complete occlusion at 180 days without major stenosis. By 1 year, complete occlusion was seen in 86.8% of aneurysms. With regard to the primary safety endpoint, 107 patients were eligible for consideration. Of these patients 5.6% had major ipsilateral stroke or neurologic death.

This large, prospective, multicenter trial provided solid evidence for the more widespread use of the PED to treat the challenging lesions of the proximal internal carotid artery.

Cavernous aneurysms Flow diversion lends itself particularly well to the cavernous segment because of its difficulty to access surgically as well as the lack of major carotid branches. In 2013, Puffer and colleagues[37] published a series of 44 consecutive patients in a prospectively maintained database. To date, this is the only study focusing exclusively on cavernous aneurysms treated with flow diversion. The mean number of flow diverters placed per patient was 2.2. Thirty-five patients were included in occlusion analysis and 71% had complete occlusion.

With regard to symptom improvement, 90% of patients presenting with symptoms had complete or significant improvement. Of note, 23% of patients developed new symptoms shortly after placement of a flow diverter, which occurred between 2 and 5 days after the procedure. These new symptoms consisted of new headache or cranial nerve deficits. Headache and cranial nerve symptoms generally resolved by 1 month; however, one patient had lasting mild cranial nerve dysfunction, limiting upgaze.

There was a 36% rate of technical complications during the procedures. These technical complications consisted of catheter-induced vasospasm, incomplete opening of the device requiring angioplasty, inability to pass the catheter across the aneurysm, vessel perforation, and groin hematoma. One patient had delayed in-stent stenosis. No patients had any clinical sequelae from these complications at last follow-up.[37]

SUMMARY

Historically, the treatment of cavernous and paraclinoid aneurysms has been a challenging task with high rates of surgical morbidity. With the rise of endovascular techniques, the morbidity has been lowered dramatically. Flow diversion has complemented coiling with higher occlusion rates and a potentially more durable treatment. Endovascular techniques are in relative infancy when compared with microsurgical techniques and it is hoped that the future will bring further advances to provide safer and more effective treatment of cavernous and paraclinoid aneurysms.

REFERENCES

1. Higashida RT, Halbach VV, Dowd C, et al. Endovascular detachable balloon embolization therapy of cavernous carotid artery aneurysms: results in 87 cases. J Neurosurg 2009;72(6):857–63. Available at: http://thejns.org/doi/abs/10.3171/jns.1990.72.6.0857. Accessed December 10, 2013.
2. van der Schaaf IC, Brilstra EH, Buskens E, et al. Endovascular treatment of aneurysms in the cavernous sinus a systematic review on balloon occlusion of the parent vessel and embolization with coils. Stroke 2002;33(1):313–8. http://dx.doi.org/10.1161/hs0102.101479.
3. Bouthillier A, van Loveren HR, Keller JT. Segments of the internal carotid artery: a new classification. Neurosurgery 1996;38(3):425–32 [discussion: 432–3].
4. Silva MN, Saeki N, Hirai S, et al. Unusual cranial nerve palsy caused by cavernous sinus aneurysms. Clinical and anatomical considerations reviewed. Surg Neurol 1999;52(2):143–8 [discussion: 148–9].
5. Day AL. Aneurysms of the ophthalmic segment. A clinical and anatomical analysis. J Neurosurg 1990;72(5):677–91. http://dx.doi.org/10.3171/jns.1990.72.5.0677.
6. Park HK, Horowitz M, Jungreis C, et al. Endovascular treatment of paraclinoid aneurysms: experience with 73 patients. Neurosurgery 2003;53(1):14–23 [discussion: 24].
7. D'Urso PI, Karadeli HH, Kallmes DF, et al. Coiling for paraclinoid aneurysms: time to make way for flow diverters? AJNR Am J Neuroradiol 2012;33(8):1470–4. http://dx.doi.org/10.3174/ajnr.A3009.
8. Tanaka Y, Hongo K, Tada T, et al. Radiometric analysis of paraclinoid carotid artery aneurysms. J Neurosurg 2002;96(4):649–53. http://dx.doi.org/10.3171/jns.2002.96.4.0649.
9. Harrigan MR, Ardelt A, Deveikis JP. Handbook of cerebrovascular disease and neurointerventional technique. Springer; 2009.
10. Nonaka T, Haraguchi K, Baba T, et al. Clinical manifestations and surgical results for paraclinoid cerebral aneurysms presenting with visual symptoms. Surg Neurol 2007;67(6):612–9. http://dx.doi.org/10.1016/j.surneu.2006.08.074 [discussion: 619].
11. White JA, Horowitz MB, Samson D. Dural waisting as a sign of subarachnoid extension of cavernous carotid aneurysms: a follow-up case report. Surg Neurol 1999;52(6):607–9 [discussion: 609–10].

12. Stiebel-Kalish H, Kalish Y, Bar-On RH, et al. Presentation, natural history, and management of carotid cavernous aneurysms. Neurosurgery 2005;57(5): 850–7 [discussion: 850–7].
13. Kupersmith MJ, Hurst R, Berenstein A, et al. The benign course of cavernous carotid artery aneurysms. J Neurosurg 1992;77(5):690–3. http://dx.doi.org/10.3171/jns.1992.77.5.0690.
14. Van Rooij WJ, Sluzewski M, Beute GN. Ruptured cavernous sinus aneurysms causing carotid cavernous fistula: incidence, clinical presentation, treatment, and outcome. AJNR Am J Neuroradiol 2006;27(1):185–9.
15. Lee AG, Mawad ME, Baskin DS. Fatal subarachnoid hemorrhage from the rupture of a totally intracavernous carotid artery aneurysm: case report. Neurosurgery 1996;38(3):596–8 [discussion: 598–9].
16. Hamada H, Endo S, Fukuda O, et al. Giant aneurysm in the cavernous sinus causing subarachnoid hemorrhage 13 years after detection: a case report. Surg Neurol 1996;45(2):143–6.
17. Wiebers DO, Whisnant JP, Huston J 3rd, et al. Unruptured intracranial aneurysms: natural history, clinical outcome, and risks of surgical and endovascular treatment. Lancet 2003;362(9378): 103–10.
18. Gonzalez LF, Walker MT, Zabramski JM, et al. Distinction between paraclinoid and cavernous sinus aneurysms with computed tomographic angiography. Neurosurgery 2003;52(5):1131–7 [discussion: 1138–9].
19. Nguyen TN, Raymond J, Guilbert F, et al. Association of endovascular therapy of very small ruptured aneurysms with higher rates of procedure-related rupture. J Neurosurg 2008;108(6):1088–92. http://dx.doi.org/10.3171/JNS/2008/108/6/1088.
20. Park HK, Horowitz M, Jungreis C, et al. Periprocedural morbidity and mortality associated with endovascular treatment of intracranial aneurysms. AJNR Am J Neuroradiol 2005;26(3): 506–14.
21. Kobayashi S, Kyoshima K, Gibo H, et al. Carotid cave aneurysms of the internal carotid artery. J Neurosurg 1989;70(2):216–21. http://dx.doi.org/10.3171/jns.1989.70.2.0216.
22. Almeida GM, Shibata MK, Bianco E. Carotid-ophthalmic aneurysms. Surg Neurol 1976;5(1): 41–5.
23. Drake CG, Vanderlinden RG, Amacher AL. Carotid-ophthalmic aneurysms. J Neurosurg 1968; 29(1):24–31. http://dx.doi.org/10.3171/jns.1968.29.1.0024.
24. Ferguson GG, Drake CG. Carotid-ophthalmic aneurysms: visual abnormalities in 32 patients and the results of treatment. Surg Neurol 1981;16(1): 1–8.
25. Fox JL. Microsurgical treatment of ventral (paraclinoid) internal carotid artery aneurysms. Neurosurgery 1988;22(1 Pt 1):32–9.
26. Javalkar V, Banerjee AD, Nanda A. Paraclinoid carotid aneurysms. J Clin Neurosci 2011;18(1):13–22. http://dx.doi.org/10.1016/j.jocn.2010.06.020.
27. Linskey ME, Sekhar LN, Hirsch WL Jr, et al. Aneurysms of the intracavernous carotid artery: natural history and indications for treatment. Neurosurgery 1990;26(6):933–7 [discussion: 937–8].
28. Dolenc V. Direct microsurgical repair of intracavernous vascular lesions. J Neurosurg 1983; 58(6):824–31. http://dx.doi.org/10.3171/jns.1983.58.6.0824.
29. Dolenc VV. Extradural approach to intracavernous ICA aneurysms. Acta Neurochir Suppl 1999;72: 99–106.
30. Galbraith JG, Clark RM. Role of carotid ligation in the management of intracranial carotid aneurysms. Clin Neurosurg 1974;21:171–81.
31. Serbinenko FA. Balloon catheterization and occlusion of major cerebral vessels. J Neurosurg 1974; 41(2):125–45. http://dx.doi.org/10.3171/jns.1974.41.2.0125.
32. Elhammady MS, Wolfe SQ, Farhat H, et al. Carotid artery sacrifice for unclippable and uncoilable aneurysms: endovascular occlusion vs common carotid artery ligation. Neurosurgery 2010;67(5):1431–7. http://dx.doi.org/10.1227/NEU.0b013e3181f076ac.
33. van Rooij WJ. Endovascular treatment of cavernous sinus aneurysms. AJNR Am J Neuroradiol 2012;33(2):323–6. http://dx.doi.org/10.3174/ajnr.A2759.
34. Arambepola PK, McEvoy SD, Bulsara KR. De novo aneurysm formation after carotid artery occlusion for cerebral aneurysms. Skull Base 2010;20(6): 405–8. http://dx.doi.org/10.1055/s-0030-1253578.
35. Dyste GN, Beck DW. De novo aneurysm formation following carotid ligation: case report and review of the literature. Neurosurgery 1989;24(1): 88–92.
36. Arnaout OM, Rahme RJ, Aoun SG, et al. De novo large fusiform posterior circulation intracranial aneurysm presenting with subarachnoid hemorrhage 7 years after therapeutic internal carotid artery occlusion: case report and review of the literature. Neurosurgery 2012;71(3):E764–71. http://dx.doi.org/10.1227/NEU.0b013e31825fd169.
37. Puffer RC, Piano M, Lanzino G, et al. Treatment of cavernous sinus aneurysms with flow diversion: results in 44 patients. AJNR Am J Neuroradiol 2013. http://dx.doi.org/10.3174/ajnr.A3826.
38. Van Rooij WJ, Sluzewski M, Slob MJ, et al. Predictive value of angiographic testing for tolerance to therapeutic occlusion of the carotid artery. AJNR Am J Neuroradiol 2005;26(1):175–8.

39. Baxter BW, Rosso D, Lownie SP. Double microcatheter technique for detachable coil treatment of large, wide-necked intracranial aneurysms. AJNR Am J Neuroradiol 1998;19(6):1176–8.
40. Raymond J, Guilbert F, Weill A, et al. Long-term angiographic recurrences after selective endovascular treatment of aneurysms with detachable coils. Stroke 2003;34(6):1398–403. http://dx.doi.org/10.1161/01.STR.0000073841.88563.E9.
41. Kole MK, Pelz DM, Kalapos P, et al. Endovascular coil embolization of intracranial aneurysms: important factors related to rates and outcomes of incomplete occlusion. J Neurosurg 2005;102(4):607–15. http://dx.doi.org/10.3171/jns.2005.102.4.0607.
42. Molyneux A, Kerr R, International Subarachnoid Aneurysm Trial (ISAT) Collaborative Group, et al. International Subarachnoid Aneurysm Trial (ISAT) of neurosurgical clipping versus endovascular coiling in 2143 patients with ruptured intracranial aneurysms: a randomized trial. J Stroke Cerebrovasc Dis 2002;11(6):304–14. http://dx.doi.org/10.1053/jscd.2002.130390.
43. Fargen KM, Hoh BL, Welch BG, et al. Long-term results of enterprise stent-assisted coiling of cerebral aneurysms. Neurosurgery 2012;71(2):239–44. http://dx.doi.org/10.1227/NEU.0b013e3182571953 [discussion: 244].
44. Murayama Y, Nien YL, Duckwiler G, et al. Guglielmi detachable coil embolization of cerebral aneurysms: 11 years' experience. J Neurosurg 2003; 98(5):959–66. http://dx.doi.org/10.3171/jns.2003.98.5.0959.
45. Roy D, Raymond J, Bouthillier A, et al. Endovascular treatment of ophthalmic segment aneurysms with Guglielmi detachable coils. AJNR Am J Neuroradiol 1997;18(7):1207–15.
46. Gurian JH, Viñuela F, Guglielmi G, et al. Endovascular embolization of superior hypophyseal artery aneurysms. Neurosurgery 1996;39(6): 1150–4 [discussion: 1154–6].
47. Thornton J, Aletich VA, Debrun GM, et al. Endovascular treatment of paraclinoid aneurysms. Surg Neurol 2000;54(4):288–99.
48. Lylyk P, Miranda C, Ceratto R, et al. Curative endovascular reconstruction of cerebral aneurysms with the pipeline embolization device: the Buenos Aires experience. Neurosurgery 2009;64(4): 632–42. http://dx.doi.org/10.1227/01.NEU.0000339109.98070.65 [discussion: 642–3]. [quiz: N6].
49. Lubicz B, Collignon L, Raphaeli G, et al. Pipeline flow-diverter stent for endovascular treatment of intracranial aneurysms: preliminary experience in 20 patients with 27 aneurysms. World Neurosurg 2011;76(1–2):114–9. http://dx.doi.org/10.1016/j.wneu.2011.02.015.
50. Becske T, Kallmes DF, Saatci I, et al. Pipeline for uncoilable or failed aneurysms: results from a multicenter clinical trial. Radiology 2013;267(3):858–68. http://dx.doi.org/10.1148/radiol.13120099.
51. Nelson PK, Lylyk P, Szikora I, et al. The pipeline embolization device for the intracranial treatment of aneurysms trial. AJNR Am J Neuroradiol 2011;32(1):34–40. http://dx.doi.org/10.3174/ajnr.A2421.
52. The treatment of traumatic arteriovenous fistula. South Med J. Available at: http://journals.lww.com/smajournalonline/Fulltext/1930/02000/The_Treatment_of_Traumatic_Arteriovenous_Fistula.4.aspx. Accessed January 27, 2014.
53. Szikora I, Berentei Z, Kulcsar Z, et al. Treatment of intracranial aneurysms by functional reconstruction of the parent artery: the Budapest experience with the pipeline embolization device. AJNR Am J Neuroradiol 2010;31(6):1139–47. http://dx.doi.org/10.3174/ajnr.A2023.
54. Byrne JV, Beltechi R, Yarnold JA, et al. Early experience in the treatment of intra-cranial aneurysms by endovascular flow diversion: a multicentre prospective study. PLoS One 2010;5(9). http://dx.doi.org/10.1371/journal.pone.0012492.

Endovascular Treatment of Supraclinoid Internal Carotid Artery Aneurysms

Biraj M. Patel, MD[a,b], Azam Ahmed, MD[a,b], David Niemann, MD[a,b,*]

KEYWORDS

• Supraclinoid • Ophthalmic • Superior hypophyseal • Blister • Dorsal wall • Anterior choroidal • Posterior communicating aneurysms

KEY POINTS

- Endovascular management of supraclinoid aneurysms have come into favor as a result of recent advances in devices, techniques, and knowledge.
- Treatment of large or giant aneurysms have been revolutionized by flow diverter technology; albeit, long-term follow-up results are eagerly awaited for their validation.
- Blister-type aneurysms are unique intracranial aneurysms and pose a significant risk to patients even after treatment because of their tenuous pathophysiology.
- Discussion of treatment options for supraclinoid internal carotid artery aneurysms among a multidisciplinary neurovascular team (cerebrovascular neurosurgeons and neurointerventionalists) should include extensive review of radiological studies, vascular anatomy, patients' comorbidities, aneurysm size and morphology, and ruptured versus unruptured presentation.

INTRODUCTION

Supraclinoid aneurysms are typically defined as intradural aneurysms that arise from the internal carotid artery (ICA) distal to the distal dural ring, or roof of the cavernous sinus, to the carotid terminus. Being intradural, these aneurysms pose a risk for subarachnoid hemorrhage and are, therefore, generally treated depending on the size of the aneurysm, patients' age, and comorbidities. The paraclinoid region is composed of complex osseous anatomy and dural attachments and is in close proximity to the optic nerve, thereby making microsurgical clipping of some aneurysms in this region technically challenging. Endovascular treatment with balloon- or stent-assisted coil embolization and, more recently, flow diversion technology is being used more frequently for treatment of paraclinoid as well as supraclinoid aneurysms.

RELEVANT ANATOMY AND PATHOPHYSIOLOGY

The anterior clinoid process projects from the posteromedial border of the lesser wing of the sphenoid bone and forms a roof over the proximal portion of the ICA. The roof of the optic canal (anterior root) and optic strut (posterior root) communicate with the body of the sphenoid bone at the medial aspect of the anterior clinoid process. The optic strut also borders the lower margin of the anterior clinoid process to the body

Disclosures: None.

[a] Department of Radiology, University of Wisconsin Hospital and Clinics, 600 Highland Avenue, Madison, WI 53705, USA; [b] Department of Neurological Surgery, University of Wisconsin Hospital and Clinics, 600 Highland Avenue, Madison, WI 53705, USA

* Corresponding author. Department of Neurological Surgery, University of Wisconsin Hospital and Clinics, 600 Highland Avenue, Madison, WI 53705.

E-mail address: d.niemann@neurosurgery.wisconsin.edu

Neurosurg Clin N Am 25 (2014) 425–435
http://dx.doi.org/10.1016/j.nec.2014.04.003
1042-3680/14/$ – see front matter

of the sphenoid bone. The anterior clinoid process harbors attachments of the falciform ligament, the anteromedial part of the tentorium, the petroclinoid (anterior and posterior) ligaments, and the interclinoid dural folds.[1]

The clinoidal segment of the ICA lies between the proximal and distal dural rings. The clinoidal ICA traverses the distal dural ring and enters the subarachnoid space. The distal dural ring is thicker at its lateral margin and tightly adheres the artery to adjacent structures. However, medially it may be incompletely attached allowing a small potential subarachnoid space, or carotid cave, abutting inferiorly and medially to the ICA. Proximal to the proximal dural ring, the ICA becomes intracavernous. From the distal dural ring to the carotid terminus, or anterior and middle cerebral artery bifurcation, is the supraclinoid region. The supraclinoid ICA courses medial to the anterior clinoid process below the optic nerve and superior/posterior to the lateral aspect of the optic chiasm. It terminates below the anterior perforated substance at the medial edge of the Sylvian fissure.[1,2]

Typically, paraclinoid and cavernous aneurysms are differentiated based on their relationship to the origin of the ophthalmic artery. This distinction is important for treatment versus no treatment decision making, as their natural history and risk of subarachnoid hemorrhage is significantly different. There is variability in the origin of the ophthalmic artery off the ICA. For instance, Horiuchi and colleagues[3] reported a prevalence of intradural origin of the ophthalmic artery of 85.7% and an extradural origin of 7.6%. They reported an interdural origin (between the 2 dural rings) of 6.7%. Among the supraclinoid aneurysms, the ophthalmic and superior hypophyseal aneurysms can be angiographically differentiated based on their projection off the ICA. The former typically projects superiorly off the parent vessel and the latter inferiorly or inferomedially.

For purposes of this article, endovascular treatment of ophthalmic, superior hypophyseal, dorsal wall blister, posterior communicating, anterior choroidal, and carotid terminus aneurysms are discussed.

NATURAL HISTORY, CLINICAL PRESENTATION, AND INDICATIONS FOR TREATMENT

Various risk factors have been associated with higher prevalence of intracranial aneurysms, including female sex, family history, cigarette smoking, excessive alcohol use, hypertension, ischemic heart disease, hyperlipidemia, autosomal dominant polycystic kidney disease, type IV Ehlers-Danlos syndrome, pituitary tumors, aortic coarctation, Graves disease, Marfan syndrome, neurofibromatosis type 1, cerebral arteriovenous malformations (flow-related aneurysms), and oral contraceptive use.[4]

There is no debate that ruptured intracranial aneurysms should be treatment promptly as it carries a high mortality rate of approximately 50% to 60%.[5] However, the decision of treatment versus no treatment is not as clear when the aneurysm is unruptured and found incidentally. In these cases, risk stratification must take into account patients' age, aneurysm size, location, and morphology.

Multiple previous large trials as well as numerous case series have made efforts to quantify risk of intracranial aneurysms. For instance, the International Study of Unruptured Intracranial Aneurysms (ISUIA) trial concluded the 5-year cumulative rupture rates for patients with aneurysms involving the anterior circulation and who did not have subarachnoid hemorrhage to be 0% for less than 7 mm, 2.6% for 7 to 12 mm, 14.5% for 13 to 24 mm, and 40.0% for greater than or equal to 25 mm.[6] In ISUIA, Posterior communicating artery (Pcomm) aneurysms were grouped with the posterior circulation aneurysms with respect to risk of rupture. The posterior circulation and posterior communicating artery aneurysms of the same size were shown to have higher risk of rupture: 2.5%, 14.5%, 18.4%, and 50.0%, respectively.[6] A systemic review by Rinkel and colleagues[7] reported an overall risk of aneurysm rupture of 1.9% per year (0.7% for unruptured aneurysms $\leq$10 mm and 4.0% for those >10 mm). A meta-analysis by Clark and colleagues[8] of patients with unruptured aneurysms found that when the ISUIA cohort was excluded, the rate of rupture for Pcomm aneurysms (0.46% annually) mimics that of anterior circulation aneurysms (0.49% annually) rather than posterior circulation aneurysms (1.9% annually). The authors' of this article tend to treat Pcomm aneurysms more aggressively.

In addition to the risk of rupture and subarachnoid hemorrhage, large or giant aneurysms, particularly in the paraclinoid/supraclinoid regions, can cause mass effect on adjacent cranial nerves resulting in visual disturbances, thereby necessitating treatment. Endovascular treatment of large or giant aneurysms with coil embolization, and more recently flow diversion, has been shown to reduce mass effect (on cranial nerve) as the aneurysm thromboses, contracts, and diminishes in pulsatility, often with resolution of associated cranial neuropathy.

Posterior communicating artery aneurysms are relatively common, accounting for 15% to 25% of all intracranial aneurysms.[9,10] Pcomm aneurysms arise at the origin of the respective vessel off the posterolateral aspect of the ICA. The laterally projecting Pcomm aneurysms can compress the oculomotor nerve against the tentorium at its superomedial aspect causing pupil-sparing cranial nerve III palsy.[11] The Pcomm harbors multiple small arterial branches supplying the optic chiasm, oculomotor nerve, ventral thalamus, mammillary bodies, tuber cinereum, hypothalamus, and internal capsule.[9,12] Hence, of course, treatment strategies should focus on maintaining antegrade flow so as to reduce the risk of ischemic injury to the diencephalon to avoid significant morbidity. In some cases, however, retrograde flow can be adequate enough to maintain perfusion of this territory, which should be confirmed with angiography or intraoperative indocyanine green (ICG) during clipping.

Anterior choroidal artery (ACh) aneurysms arise at the origin of the respective vessel off the posterolateral aspect of the ICA. Although the ACh artery is relatively small in caliber, it supplies eloquent territories, including the posterior two-thirds of the posterior limb internal capsule, optic tract, cerebral peduncle, uncus, optic radiations, lateral geniculate body, amygdala, anterior hippocampus, fornix, pulvinar, and globus pallidus. The preservation of this vessel (or vessels, if duplicate variant anatomy) during microsurgical clipping or endovascular treatment of an aneurysm is important and may be challenging in certain circumstances, with morbidity reported at 6% to 33% and mortality at 10% to 29%.[13–15] Morbidity can be as severe as ACh syndrome, which presents with contralateral hemiplegia, dysarthria, lethargy, and occasionally sensory and vision loss.[15]

Blister, or dorsal wall, aneurysms that arise from nonbranching sites of the supraclinoid ICA are rare but devastating causes of a subarachnoid hemorrhage. These aneurysms are most often tenuous because of their small size, very broad necks, and fragile walls. Pathology studies have shown blister aneurysms to be more like pseudoaneurysms than saccular aneurysms. They have been shown to have focal wall laceration causing ulceration and separation of the internal elastic lamina and media. The focal defect is covered with thin fibrous tissue and clot, lacking a collagen layer, making them much more prone to intraoperative and perioperative rupture.[16,17]

Although aneurysm size is a main factor based on previous trials, other factors, such as the aspect ratio, presence of daughter sac, and psychosocial issues, also contribute to the decision to treat. In addition to the aforementioned factors, the authors' also take into account their individual philosophies and experiences in the treatment decision-making process.

DIAGNOSIS AND TREATMENT PLANNING

Because of the complex anatomy in this region, cross-sectional imaging, such as magnetic resonance angiography (MRA) or computed tomographic angiography (CTA), is often limited in classifying aneurysms, especially large or giant variants. Digital subtraction angiography (DSA) including 3-dimensional (3D) rotational dual-volume angiography with multiplanar reformations remains the gold standard modality and is widely used to classify intradural versus extradural aneurysms as well as to evaluate the size, morphology, and bony relationship of the aneurysm as part of treatment (open skull base surgery or endovascular) planning. Intraprocedural use of flat detector CT (FDCT) may be beneficial to evaluate the anatomy of the device and its relationship to the vasculature (see **Fig. 2**).

CTA with 3D reconstructions can also be useful to examine the aneurysm relationship to the bony skull base anatomy, which is particularly helpful for open surgical approaches. CTA also allows for making accurate measurements of aneurysms and parent vessels. For treatment planning and virtual surgery, the authors' usually start with CTA of the head and neck to assess the endovascular route, aneurysm morphology, and measurements of the aneurysm and parent vessel.

MR imaging (MRI) and MRA are useful in evaluating the true size of thrombosed aneurysms as well as evaluating potential mass effect on adjacent structures and aneurysm wall calcification. Additionally, MRI is useful preemptively for ventriculoperitoneal shunt placement in patients with hydrocephalus with transependymal cerebrospinal fluid flow in the setting of subarachnoid hemorrhage, especially before stenting or flow diverter placement requiring dual antiplatelet therapy.

Aneurysm Classification

Various classifications have been proposed for paraclinoid/supraclinoid aneurysms.[18] The authors' of this article prefer a simplistic classification of these aneurysms, which is based on the close proximity to the respective arterial branch off of the ICA (ie, ophthalmic, superior hypophyseal, posterior communicating, anterior choroidal, and carotid terminus aneurysms). Also noteworthy in the supraclinoid region are rare but significant blister aneurysms, which arise from nonbranching portions of the dorsal, or anterior, wall of the ICA.

ENDOVASCULAR CONSIDERATIONS

Until the advent of endovascular strategies for treatment of intracranial aneurysms in the paraclinoid/supraclinoid regions, open surgery was the mainstay treatment option and still may remain the primary option depending on the patients' age, aneurysm location, size, and morphology.

The complex anatomy surrounding the paraclinoid ICA can make microsurgical treatment of aneurysms in this region technically challenging, requiring clinoid drilling and difficulty acquiring proximal control, which adds risk to clipping procedures. Endovascular treatment is increasingly used because of technological advancements. However, in certain supraclinoid ICA aneurysms, surgical clipping can be a more straightforward option.

There have been significant advances in technology for endovascular management of intracranial aneurysms over the decades, whether it be softer coils, improved stents and stent deployment systems, parent vessel flow diversion technology, or endosaccular flow diversion technology (not yet available in the United States). Advances in guide catheter technology allow operators to negotiate difficult arch types, tortuous great vessels, cervical tonsillar loops, and so forth.

The International Subarachnoid Aneurysm Trial Collaborative Group published the first prospective randomized trial comparing surgical clipping versus endovascular coiling in 2143 patients with ruptured intracranial aneurysms. The results demonstrated the following rates of dependency or death at 1 year: 23.7% (endovascular arm) versus 30.6% (surgical arm), with relative and absolute risk reduction of 22.6% and 6.9%, respectively.[19]

In regard to unruptured aneurysms, prospective ISUIA data demonstrated the 1-year combined morbidity and mortality rate for group 1 (those without a history of subarachnoid hemorrhage (SAH) from a different aneurysm) to be 12.6% (surgical arm) versus 9.8% (endovascular arm), with a 22.3% relative risk reduction. For group 2 (those with a history of SAH from a different aneurysm that was repaired), the results were 10.1% (surgical arm) versus 7.1% (endovascular arm), with a 29.7% relative risk reduction.[5]

Ophthalmic ICA/Superior Hypophyseal Aneurysms

As previously mentioned, because of their intricate intracranial location, paraclinoid aneurysms are often treated by endovascular means.

However, because of their relationship with the tortuosity of internal carotid artery, ophthalmic ICA and superior hypophyseal aneurysms can be challenging to treat by endovascular coil embolization. Microcatheterization of such aneurysms require navigation around the anterior genu of the ICA followed immediately by an acute turn into the aneurysm neck. For the same reason, stenting of this segment can also be technically challenging and result in kinking around turns. Nevertheless, with improvement in current access devices, these tasks are quite feasible.

A significant drawback of coil embolization is insufficient aneurysm packing resulting in a higher risk of recurrence rates compared with surgical clipping. Although with the use of adjunctive techniques, such as balloon- or stent-assisted coil embolization, recurrence rates can be otherwise lowered. In the setting of subarachnoid hemorrhage, the latter is avoided as it requires dual antiplatelet therapy, which can complicate external ventricular drain placement, if clinically required (**Fig. 1**).

Large or Giant Aneurysms

Large (>15–24 mm) or giant (>25 mm) aneurysms are associated with high morbidity/mortality during surgical management.[20–22] Hence, endovascular strategies are often preferred for the management of these complex lesions, with a relatively low morbidity/mortality.[23–26] Depending on clinical presentation, aneurysm location and anatomy, time since SAH, robustness of collateral circulation, and presence of intra-aneurysmal thrombus, various endovascular strategies can be used for the management of large or giant aneurysms.[27]

Vessel deconstruction or parent vessel occlusion with coils is a relatively quick, safe, and simple technique to curtail flow into the aneurysm. However, parent vessel preservation is preferred as a result of recent technological advances. Occlusion of the ICA has been widely used for the treatment of large or giant ophthalmic ICA aneurysms.[28–31] It has been used for supraclinoid ICA including carotid terminus aneurysms when there is an absent posterior communicating artery and collateral flow is only via the anterior communicating artery.[27] Vessel deconstruction is an effective way for eliminating inflow into the aneurysm, thereby eliminating the risk of aneurysm rupture. Although depending on the patients' circle of Willis collaterals, this may not be tolerated neurologically. Therefore, balloon test occlusion of the ipsilateral ICA can be performed in conjunction with serial clinical neurologic examinations, intraprocedural electroencephalogram monitoring, and nuclear medicine single-photon emission computed tomography as well as hypotension challenge to evaluate the extent of collaterals and accurately predict the tolerability of vessel deconstruction.

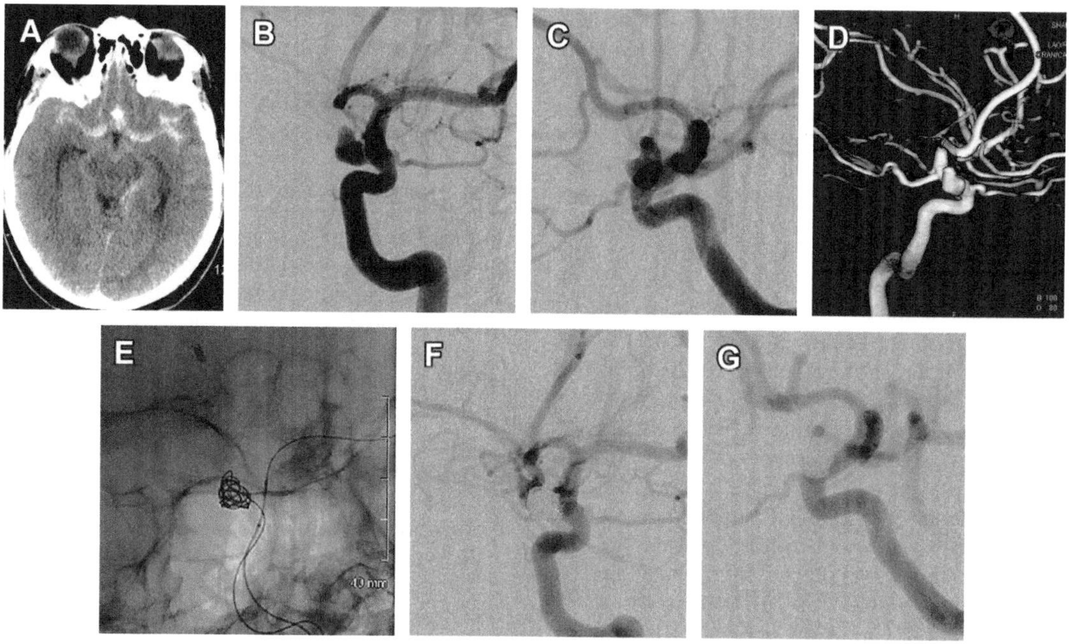

Fig. 1. A 32-year-old man found to have subarachnoid hemorrhage (*A*) secondary to ruptured left superior hypophyseal aneurysm. (*B–D*) Working projection DSA and 3D volume-rendered images demonstrate a multilobulated 5 × 6-mm saccular superior hypophyseal aneurysm. (*E*) Unsubtracted spot fluoroscopic image shows the uninflated balloon across the neck of the aneurysm before coil delivery. (*F, G*) Immediate, post–balloon-assisted coil embolization DSA images in working projections demonstrate no significant residual aneurysm.

Balloon- or stent-assisted coil embolization has been widely used for endovascular management of large or giant aneurysms, which typically have wide necks. Stent placement should be avoided in the setting of subarachnoid hemorrhage because of a need for dual antiplatelet medications. Therefore, the initial treatment plan should focus on dome protection with balloon-assisted coiling in the acute setting, followed by repeat, more aggressive coil embolization with stent assistance in a nonacute setting.

Despite immediate posttreatment angiographically satisfying result, these types of aneurysms have high recurrence rates secondary to coil compaction, coil migration into intraluminal thrombus, or dissolution of intraluminal thrombus resulting in luminal enlargement.[25–27] For this reason, routine follow-up is necessary to plan prompt retreatment if necessary.

Intraluminal embolization with Onyx HD-500 (ev3, Irvine, CA) has been proposed for the treatment of large or giant aneurysms. This treatment requires balloon occlusion of the parent vessel in order to seal the aneurysm neck during Onyx injection into the aneurysm lumen. A multicenter prospective observational study, Cerebral Aneurysm Multicenter European Onyx trial, by Molyneux and colleagues[32] reported an 8.3% incidence of permanent neurologic morbidity, including 2 procedural deaths. There was prolonged procedure time up to 6 hours. There was delayed occlusion of the carotid artery with an incidence of 9%. The complete occlusion rate of large and giant aneurysms was 72% at the 12-month follow-up, whereas the retreatment rate was 11%. Because of a relatively high complication rate and no proven benefit over coil embolization, this strategy is now used less, especially with advances in flow diversion technology.

Flow diversion for treatment of large/giant aneurysms

In April 2011, the Food and Drug Administration (FDA) approved the Pipeline Embolization Device (PED) (Covidien/ev3, Irvine, CA), which has since revolutionized the treatment of large or giant wide-necked intracranial aneurysms involving the ICA from the petrous to the superior hypophyseal segments. Other flow diverters, such as Surpass (Stryker, Fremont, CA), FRED (MicroVention, Tustin, CA), and Silk (Balt Extrusion, Montmorency, France), are used abroad and are awaiting FDA approval.

Previous in vitro studies[33–35] and a canine aneurysm model[34] have demonstrated changes in intra-aneurysmal flow patterns as a result of stent placement, resulting in flow diversion away from the aneurysm. Based on these studies, low porosity devices, such as the aforementioned flow diverters, were developed. Using experimental rabbit models, Kallmes and colleagues[36,37] demonstrated a high rate of complete or near-complete occlusion with preservation of the parent vessel and smaller side branches and no evidence of distal thromboemboli. Furthermore, histopathologic analysis of the explants demonstrated neointimal layer covering the device struts and the aneurysm neck while preserving the ostia of smaller side branches.[36,37] Diminishment of intra-aneurysmal flow results in thrombosis, which eventually regresses resulting in progressive reduction in the size of the aneurysm sac.

The Pipeline for Uncoilable or Failed Aneurysms trial was a multicenter, prospective, single-arm trial to evaluate the safety and efficacy of PED in the treatment of complex intracranial aneurysms. One hundred seven out of 108 patients (99.1%) underwent successful placement of the PED. The mean aneurysm size was 18.2 mm, with 20.4% being giant (>25 mm) aneurysms. The primary effectiveness end point (complete occlusion of aneurysm without >50% stenosis of parent vessel or need for adjunctive treatment on 180-day angiogram) was found to be 73.6%. Major ipsilateral stroke or death secondary to neurologic sequela was seen in 6 out of 107 (5.6%) patients treated.[38] Intraparenchymal hemorrhage remote from the aneurysm site was noted in 5 out of 107 (4.7%) patients. This complication has also been reported previously after treatment of intracranial aneurysms with stent-assisted coiling.[39] It has been theorized previously that this phenomenon may be related to intraprocedural embolization (thrombus, catheter coating, and so forth) resulting in microinfarctions with subsequent hemorrhagic transformation or a sequela of hemodynamic alterations after flow diversion.[38,40]

In a recent retrospective matched-pair analysis comparing PED with standard endovascular strategies for the treatment of paraclinoid aneurysms (which included ophthalmic ICA and superior hypophyseal aneurysms), Lanzino and colleagues[41] found a much higher rate of complete angiographic obliteration of aneurysms with the PED. The complication rate remained similar between the 2 groups.

Although the immediate and midterm follow-up studies are encouraging for the efficacy and safety of flow diverters for the treatment of large or giant aneurysms, long-term follow-up studies are imperative for validating them as the first-line treatment of such aneurysms.

In the authors' experience, meticulous technique and perioperative management including close hemodynamic monitoring can limit complications. Furthermore, with intradural aneurysms, aggressive flow diversion (multiple PEDs as well as coiling) may limit the risk of an aneurysm rupture while neointimal layer formation ensues along the device (**Figs. 2** and **3**).

Blister or Dorsal Wall ICA Aneurysm

As discussed earlier, blister or dorsal wall ICA aneurysms are challenging to treat via open surgery as well as endovascular strategies. Aneurysm wrapping and clipping have been used as a means of an open surgical treatment technique, but these techniques have been associated with high post-operative growth and rehemorrhage rates.[42–47] A more durable surgical treatment of this type of aneurysm is ICA trapping with or without extracranial/intracranial (EC/IC) bypass, which is the authors' preferred strategy.

Several endovascular strategies have been described for the treatment of these unstable lesions. Vessel deconstruction or parent vessel occlusion, preceded by balloon test occlusion (BTO), is an effective way for eliminating inflow into the aneurysm, thereby eliminating the risk of aneurysm rupture, with or without EC/IC bypass. In the setting of SAH, parent vessel occlusion can cut off direct access for intra-arterial treatment of refractory vasospasm should patients need it.

Vessel reconstruction with stenting, with or without coil embolization, has also been described. It is plausible that a stent across the aneurysmal/pseudoaneurysmal segment of the ICA diverts flow, thereby altering hemodynamic shear stress to the aneurysm/pseudoaneurysm wall.[48] Additionally, the stent offers a scaffolding to promote endothelialization across the aneurysm neck.

Multiple small case series reports have demonstrated favorable outcomes with stent-assisted coil embolization and/or stent-within-stent reconstruction[47,49–52] as well as with flow diversion.[53] Coil embolization in addition to stenting is often not a good option as these aneurysms generally lack a saccular component. When there is a saccular component, it often represents a pseudoaneurysm, which can rupture during microcatheterization or coil introduction resulting in intraprocedural hemorrhage.

Because of their tenuous nature, regardless of the treatment strategy used, a very-short-interval follow-up with cerebral angiogram is recommended.

Posterior Communicating Aneurysms

Wirth[54] found that Pcomm aneurysms had the lowest operative morbidity compared with

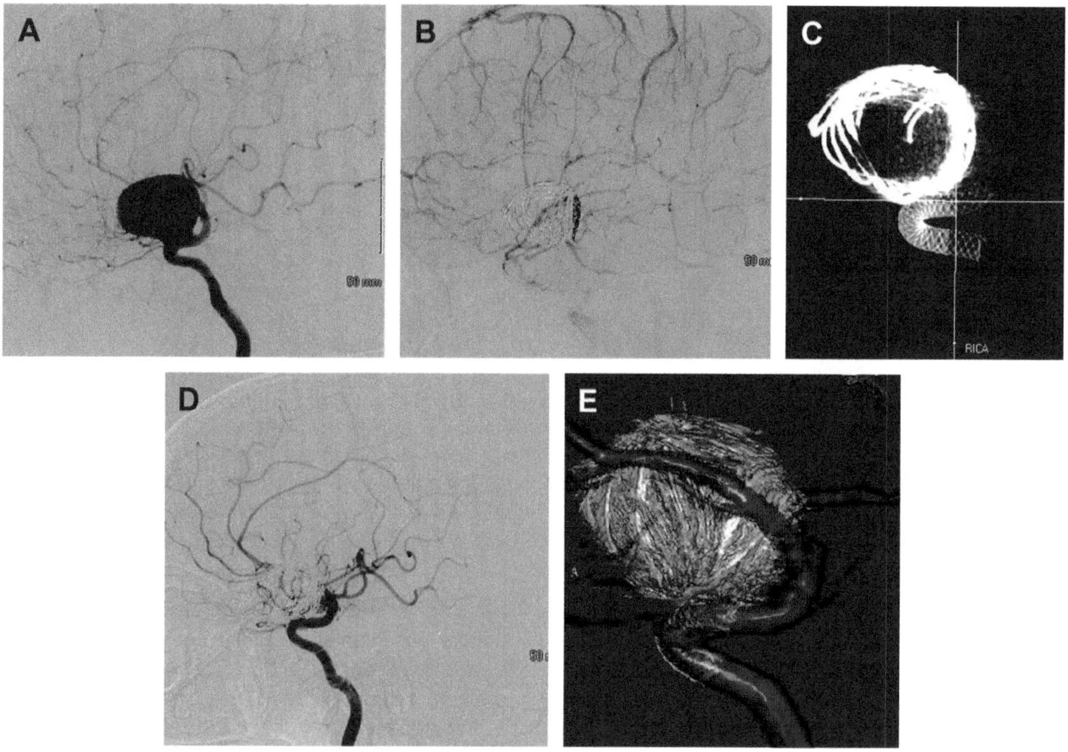

Fig. 2. A 56-year-old woman with history of a giant right ophthalmic ICA aneurysm (*A*) as seen on lateral DSA. (*B*) Lateral DSA immediately following placement of 2 PEDs and coil embolization demonstrates small amount of contrast with stasis in the aneurysm sac. (*C*) Intraprocedural FDCT demonstrating device anatomy and its relationship to the vasculature. One-year follow-up (*D*) lateral angiogram and (*E*) 3D volume-rendered image demonstrate obliteration of the aneurysm.

aneurysms in other locations (5% vs 8% middle cerebral artery, 12% ICA, 16% anterior communicating artery). These aneurysms are still often clipped depending on morphology and the clinical situation.

In contrast to paraclinoid ICA aneurysms, Pcomm aneurysms pose a lesser challenge during microcatheterization. Microcatheterization of paraclinoid ICA aneurysms require navigation around the anterior genu of the ICA followed immediately by an

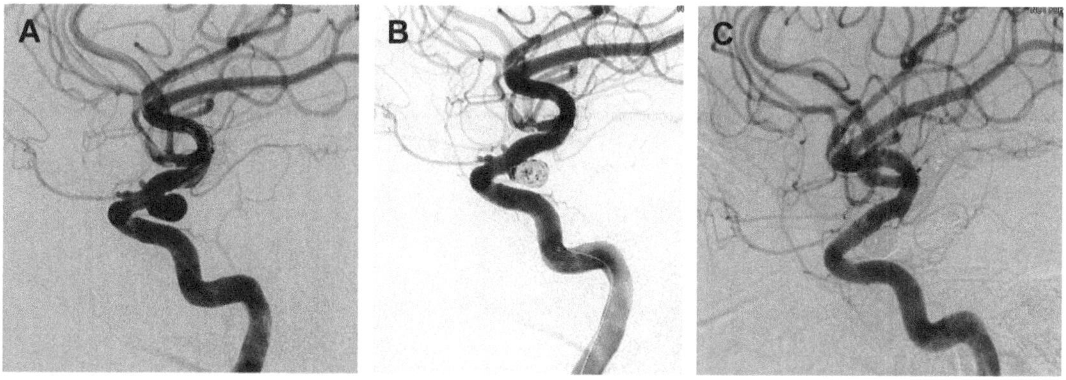

Fig. 3. A 46-year-old woman incidentally found to have multiple intracranial aneurysms during work-up for headaches. (*A*) Initial lateral DSA image demonstrates a 5- to 6-mm saccular aneurysm projecting posteriorly from the communicating segment of the left ICA as well as a very small ophthalmic ICA aneurysm. (*B*) Immediate post-PED placement and coil embolization lateral DSA images demonstrate Raymond class III aneurysm occlusion with persistent opacification of the smaller aneurysm. (*C*) Sixteen-month follow-up lateral DSA image demonstrates no residual ICA aneurysms.

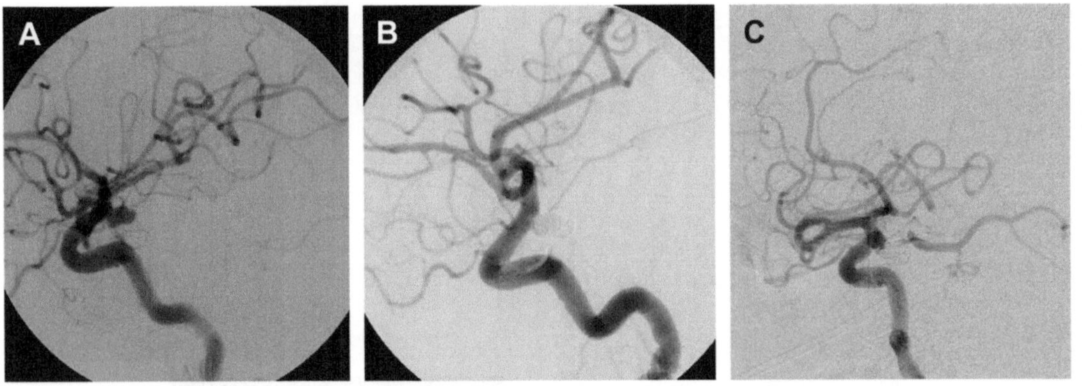

Fig. 4. A 52-year-old woman with history of clipping of a ruptured right posterior communicating artery aneurysm, followed by coil embolization of a de novo left posterior communicating artery aneurysm 10 years later that presented with carnial nerve (CN) III palsy. (*A*) Precoiling lateral DSA image demonstrates a lobulated 4- to 5-mm saccular aneurysm projecting posteriorly from the communicating segment of the left ICA. (*B*) Immediate postcoiling lateral DSA image demonstrates no significant residual sac opacification. (*C*) Nine-year follow-up lateral DSA image demonstrates no significant recurrence, with resolution of the associated cranial neuropathy.

acute turn into the aneurysms neck, whereas the neck of a Pcomm aneurysm is in direct trajectory of the relatively straight communicating segment of the ICA. Depending on a narrow or wide neck, these aneurysms can typically be treated with coiling alone or balloon/stent-assisted coiling, respectively (**Figs. 4** and **5**). Although cranial neuropathies often improve faster or more completely with open surgical treatment, endovascular treatment can also result in their improvement.

Anterior Choroidal Aneurysms

Surgical clipping of anterior choroidal aneurysms, particularly large aneurysms, can be challenging because of the usually small caliber of the aforementioned branching vessel and the eloquent territory it supplies. Furthermore, this small-caliber vessel is often kinked by the aneurysm or is adherent to the aneurysm, making dissection difficult. Multiple case series reports have published ischemic complications after ACh aneurysm clipping ranging in 4.5% to 16.0%.[13,15] A recent single-center retrospective study performed by Bohnstedt and colleagues[13] demonstrated a 12% incidence of postoperative ischemia from surgical treatment of ACh aneurysms, despite utilization of intraoperative monitoring, such as Doppler sonography, intraoperative DSA, and ICG angiography, in 40% of the cases (33 of 83). Repeated temporary clipping of the aneurysm and temporary clipping of the parent vessel for proximal control is associated with the risk of postoperative ischemia.[13] Therefore, very careful

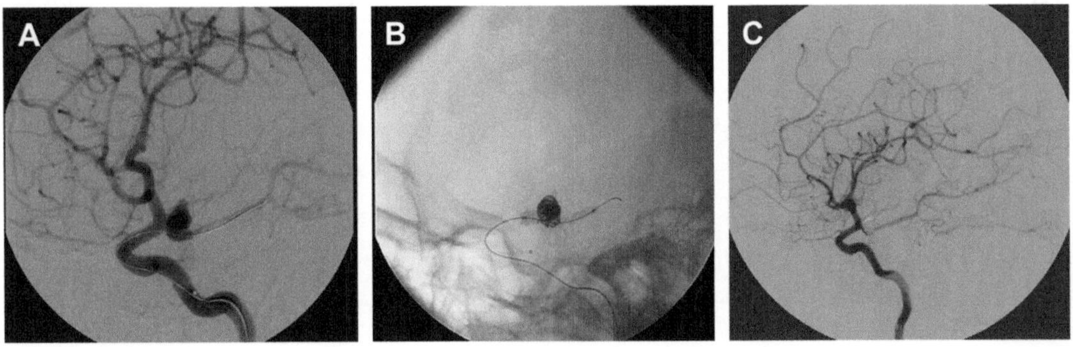

Fig. 5. A 61-year-old woman who presented with SAH secondary to a ruptured right Pcomm aneurysm. (*A*) Pretreatment lateral DSA demonstrates a 7- to 8-mm saccular aneurysm projecting posteriorly from the communicating segment of the right ICA. (*B*) Unsubtracted spot fluoroscopic image demonstrates down-the-barrel balloon remodeling within the posterior communicating artery during coil embolization. (*C*) Postcoiling lateral DSA demonstrates no significant residual sac opacification and preservation of antegrade flow within the posterior communicating artery.

microdissection and clipping are necessary if operative management is required.

Endovascular coil embolization of ACh aneurysms has been associated with a 5.5% risk of ischemia.[55] Although there is a risk of losing antegrade flow in the vessel from both open and endovascular procedures, endovascular treatment of these aneurysms may provide an advantage in that it allows for continuous angiographic surveillance of parent vessel patency.[56]

Carotid Terminus Aneurysms

Carotid terminus aneurysms are bifurcation aneurysms and, therefore, treated based on their morphology. Endovascularly, these are generally treated with coil embolization with or without balloon assistance in ruptured cases. Stent-assisted coil embolization can also be useful in cases of unruptured, wide-neck aneurysms. Close proximity of perforators at the carotid bifurcation can sometimes be a challenge during surgical clipping.

SUMMARY

Endovascular management of intracranial aneurysms has advanced significantly over the last couple decades and continues to evolve, including aneurysms within the subgroup of supraclinoid ICA (superior hypophyseal, posterior communicating, anterior choroidal, dorsal wall/blister, and carotid terminus). Although open surgical management of aneurysms in the paraclinoid region is made challenging by the complex anatomy, the supraclinoid region poses less difficulty. For this reason, endovascular treatment is generally favored for the former group of aneurysms. Advances in neuroendovascular access devices and stent/flow diversion technology are increasingly used for vessel reconstruction.

REFERENCES

1. De Jesús O, Sekhar LN, Riedel CJ. Clinoid and paraclinoid aneurysms: surgical anatomy, operative techniques, and outcome. Surg Neurol 1999; 51(5):477–87.
2. Gibo H, Lenkey C, Rhoton AL Jr. Microsurgical anatomy of the supraclinoid portion of the internal carotid artery. J Neurosurg 1981;55(4):560–74.
3. Horiuchi T, Tanaka Y, Kusano Y, et al. Relationship between the ophthalmic artery and the dural ring of the internal carotid artery. Clinical article. J Neurosurg 2009;111(1):119–23.
4. Zipfel GJ, Dacey RG. Update on the management of unruptured intracranial aneurysms. Neurosurg Focus 2004;17(5):E2.
5. Chen PR, Frerichs K, Spetzler R. Natural history and general management of unruptured intracranial aneurysms. Neurosurg Focus 2004;17(5):E1.
6. Wiebers DO, Whisnant JP, Huston J 3rd, et al. Unruptured intracranial aneurysms: natural history, clinical outcome, and risks of surgical and endovascular treatment. Lancet 2003;362(9378):103–10.
7. Rinkel GJ, Djibuti M, Algra A, et al. Prevalence and risk of rupture of intracranial aneurysms: a systematic review. Stroke 1998;29(1):251–6.
8. Clarke G, Mendelow AD, Mitchell P. Predicting the risk of rupture of intracranial aneurysms based on anatomical location. Acta Neurochir 2005;147: 259–63.
9. Golshani K, Ferrell A, Zomorodi A, et al. A review of the management of posterior communicating artery aneurysms in the modern era. Surg Neurol Int 2010;1:88.
10. Morita A, Kirino T, Hashi K, et al. The natural course of unruptured cerebral aneurysms in a Japanese cohort. N Engl J Med 2012;366(26):2474–82.
11. Motoyama Y, Nonaka J, Hironaka Y, et al. Pupil-sparing oculomotor nerve palsy caused by upward compression of a large posterior communicating artery aneurysm. Case report. Neurol Med Chir (Tokyo) 2012;52(4):202–5.
12. He W, Gandhi CD, Quinn J, et al. True aneurysms of the posterior communicating artery: a systematic review and meta-analysis of individual patient data. World Neurosurg 2011;75(1):64–72.
13. Bohnstedt BN, Kemp WJ 3rd, Li Y, et al. Surgical treatment of 127 anterior choroidal artery aneurysms: a cohort study of resultant ischemic complications. Neurosurgery 2013;73(6):933–40.
14. Yasargil MG, Yonas H, Gasser JC. Anterior choroidal artery aneurysms: their anatomy and surgical significance. Surg Neurol 1978;9(2):129–38.
15. Friedman JA, Pichelmann MA, Piepgras DG, et al. Ischemic complications of surgery for anterior choroidal artery aneurysms. J Neurosurg 2001; 94(4):565–72.
16. Abe M, Tabuchi K, Yokoyama H, et al. Blood blister-like aneurysms of the internal carotid artery. J Neurosurg 1998;89(3):419–24.
17. Ishikawa T, Nakamura N, Houkin K, et al. Pathological consideration of a "blister-like" aneurysm at the superior wall of the internal carotid artery: case report. Neurosurgery 1997;40(2):403–5.
18. Javalkar V, Banerjee AD, Nanda A. Paraclinoid carotid aneurysms. J Clin Neurosci 2011;18(1):13–22.
19. Molyneux A, Kerr R, Stratton I, et al. International Subarachnoid Aneurysm Trial (ISAT) of neurosurgical clipping versus endovascular coiling in 2143 patients with ruptured intracranial aneurysms: a randomised trial. Lancet 2002;360(9342):1267–74.
20. Lozier AP, Kim GH, Sciacca RR, et al. Microsurgical treatment of basilar apex aneurysms: perioperative

and long-term clinical outcome. Neurosurgery 2004;54:286–96.
21. Sullivan BJ, Sekhar LN, Duong DH, et al. Profound hypothermia and circulatory arrest with skull base approaches for treatment of complex posterior circulation aneurysms. Acta Neurochir (Wien) 1999; 141:1–11.
22. Ogilvy CS, Carter BS. Stratification of outcome for surgically treated unruptured intracranial aneurysms. Neurosurgery 2003;52:82–7.
23. Lempert TE, Malek AM, Halbach VV, et al. Endovascular treatment of ruptured posterior circulation cerebral aneurysms. Clinical and angiographic outcomes. Stroke 2000;31:100.
24. Lozier AP, Connolly ES Jr, Lavine SD, et al. Guglielmi detachable coil embolization of posterior circulation aneurysms: a systematic review of the literature. Stroke 2002;33:2509–18.
25. Sluzewski M, Menovsky T, van Rooij WJ, et al. Coiling of very large or giant cerebral aneurysms: long-term clinical and serial angiographic results. AJNR Am J Neuroradiol 2003;24:257–62.
26. Gruber A, Killer M, Bavinzski G, et al. Clinical and angiographic results of endosaccular coiling treatment of giant and very large intracranial aneurysms: a 7-year, single-center experience. Neurosurgery 1999;45:793–803.
27. van Rooij WJ, Sluzewski M. Endovascular treatment of large and giant aneurysms. AJNR Am J Neuroradiol 2009;30(1):12–8.
28. van der Schaaf IC, Brilstra EH, Buskens E, et al. Endovascular treatment of aneurysms in the cavernous sinus: a systematic review on balloon occlusion of the parent vessel and embolization with coils. Stroke 2002;33:313–38.
29. Larson JJ, Tew JM Jr, Tomsick TA, et al. Treatment of aneurysms of the internal carotid artery by intravascular balloon occlusion: long-term follow-up of 58 patients. Neurosurgery 1990;36:23–30.
30. van Rooij WJ, Sluzewski M, Slob MJ, et al. Predictive value of angiographic testing for tolerance to therapeutic occlusion of the carotid artery. AJNR Am J Neuroradiol 2005;1:175–8.
31. Lubicz B, Gauvrit JY, Leclerc X, et al. Giant aneurysms of the internal carotid artery: endovascular treatment and long-term follow-up. Neuroradiology 2003;45:650–5.
32. Molyneux AJ, Cekirge S, Saatci I, et al. Cerebral Aneurysm Multicenter European Onyx (CAMEO) trial: results of a prospective observational study in 20 European centers. AJNR Am J Neuroradiol 2004;25:39–51.
33. Geremia G, Haklin M, Brennecke L. Embolization of experimentally created aneurysms with intravascular stent devices. AJNR Am J Neuroradiol 1994;15:1223–31.
34. Wakhloo AK, Schellhammer F, de Vries J, et al. Self-expanding and balloon-expandable stents in the treatment of carotid aneurysms: an experimental study in a canine model. AJNR Am J Neuroradiol 1994;15:493–502.
35. Turjman F, Acevedo G, Moll T, et al. Treatment of experimental carotid aneurysms by endoprosthesis implantation: preliminary report. Neurol Res 1993;15:181–4.
36. Kallmes DF, Ding YH, Dai D, et al. A new endoluminal, flow-disrupting device for treatment of saccular aneurysms. Stroke 2007;38:2346–52.
37. Kallmes DF, Ding YH, Dai D, et al. A second-generation, endoluminal, flow-disrupting device for treatment of saccular aneurysms. AJNR Am J Neuroradiol 2009;30:1153–8.
38. Becske T, Kallmes DF, Saatci I, et al. Pipeline for uncoilable or failed aneurysms: results from a multicenter clinical trial. Radiology 2013;267(3):858–68.
39. Fiorella D, Albuquerque FC, Woo H, et al. Neuroform stent assisted aneurysm treatment: evolving treatment strategies, complications and results of long term follow-up. J Neurointerv Surg 2010;2(1): 16–22.
40. Cruz JP, Chow M, O'Kelly C, et al. Delayed ipsilateral parenchymal hemorrhage following flow diversion for the treatment of anterior circulation aneurysms. AJNR Am J Neuroradiol 2012;33(4): 603–8.
41. Lanzino G, Crobeddu E, Cloft HJ, et al. Efficacy and safety of flow diversion for paraclinoid aneurysms: a matched-pair analysis compared with standard endovascular approaches. AJNR Am J Neuroradiol 2012;33(11):2158–61.
42. Kurokawa Y, Wanibuchi M, Ishiguro M, et al. New method for obliterative treatment of an anterior wall aneurysm in the internal carotid artery: encircling silicone sheet clip procedure: technical case report. Neurosurgery 2001;49:469–72.
43. Lee JW, Choi HG, Jung JY, et al. Surgical strategies for ruptured blister-like aneurysms arising from the internal carotid artery: a clinical analysis of 18 consecutive patients. Acta Neurochir 2009;151: 125–30.
44. McLaughlin N, Laroche M, Bojanowski MW. Surgical management of blood blister–like aneurysms of the internal carotid artery. World Neurosurg 2010;74:483–93.
45. Meling TR, Sorteberg A, Bakke SJ, et al. Blood blister-like aneurysms of the internal carotid artery trunk causing subarachnoid hemorrhage: treatment and outcome. J Neurosurg 2008;108: 662–71.
46. Mitha AP, Spetzler RF. Blister-like aneurysms: an enigma of cerebrovascular surgery. World Neurosurg 2010;74:444–5.

47. Walsh KM, Moskowitz SI, Hui FK, et al. Multiple overlapping stents as monotherapy in the treatment of 'blister' pseudoaneurysms arising from the supraclinoid internal carotid artery: a single institution series and review of the literature. J Neurointerv Surg 2014;6(3):184–94.
48. Canton G, Levy DI, Lasheras JC, et al. Flow changes caused by the sequential placement of stents across the neck of sidewall cerebral aneurysms. J Neurosurg 2005;103:891–902.
49. Lee BH, Kim BM, Park MS, et al. Reconstructive endovascular treatment of ruptured blood blister-like aneurysms of the internal carotid artery. J Neurosurg 2009;110:431–6.
50. Gaughen JR, Hasan D, Dumont AS, et al. The efficacy of endovascular stenting in the treatment of supraclinoid internal carotid artery blister aneurysms using a stent-in-stent technique. Am J Neuroradiol 2010;31:1132–8.
51. Meckel S, Singh TP, Undren P, et al. Endovascular treatment using predominantly stent-assisted coil embolization and antiplatelet and anticoagulation management of ruptured blood blister-like aneurysms. Am J Neuroradiol 2011;32:764–71.
52. Fiorella D, Albuquerque FC, Deshmukh VR, et al. Endovascular reconstruction with the Neuroform stent as monotherapy for the treatment of uncoilable intradural pseudoaneurysm. Neurosurgery 2006;59:291–300.
53. Çinar C, Oran I, Bozkaya H, et al. Endovascular treatment of ruptured blister-like aneurysms with special reference to the flow-diverting strategy. Neuroradiology 2013;55(4):441–7.
54. Wirth FP. Surgical treatment of incidental intracranial aneurysms. Clin Neurosurg 1986;33:125–35.
55. Piotin M, Mounayer C, Spelle L, et al. Endovascular treatment of anterior choroidal artery aneurysms. AJNR Am J Neuroradiol 2004;25(2):314–8.
56. Kim BM, Kim DI, Shin YS, et al. Clinical outcome and ischemic complication after treatment of anterior choroidal artery aneurysm: comparison between surgical clipping and endovascular coiling. AJNR Am J Neuroradiol 2008;29(2):286–90.

Endovascular Management of Anterior Communicating Artery Aneurysms

Daniel S. Ikeda, MD, Evan S. Marlin, MD,
Andrew Shaw, MD, Eric Sauvageau, MD,
Ciarán J. Powers, MD, PhD*

KEYWORDS

• Anterior communicating artery aneurysms • Endovascular techniques • Intracranial aneurysms
• Neurosurgery • Subarachnoid hemorrhage

KEY POINTS

- The anterior communicating artery (AComA) is a common location for ruptured and unruptured aneurysms and represents a vascular location with wide anatomic variability.
- Current data from both prospective and retrospective analyses have demonstrated endovascular treatment of ruptured and unruptured aneurysms as a safe and durable treatment compared with the previous standard of care, aneurysm clipping.
- Although not all AComAAs are suitable for endovascular treatment, technological advances, including balloon-assisted coil embolization (BACE) and stent-assisted coil embolization (SACE), have broadened indications.
- Experience and advancements in endovascular care of intracranial aneurysms have increased the ability for physicians to treat patients, but reduction of perioperative complications, including thromboembolic stroke and intraprocedural hemorrhage, remain an area for improvement.

INTRODUCTION

AComAAs represent a common location of intracranial aneurysms in the ruptured and unruptured patient population (**Fig. 1**). Many large series find that AComAAs represent the most common location, up to 40%, of ruptured intracranial aneurysms in adults.[1–3] Similar representation of AComAAs is found in trials of unruptured aneurysms.[4,5] The anatomy of the AComA complex can be variable, with many permutations requiring physicians to tailor the treatment, surgically or endovascularly, depending on the anatomy.[6–8]

With the results of the International Subarachnoid Aneurysm Trial (ISAT) published in 2002, the treatment of intracranial aneurysms has preferentially shifted toward endovascular treatment at most institutions.[3,9,10] Although there remains a large role for open surgical clipping, the endovascular trend has further been facilitated by physician experience and novel technical developments, which have broadened indications of endovascular treatment.[11–14] Given the increasing options in endovascular treatments, coupled with open vascular clipping, patient care can often be individualized to minimize risk to the patient.

Disclosures: None.
Department of Neurological Surgery, The Ohio State University Wexner Medical Center, 410 West 10th Avenue, Columbus, OH 43210, USA
* Corresponding author. Department of Neurological Surgery, The Ohio State University Wexner Medical Center, N-1018 Doan Hall, 410 West 10th Avenue, Columbus, OH 43210.
E-mail address: ciaran.powers@osumc.edu

http://dx.doi.org/10.1016/j.nec.2014.04.004

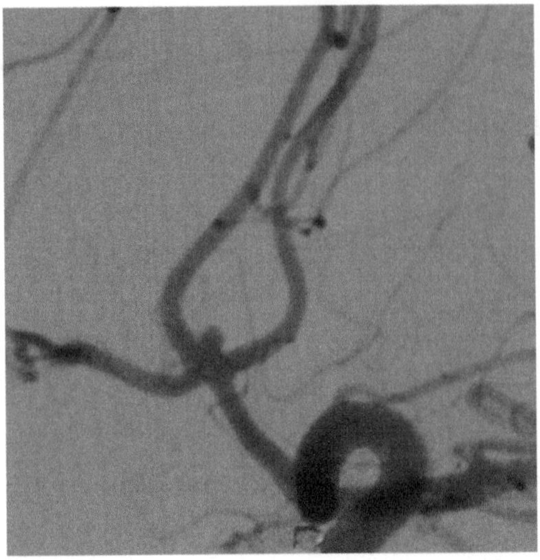

Fig. 1. AComAA. Typical appearance of an AComAA found incidentally.

This article discusses the anatomic variability associated with the AComA complex and anterior cerebral arteries (ACAs) and the presentation of AComAAs. Furthermore, the evidence for endovascular treatment of AComAAs is reviewed. Finally, how technological advancements that have broadened the scope of treatment is discussed and possible future advancements described.

ANATOMY OF THE ANTERIOR CEREBRAL AND ANTERIOR COMMUNICATING ARTERIES

The normal ACA is often divided into 5 anatomic segments starting at carotid bifurcation.[15–17] The A1 segment, or precommunicating segment, extends from the bifurcation of the internal carotid artery (ICA) to join the AComA. The precommunicating segment joins the AComA in a majority of cases (70%).[15] The average length of the A1 segment is approximately 13 mm.[17] Tortuosity in the precommunicating segment can make navigation of the microcatheter difficult en route to aneurysm treatment. The A2 (infracallosal) segment extends from the A1-AComA junction to the genu of the corpus callosum. The A3 (precallosal) segment extends around the callosal genu. The A4 (supracallosal) and A5 (postcallosal) segments course above the corpus callosum. There are several variations to the distal ACAs, including the unpaired azygous artery, bihemispheric ACA, and triplicated vessels (**Fig. 2**).[17,18]

Larger branches of the distal ACA include the orbitofrontal, frontopolar, and other cortical branches. In general these branches have little significance in planning for endovascular treatment of an AComAA. The pericallosal artery is the terminal branch of the ACA, extending from the A2 to A5.[15] Its largest branch is the callosomarginal artery, which often arises near the genu of the corpus callosum and courses in the cingulate sulcus. The pericallosal or callosomarginal arteries can be catheterized distally to assist in tracking a guide catheter to the petrosal segment of the ICA for more proximal support.

Critical arteries, especially susceptible to injury during endovascular or surgical treatment of AComAAs, are the perforating arteries of the ACA. On average, there are 8 basal perforating arteries, or medial lenticulostriate arteries, that arise from the A1, A2, and AComA.[17] They supply the anterior hypothalamus, optic chiasm, lamina terminalis, medial portion of the anterior commissure, pillars of the fornix, anterior perforated substance, and

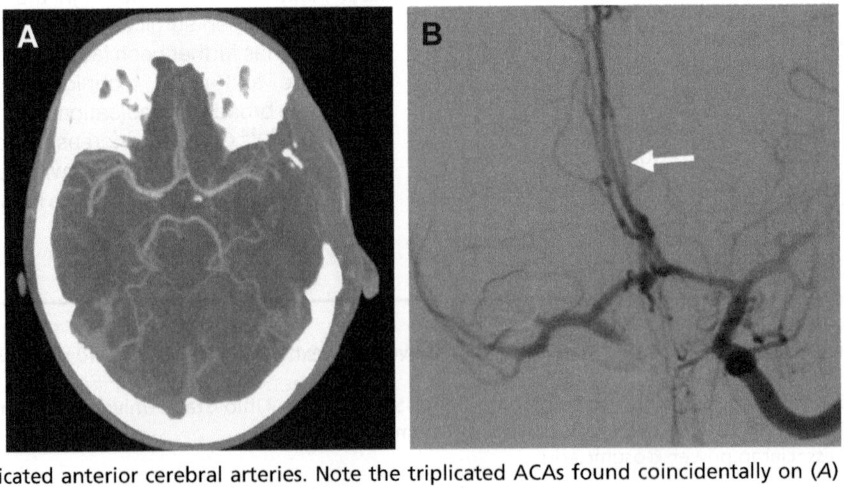

Fig. 2. Triplicated anterior cerebral arteries. Note the triplicated ACAs found coincidentally on (*A*) CTA and (*B*) DCA in a patient with an AVM (*white arrow*).

anterior third ventricle. One large perforating artery, and most consistent, is the recurrent artery of Heubner. Arising from the proximal A2 in a majority of cases, it doubles back over the parent ACA above the carotid bifurcation and into the medial sylvian fissure where it enters the anterior perforated substance. The recurrent artery supplies the anterior caudate, adjacent internal capsule, anterior putamen and globus pallidus, and the uncinate fasciculus.[19,20] Although a malpositioned clip during open aneurysm surgery can injure or occlude the recurrent artery causing significant neurologic deficits, a similar catastrophe can occur from microcatheter or microwire injury during endovascular treatment.

In normal anatomy, the bilateral A1 segments are connected by the AComA with equal contribution. Although it can be difficult to identify angiographically by standard views, the average AComA diameter averages approximately 1 mm and usually measures between 2 and 3 mm long.[17] There is significant variability in the ACA-AComA complex with greater than one-half of specimens having an imbalance of A1 contribution in one cadaveric study.[15] A true hypoplastic A1, or A1 segment measuring less than 1.5 mm in diameter, however, is present in only 10% of cases.[21,22] The larger the degree asymmetry between A1 segments, the higher the diameter and vascular compensation necessitated of the AComA (**Fig. 3**). This asymmetry can lead to alterations in hemodynamics and delayed aneurysm formation, because AComAAs have a high rate (up to 85%) of A1 hypoplasia.[23,24] This pathophysiology has also been suggested in the de novo development of AComA in the setting of carotid occlusion (**Fig. 4**).[25,26]

Other common variations of the AComA include fenestrations, complete duplications, or triplications. In general, anatomic studies identify more of such anatomic variations (up to 40%) than are found on diagnostic cerebral arteriography (DCA).[15,27,28] Three-dimensional rotational angiography (3DRA) can increase angiographers'

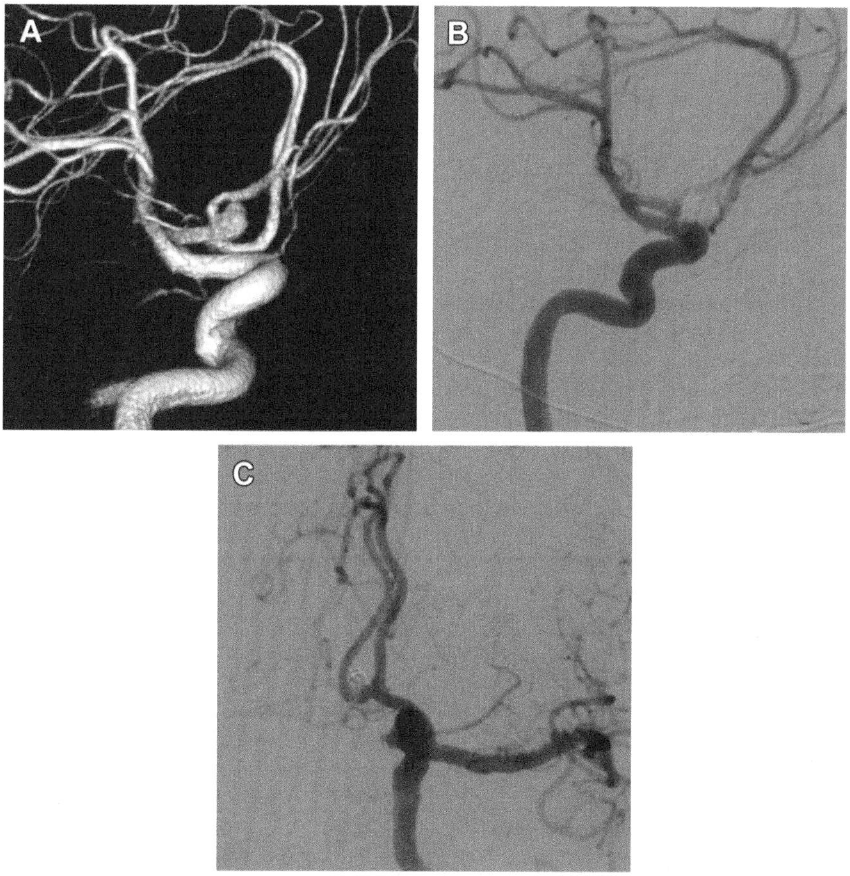

Fig. 3. Atretic contralateral A1. Atretic or hypoplastic contralateral A1s are thought to be more frequently encountered in patients with AComAAs, (*A*) as in this patient (3DRA) with an atretic left A1 who underwent (*B*) successful clip obliteration of her AComAA (DCA). (*C*) Similarly, another patient with a hypoplastic right A1 underwent successful coil embolization for his ruptured aneurysm (DCA).

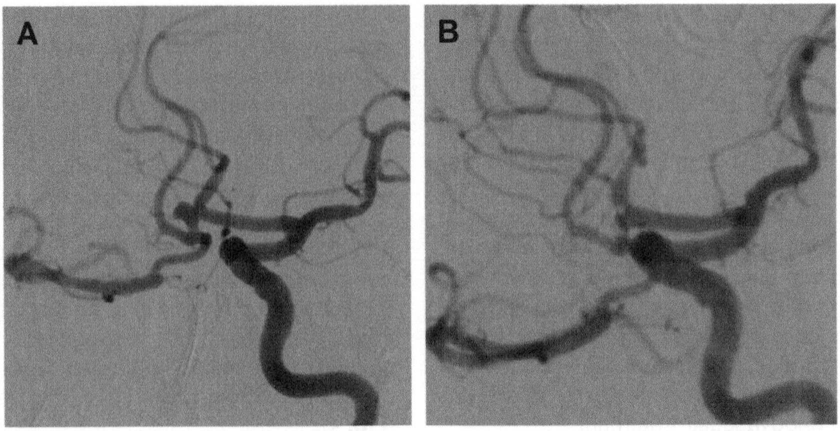

Fig. 4. Contralateral ICA occlusion. This patient presented with a ruptured AComAA in the setting of a chronically occluded right ICA. (*A*) Pre- and (*B*) postclip occlusion arteriograms demonstrate the cross-filling of the right hemisphere from the left ICA.

ability to visualize fenestrations.[27] Although some investigations have found an increased incidence of AComAAs associated with fenestrations, these findings have not been consistent.[8,27,28] Such anatomic variations have little impact during surgical or endovascular treatment. They do, however, underline the necessity to have an adequate working view during endovascular treatment.

CLINICAL PRESENTATION, DIAGNOSIS, AND DECISION TO TREAT

As with all intracranial aneurysms, ruptured AComAAs can have variable features at presentations, with some patients only complaining of mild headache and other unfortunate patients presenting with severe neurologic injury or death (**Fig. 5**).[3,9,29,30] Many unruptured AComAAs present as an incidental finding from unrelated symptoms. Unlike posterior communicating artery or posterior circulation aneurysms, AComAAs are not typically associated with symptomatology from local mass effect. There are, however, a few exceptions in the literature.[31–35] In a large series of giant AComAAs, lesions greater than 3.5 cm were associated with dementia from local mass effect.[31] Visual symptoms or loss from mass effect on the optic apparatus is a well-described phenomenon of large, inferiorly projecting aneurysms.[31,32,34] More peculiar symptoms of Korsakoff psychosis and pulsatile tinnitus have been reported.[33,35]

The detection of intracranial aneurysms with the use of noninvasive imaging has improved significantly over the past 2 decades.[36–40] CT angiography (CTA) has been described as having a sensitivity of 99% for aneurysms 3 mm or larger and having a high sensitivity (97%) and specificity (100%) for AComAAs.[41] Magnetic resonance angiography (MRA) has similarly been shown to have a high sensitivity and specificity in detecting intracranial aneurysms.[38–40] Although not statistically significant ($P = .054$), one study found a strong trend toward improved diagnosis with higher-resolution (3T) MRA.[39]

Noninvasive angiographic imaging has improved in detecting intracranial aneurysms, but DCA remains the gold standard. There is some evidence that suggests advanced 3-D CTA reconstructions can be useful in determining an endovascular or surgical treatment of intracranial aneurysms, and some institutions have prescribed to this method of triage.[42] Many institutions, including the authors', however, continue to use DCA with 3DRA as the standard in decision making.

The poor natural history after a ruptured intracranial aneurysm necessitates treatment of the overwhelming majority of patients. With a rehemorrhage rate of 50% at 6 months, the decision is often not whether to treat but how to treat.[43,44] Medical and surgical advancements have improved mortality after aneurysmal subarachnoid hemorrhage (SAH). In their 1968 article, Hunt and Hess[29] found an overall mortality of 35% after admission to the hospital. In contrast, modern studies consistently demonstrated disability and mortality rates with significant improvement, such as the ISAT, which found a 5-year mortality rate of 11.9% regardless of treatment.[45]

In the subset of anterior circulation aneurysms, patients with AComAAs often fair better overall compared with their posterior circulation counterparts.[46] In ISAT and the recent Barrow Ruptured Aneurysm Trial (BRAT), endovascular management of ruptured aneurysms was found to benefit

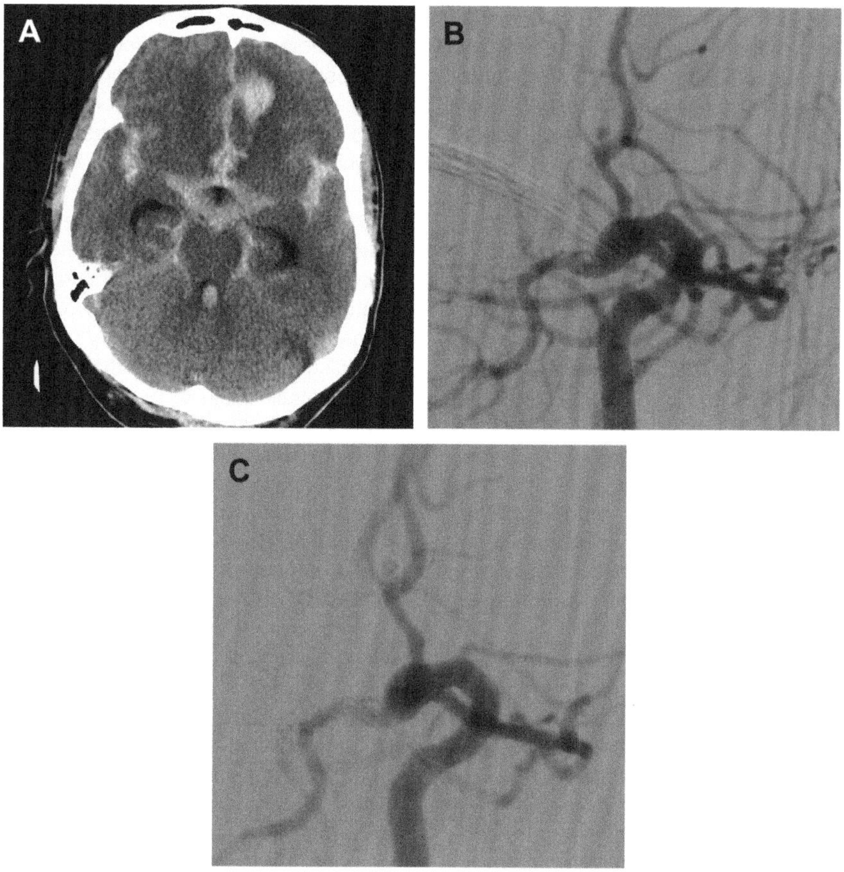

Fig. 5. AComAA presenting with SAH. (*A*) A head CT showing typical appearance of Fisher grade 3 SAH with a left gyrus rectus hemorrhage. (*B*) Pre- and (*C*) postcoiling DCA of a small AComAA.

patients in reducing risk of severe morbidity and mortality,[9,30] although 5-year evidence from ISAT and 3-year evidence from the BRAT showed no benefit in outcomes in patients with aneurysms of the anterior circulation treated by either modality.[45,47] In the setting of rupture, early intervention to secure the aneurysm allows for critical care and neurosurgical physicians to prevent rehemorrhage, aggressive treatment of vasospasm, and prevention of delayed cerebral ischemia.

In cases of incidental or unruptured aneurysms, the decision for treatment is often based on many factors. The International Study of Unruptured Intracranial Aneurysms (ISUIA) was the first large-scale, prospective study looking at the natural history of unruptured aneurysms as well as the risks of treatment.[4,48] Although prior studies found rupture risks as high as 32%, ISUIA along with the Unruptured Cerebral Aneurysm Study from Japan found lower risks of rupture for most aneurysms.[49] Factors found to increase the risk of rupture were size (greater than 7 mm), unusual shape or protrusion coming from aneurysm dome, posterior circulation location, previous personal history of SAH, and SAH in a first-degree relative.[48,49] Another arm of ISUIA compared risks of treatment with risks of the natural history, finding the morbidity and mortality for surgical and endovascular treatment greatly exceeding the 7.5-year risk of rupture in patients without a prior history of SAH in aneurysms smaller than 10 mm.[4] The impact of ISUIA has led some centers to recommend treatment of aneurysms of the anterior circulation, including AComAAs, larger than 7 mm and to conservatively manage smaller lesions. A recent study of 932 patients, however, found AComA and distal ACA aneurysms greater than 4 mm to have risks of rupture similar to posterior circulation these aneurysms should be considered for treatment.[5]

ENDOVASCULAR TREATMENT OF ANTERIOR COMMUNICATING ARTERY ANEURYSMS

History

Although initially performed through a craniotomy, reports of aneurysm embolization were described as early as 1962.[50,51] With poor results of this method of embolization, coupled with advancements in microsurgical clip reconstruction, embolization did not become popular until the early 1990s. At this time, advances in catheter technology had already been made to make cerebral catheterization safer.

In 1991, Guglielmi[52,53] reported the experimental results and clinical application of electrolytically detachable platinum coils for aneurysm embolization. Initially, endovascular treatment was geared toward the treatment of posterior circulation lesions, such as basilar apex aneurysms, because surgery for these lesions was associated with higher morbidity then their anterior circulation counterparts.[54] In the largest series of endovascularly treated aneurysms of its time, only 43% of the aneurysms treated were of the anterior circulation.[55] With more than 97% of the aneurysms treated in ISAT found in the anterior circulation, greater benefit was generalized to aneurysms arising from the AComA.[9]

After the publication of ISAT, the field of endovascular neurosurgery expanded, with technological advancements allowing physicians to treat aneurysms thought previously uncoilable. These include BACE, SACE, embolization with Onyx HD-500 (eV3 Neurovascular, Irvine, California), flow-diverting stents, and, most recently, the Woven EndoBridge (WEB) aneurysm embolization system (Sequent Medical, Aliso Viejo, California).[56,57] Furthermore, microcatheter techniques have evolved and coil technology has improved to aid in primary aneurysm coiling. These advancements have assisted in the treatment of patients who may not be surgical candidates but harbor aneurysms, which were historically difficult to treat endovascularly. **Table 1** summarizes the results of studies dedicated to the treatment of AComAAs treated endovascularly over the past 10 years.

General Techniques and Principles

Several basic principles and steps help ensure safe interventional procedures. Although some institutions perform aneurysm embolization in conscious patients, the authors perform interventional procedures under general endotracheal anesthesia. Prior to starting the procedure, the patient should have 2 peripheral intravenous lines, a Foley catheter, and an arterial line for monitoring of periprocedural blood pressure. Blood pressure monitoring with arterial lines in the immediate postoperative period is beneficial. All sheaths, guide catheters, and microcatheters are continually flushed with heparinized saline. Generally, the authors begin the procedure with a micropuncture needle and ultimately upsize to a 6-French (F) short sheath unless femoral access is tortuous or arch anatomy is unfavorable, in which case, a long sheath or 6F shuttle is used.

Once access is obtained, 70 U/kg of heparin are administered for an activated clotting time (ACT) goal of 250 seconds. The authors use ACT point-of-care testing through the duration of the procedure to ensure adequate anticoagulation. Meticulous attention to ACT can help prevent disastrous thromboembolic and hemorrhagic complications. It is critical that protamine is immediately available in case of intraoperative rupture. An appropriate guide catheter and selector catheter are used to access the vessel of interest. The ICA ipsilateral to the dominant A1 is catheterized. In cases where the A1s are codominant, the A1 with the straightest course to the aneurysm should be catheterized.

For AComAAs, proximal support is paramount. The authors often use the use of the Neuron 070 (Penumbra, Alameda, California) as a guide catheter and advance it as far as the distal petrous or proximal cavernous ICA segment. In cases of significant cervical ICA tortuosity, the authors often use of the Navien catheter (eV3 Neurovascular). Once treatment projections are chosen, 10 mg of intra-arterial verapamil are given to prevent catheter-induced vasospasm. If the guide catheter cannot be advanced to the petrous segment initially, it is advanced to the desired position over a microcatheter that is supported in a distal A2 or M2 segment.

If stenting is planned prior to treatment, dual antiplatelet therapy with aspirin, 325 mg daily, and clopidogrel, 75 mg daily, is initiated 7 days prior to treatment. Clopidogrel therapy is stopped 3 months after stent placement, whereas aspirin therapy is often continued indefinitely. Some patients are unresponsive to clopidogrel inhibition and are at greater risk for suffering a periprocedural thromboembolic event, because the target moiety of platelets, $P2Y_{12}$, has been shown to have a variable response to clopidogrel.[68,69] The real-time evaluation of platelet inhibition with the VerifyNow $P2Y_{12}$ assay is a measure many physicians use to guide therapy.[70] No standard of care has been established, however, regarding the medication regimen to be used in patients found unresponsive to standard clopidogrel inhibition. At the authors' institution, the daily dose of clopidogrel is doubled, to 150 mg in divided doses, whereas other investigators have advocated the addition of cilostazol or ticlopidine to standard clopidogrel therapy. In settings where a stent needs to be placed without preoperatively medicating, a loading dose of aspirin, 325 mg, and clopidogrel, 300 to 600 mg, is given.

For aneurysms requiring stenting or with significant coil mass exposed at the neck, a heparin infusion, at 8 U/kg/h, is often used overnight to prevent delayed thromboembolic complications. If delayed thromboembolism occurs, an abciximab infusion is initiated for 24 hours and daily clopidogrel dose is increased. A postoperative blood pressure goal of less than 160 mm of Hg is strictly enforced.

Treatment

Primary coiling

The largest study of endovascular versus open surgical treatment of aneurysms was designed for aneurysms that could be coiled primarily.[9] Generally, this technique is reserved for aneurysms with a favorable dome-to-neck ratio (2 or greater). Aneurysms with a neck diameter of 7 mm or greater are often difficult to treat by standard coiling without BACE or SACE. The options for endovascular neurosurgeons and interventionalists have significantly increased in recent years, with greater selection in coils and microcatheters. In general, once a microcatheter is securely within the aneurysm, a framing coil sized to the smallest dimension of the aneurysm or the mean value of the height, width, and depth can be used. Oversizing the first framing coil is thought to cause unnecessary wall tension and is generally avoided.

Contemporary framing coils are designed with larger and smaller loops with the smaller loops intended to break inside the aneurysm and the larger coils to form the basket. Once a farming coil is securely placed, subsequent coils should be filling coils or smaller framing coils. Most standard coils find adequate aneurysm embolization with a packing density of approximately 30%, although some coils boast a more robust percentage of obliteration.[71,72] Regardless of packing density, respecting the lumen of the parent vessel and not allowing coils to herniate from the aneurysm are basic tenets of aneurysm embolization.

Before ISAT, the published experience of endovascular treatment of cerebral aneurysms was fairly poor. One study found a significant difference of angiographic obliteration of ACA (including AComA) aneurysms compared with microsurgical ligation.[73] The same investigators found better endovascular results in the treatment of posterior circulation aneurysms only. Another early prospective study found better results of aneurysmal obliteration in clipping (93.2%) versus coiling (56.1%) and a lower risk of permanent injury related to treatment of anterior circulation aneurysms including neurologic injury and death (1.7% vs 7.5%).[74] With further experience and improved endovascular techniques and technologies, primary aneurysm coiling is now the preferred method of treatment at most centers when the geometry of the aneurysm is favorable.

When BACE and SACE cannot be performed, the dual catheter technique can be attempted for wide-necked AComAAs.[75,76] That is, with 2 microcatheters in the aneurysm, coils are alternatively deployed from each catheter while only detaching after 2 coils are fully introduced into the aneurysm and have demonstrated stability in the coil mass. Theoretically, this improves packing density while ensuring the coil mass does not herniate through the fundus of the aneurysm. A similar technique used at the authors' institution is bringing a second microcatheter into the lumen of the distal A2. When coiling the aneurysm through the primary microcatheter, the second microcatheter serves to protect the A2 from unintended occlusion or stenosis from the coil mass. This is especially helpful when the origin of the A2 is incorporated into the neck of the aneurysm and a balloon or stent is not desired, as in cases of tortuous proximal anatomy or in cases of ruptured aneurysms (**Fig. 6**).

Complications related to primary coiling of AComAAs include thromboembolic events, intraoperative rupture, failure to completely obliterate angiographically, coil malposition, and delayed coil compaction or aneurysm recurrence. A large meta-analysis of 1552 AComA found a procedure-related morbidity of 6%.[77] A higher rate of mortality was found in ruptured aneurysms (4%) compared with unruptured aneurysms (2%). Although attention to ACT and technical prudence can limit most complications, delayed coil compaction and aneurysm recurrence are not seen until months or years later. Treated aneurysms with large volumes (greater than 600 mm^3) and lower packing density of coils (less than 20%) have a higher rate of recurrence (as high as 30.1%).[78] Although the risk of rebleeding after aneurysm coiling is low (1%–2%), significant morbidity and mortality are associated with rehemorrhages.[77,79] Retreatment after aneurysm coiling has been found safe with morbidity and mortality rates as low as 0%.[80–82] Aneurysm regrowth, however, a separate cause from coil compaction, has been found difficult to treat endovascularly (**Fig. 7**).[82,83] Surgical treatment is recommended for anterior circulation aneurysms, including those of the AComA, in this setting.[82]

Balloon-assisted coiling

First described in 1997, the technique of BACE proposed benefits of treating wide-necked

Table 1
Summary of studies of endovascular treatment of AComA aneurysms

Author, Year	Study Design	Aneurysms Treated: Total	Aneurysms Treated: Ruptured	Complete Obliteration[a] (%)	Procedure-Related Complications (%): Thromboembolic	Procedure-Related Complications (%): Intraoperative Rupture	Procedure Morbidity and Mortality (%)	Key Points
Elias et al,[58] 2003	Prospective	30	30	56.7	N/A	N/A	N/A	Favorable outcomes achieved in younger, good-grade SAH females.
Proust et al,[59] 2003	Prospective	37	36	78.4	10.8	2.7	13.5	Endovascular treatment may be preferred in AComAAs when the fundus is oriented posteriorly.
Birknes et al,[60] 2006	Retrospective	123	113	77.5	0.8	3.3	N/A	Predicting successful aneurysm embolization may be dictated by aneurysm morphology.
Guglielmi et al,[61] 2009	Retrospective	306	236	45.5	N/A	3.0	4.5	There is less risk to perforating blood vessels when treating AComAAs endovascularly compared with surgery.
Songsaeng et al,[62] 2010	Retrospective	96	7	62.5	N/A	N/A	N/A	Statistically significant increased rate of recurrence with unilateral A1 aplasia.
Finitsis et al,[63] 2010	Prospective	268	234	29.5	8.1	4.3	9.1	The risk of aneurysm recurrence was significantly more frequent in ruptured aneurysms and larger aneurysms (>4 mm).

Raslan et al,[64] 2011	Retrospective	44	43	72.7	6.8	11.4	11.4	Long-term occlusion rates can be achieved with SACE in the setting of SAH with no patients requiring retreatment in their series.
Choi et al,[65] 2011	Retrospective	45	45	N/A	0	2.2	0	Morphologic features of AComAAs (size, neck, dome-to-neck ratio, multiple lobulations, and vessel incorporation) need to be considered in deciding for a surgical or endovascular treatment.
Schuette et al,[66] 2011	Retrospective	347	277	N/A	N/A	5.2	N/A	Smaller AComAAs (<4 mm) and treatment in the setting of SAH pose increased risk for intraoperative rupture
Johnson et al,[67] 2013	Retrospective	64	5	70.9	0	1.6	1.6	SACE was found safe and durable treatment of AComAAs <15 mm.
Huang et al,[14] 2013	Retrospective	27	27	74.1	0	3.7	0	SACE was found safe in the acutely ruptured setting for wide-necked AComAAs.

[a] Complete obliteration varies depending on the original study investigators' metric for measurement. Some studies used the Raymond classification to determine complete occlusion, whereas others used a percentage of angiographic obliteration to define *complete obliteration* (ie, >90%).

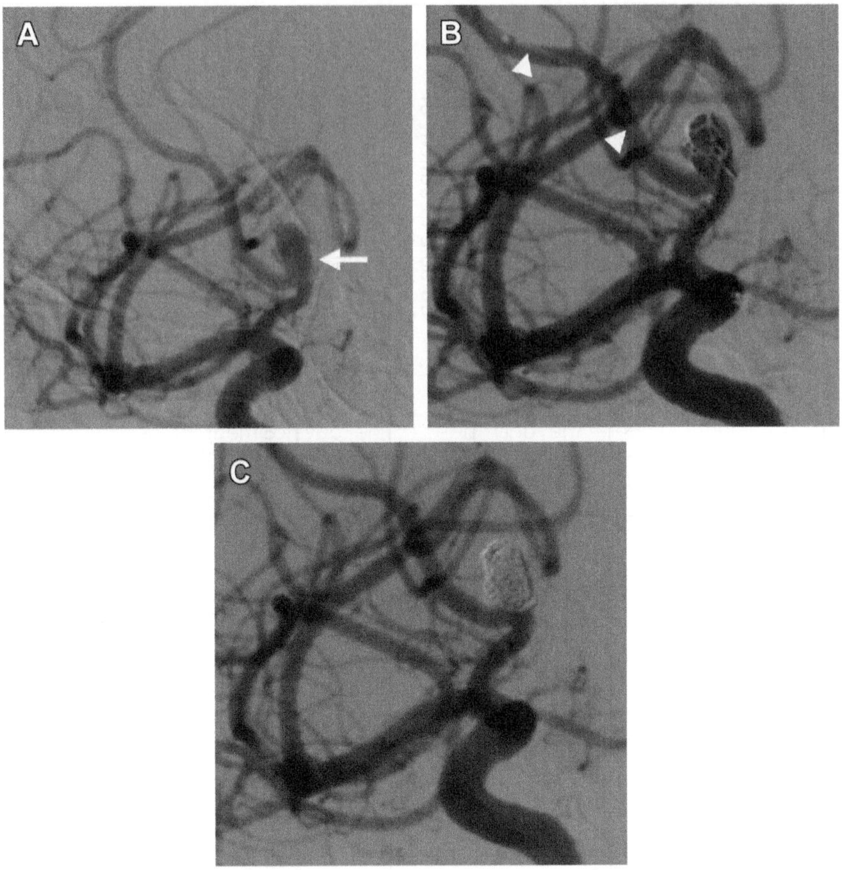

Fig. 6. Primary coiling with second microcatheter A2 protection. (*A*) This patient with an unruptured AComAA (*white arrow*) was treated with a (*B*) second microcatheter protecting the origin of the right A2 (*white arrowheads*). (*C*) A postcoil DCA shows successful coil embolization.

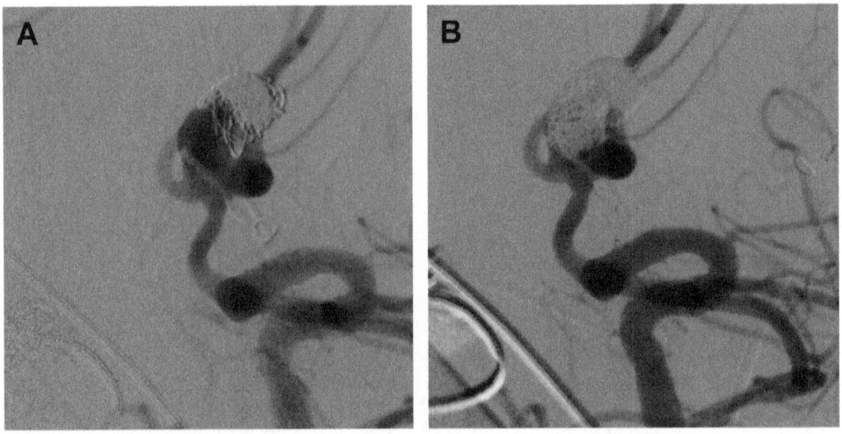

Fig. 7. Aneurysm coil compaction and regrowth. This patient presented with a ruptured wide-necked AComAA. She was initially coiled, although after a follow-up arteriogram demonstrated coil compaction, she underwent attempted clip reconstruction. Another follow-up DCA (*A*) demonstrated aneurysm regrowth. The patient refused further open surgical options and aneurysm coiling was attempted (*B*), although the aneurysm neck remained after coiling.

aneurysms by stabilizing the microcatheter within the aneurysm, forcing the coils to conform to the shape of the aneurysm, and protecting the parent vessel from coil mass herniation.[84–86] BACE is especially helpful in the treatment of ruptured, wide-necked AComAAs because dual antiplatelet therapy with SACE is not desirable in this setting.

Initially, low compliance balloons, such as the HyperGlide (eV3 Neurovascular) balloon-mounted microcatheter, were developed and helped BACE become widely accepted as a safe treatment strategy.[87,88] These balloons, however, were unable to contour to the unique AComA complex many of these aneurysms possess. More compliant devices, such as the HyperForm (eV3 Neurovascular) and TransForm (Stryker Neurovascular, Fremont, California) balloons, have been developed and are particularly useful in protecting wide-necked AComAAs with A2s emanating from the neck of the lesion (**Fig. 8**).

Contemporary studies have demonstrated BACE as a safe and durable treatment of ruptured and unruptured AComAAs. Chalouhi and colleagues[89] found no permanent morbidity or mortality related to the treatment of 76 consecutive patients treated with BACE, 25% of which were AComAAs. In a series of more than 800 patients (385 AComAAs) treated with BACE, Cekirge and colleagues[90] found a total aneurysm occlusion rate of 87.6% at 2-year follow-up with a 1.4% rate of procedure-related morbidity and mortality.

Another proposed benefit of BACE during aneurysm treatment is hemostasis or temporary parent vessel occlusion in the event of intraprocedural aneurysm rupture.[91] Although this is intuitive, some investigators argue that BACE may increase the risk of intraprocedural rupture secondary to increased microcatheter manipulation and increased pressure within the aneurysm when the balloon is inflated.[85] Some investigators have also found an increased risk of thromboembolic complications in BACE (9.8%) compared with standard coiling (2.2%).[92] This has not been found, however, in larger, prospective studies with comparable thromboembolic rates found.[93–95]

Stent-assisted coiling

In 1998, the first reported case of successful SACE was published.[96] SACE can be performed as a "stent, then coil" procedure (as 1 or 2 stages) or as a failsafe "coil, then stent" option when parent artery protection from a herniating coil mass is necessary after attempted primary coiling or BACE. Initially, SACE was used primarily for proximal intracranial aneurysms, such as those in the cavernous or ophthalmic ICA segments. Further operator experience and advancements in stent technology, including open cell stent designs (such as the Neuroform or Neuroform EZ, Stryker Neurovascular), have allowed for SACE in more distal, tortuous vessels such as the AComA segment.

The variable anatomy of the AComA allows for surgeons or interventionalists to place the stent in several different configurations. Stenting from the ipsilateral A1 to the contralateral A2 often allows for the easiest scenario of deployment while maximizing aneurysm neck coverage by the stent (**Fig. 9**). Sometimes the anatomy of the AComA is more favorable for a stent to be deployed from ipsilateral A1 to contralateral A1 or ipsilateral A2. More complex SACE techniques have been described, such as the Y-stent technique, where the first stent is usually delivered from ipsilateral A1 to ipsilateral A2 and then a second stent is placed from ipsilateral A1 to contralateral A2.[97,98] The X-configured SACE has been reported

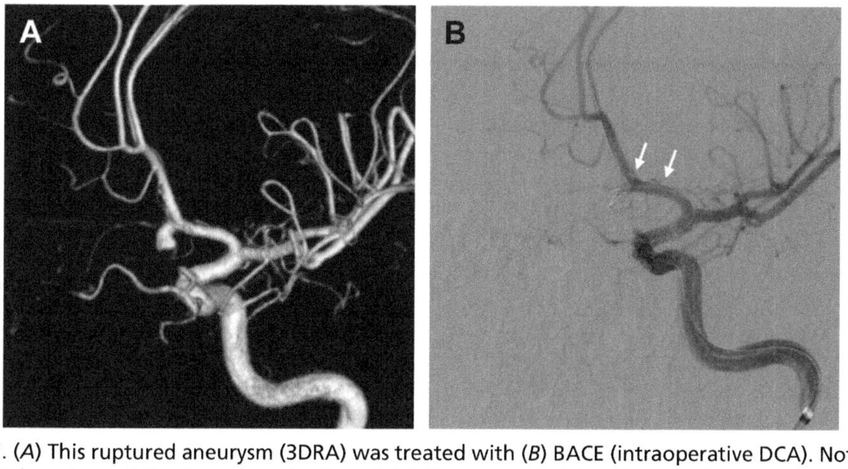

Fig. 8. BACE. (*A*) This ruptured aneurysm (3DRA) was treated with (*B*) BACE (intraoperative DCA). Note the proximal and distal markers of the HyperForm balloon (eV3 Neurovascular) (*white arrows*).

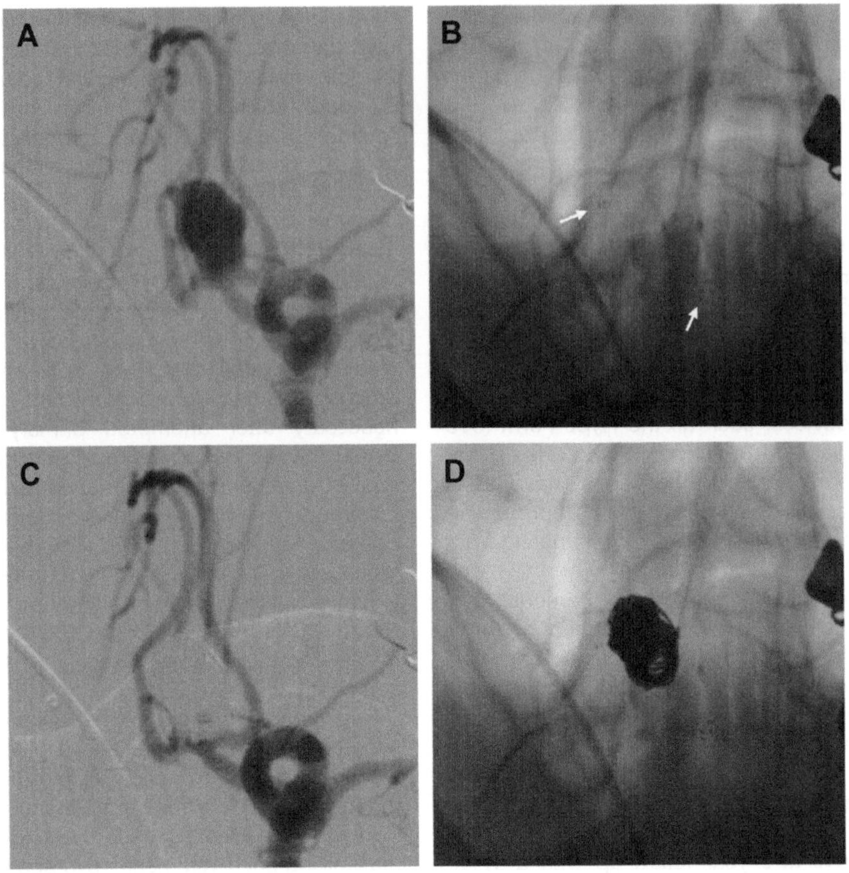

Fig. 9. SACE. (*A*) This wide-necked, unruptured AComAA was treated with (*C*) SACE. (*B*) Unsubtracted images demonstrate the stent delivered from contralateral A2 to ipsilateral A1 (*white arrows*) and the (*D*) final coil mass.

successfully in a few cases.[13,99,100] In Lazzaro and Zaidat's[101] case, two 4.5 mm × 22 mm Enterprise stents (Cordis endovascular, Miami Lakes, Florida) were sequentially deployed from the ipsilateral A1 to the contralateral A2. Although the Enterprise stent is a closed-cell design, the investigators reported no in-stent stenosis at the expected waist in follow-up.

Contemporary studies of SACE have shown a low procedural morbidity with high rates of long-term aneurysm occlusion (approximately 90%).[102–104] AComAAs are often underrepresented in such studies, because most aneurysms that are candidates for SACE are surgically accessible. In a series of 554 aneurysms treated with SACE, Chalouhi and colleagues[102] reported only 7 (1.5%) aneurysms were of the AComA. In 2009, Huang and colleagues[14] reported their experience of 21 patients with ruptured AComAAs treated with SACE. Only 1 patient died in their series, and the death was attributed to complications of the initial SAH. They reported no thromboembolic complications. One intraoperative rupture occurred, which was successfully stopped with further coiling, and the patient recovered without neurologic sequela. Only 1 recanalization was found at follow-up. In 2011, Raslan and colleagues[64] reported their series of 44 patients treated with SACE for AComAAs. All but one aneurysm was incidental. The investigators found complete occlusion, a dog-ear remnant, or minimal neck remnant in 87.9% (29/33) patients at long-term follow-up. Five of the 44 (11%) patients suffered severe, procedure-related disability, including 2 hemorrhagic and 3 thromboembolic complications. The investigators report that all complications occurred early in their experience and that refinements in antiplatelet regimens and device experience have limited their complications.

Performing SACE in the setting of SAH is a concern for many practitioners. In a series of 65 patients (9 with AComAAs) with SAH treated with SACE, the investigators found a good outcome in 63.1% of patients, and 15.4% of patients suffered major bleeding or thromboembolic complications during treatment, including 3 fatal hemorrhages.[105] Although surgical craniotomy with aneurysm clipping is preferable in most patients with ruptured, wide-necked AComAAs, SACE is feasible and may be considered in some situations.

Flow-diverting stents

Flow-diverting stents, a new technology initially developed for the treatment of large carotid aneurysms, have demonstrated a similar procedural safety profile, superior rates of complete obliteration, and need for retreatment when compared with standard coiling.[106,107] Increased aneurysm neck coverage and decreased porosity of the stent cause hemostasis and thrombosis within the aneurysm and eventually scaffolding for neointimal growth across the neck of the aneurysm. The current iteration of the only Food and Drug Administration–approved device, the Pipeline Embolization Device (eV3 Neurovascular), requires the use of 2.8/3.2F delivery catheter, such as the Marksman catheter (eV3 Neurovascular), which is stiffer and less trackable then standard coiling microcatheters used for AComAA treatment. Although a case report of successful treatment of an AComA blister-like aneurysm has been reported, the current device technology, the unique anatomy of the AComA complex, and the unknown long-term effects of flow diversion on side branches or small perforating arteries limit the use of flow-diversion stents for AComAAs.[108] Additionally, use of the Pipeline Embolization Device for aneurysms distal to the posterior communicating artery is off-label.

Intrasaccular WEB aneurysm embolization system

The concept of intrasaccular flow disruption for wide-necked bifurcation aneurysms has been recently studied and is in use in parts of Europe.[109,110] The WEB aneurysm embolization device is a braided wire deployed intrasaccularly causing prompt aneurysm obliteration. Its use does not require concomitant antiplatelet treatment and can be used in the setting of ruptured aneurysms. The WEB may develop as a treatment alternative to BACE and SACE in wide-necked AComAAs that cannot be clipped. In a study of 21 patients (5 with AComAAs), there were no treatment failures, with 5 patients requiring an additional endovascular treatment with supplemental coiling or stenting and 1 thromboembolic complication.[110] The initial reports of this device are promising, but larger studies are needed to identify WEB's role in the treatment of AComAAs.

Follow-Up Considerations

Aneurysm recanalization or recurrence is a concern for any modality of endovascular treatment of AComAAs. At the authors' institution, a DCA with 3DRA is performed 6 months after initial treatment. A baseline MRA is performed at this time; 3T MRA has been shown to have a nearly 91% concordance rate with traditional DCA.[111] CTA is avoided secondary to the artifact produced. For ruptured aneurysms, noninvasive diagnostic imaging is obtained 1 year later, then annually for 2 years, and then once every 2 to 5 years. For nonruptured aneurysms, noninvasive imaging is obtained after 1 year. If there is no recurrence, they are typically discharged with follow-up as needed. Aneurysm remnants or recurrences are treated on a case-by-case basis.

In regards to antiplatelet therapy, patients receiving stents remain on dual antiplatelet therapy for a minimum of 3 months. After 3 months, if a patient is asymptomatic and without any thromboembolic complications, clopidogrel is held and full-dose aspirin is continued. Full-dose aspirin is transitioned to 81 mg indefinitely at 6 months if occlusion remains complete.

SUMMARY

Aneurysms of the AComA represent a common and anatomically heterogeneous group of lesions for neurosurgeons and interventionalists. Endovascular technology and methods have advanced significantly in the past 2 decades. Randomized controlled trials have demonstrated benefit for patients with ruptured aneurysms to be treated with primary coil embolization. Further advancements in BACE and SACE have broadened the scope of endovascular practice and have paved the way for treatment of aneurysms once thought uncoilable.

Newer treatments, such as FDS and intrasaccular flow disruption, have shown promise, but their role regarding AComAAs has not been fully defined and experience remains modest. Future advancements to decrease rates of procedural complications, such as thromboembolism, but increase rates of permanent total occlusion are welcomed. With a full armamentarium of surgical and endovascular techniques, we are entering an age of medicine where care can be uniquely specified to benefit patients on an individual level.

REFERENCES

1. Hernesniemi J, Dashti R, Lehecka M, et al. Microneurosurgical management of anterior communicating artery aneurysms. Surg Neurol 2008;70: 8–28 [discussion: 29].
2. Kassell NF, Torner JC, Jane JA, et al. The International Cooperative Study on the timing of aneurysm surgery. Part 2: surgical results. J Neurosurg 1990; 73:37–47.

3. Molyneux AJ, Kerr RS, Yu LM, et al. International subarachnoid aneurysm trial (ISAT) of neurosurgical clipping versus endovascular coiling in 2143 patients with ruptured intracranial aneurysms: a randomised comparison of effects on survival, dependency, seizures, rebleeding, subgroups, and aneurysm occlusion. Lancet 2005; 366:809–17.
4. Wiebers DO, Whisnant JP, Huston J 3rd, et al. Unruptured intracranial aneurysms: natural history, clinical outcome, and risks of surgical and endovascular treatment. Lancet 2003;362:103–10.
5. Bijlenga P, Ebeling C, Jaegersberg M, et al. Risk of rupture of small anterior communicating artery aneurysms is similar to posterior circulation aneurysms. Stroke 2013;44:3018–26.
6. Makowicz G, Poniatowska R, Lusawa M. Variants of cerebral arteries - anterior circulation. Pol J Radiol 2013;78:42–7.
7. Sanders WP, Sorek PA, Mehta BA. Fenestration of intracranial arteries with special attention to associated aneurysms and other anomalies. AJNR Am J Neuroradiol 1993;14:675–80.
8. San-Galli F, Leman C, Kien P, et al. Cerebral arterial fenestrations associated with intracranial saccular aneurysms. Neurosurgery 1992;30:279–83.
9. Molyneux A, Kerr R, Stratton I, et al. International Subarachnoid Aneurysm Trial (ISAT) of neurosurgical clipping versus endovascular coiling in 2143 patients with ruptured intracranial aneurysms: a randomised trial. Lancet 2002;360:1267–74.
10. Gnanalingham KK, Apostolopoulos V, Barazi S, et al. The impact of the international subarachnoid aneurysm trial (ISAT) on the management of aneurysmal subarachnoid haemorrhage in a neurosurgical unit in the UK. Clin Neurol Neurosurg 2006; 108:117–23.
11. Malek AM, Halbach VV, Phatouros CC, et al. Balloon-assist technique for endovascular coil embolization of geometrically difficult intracranial aneurysms. Neurosurgery 2000;46:1397–406 [discussion: 1406–7].
12. Shapiro M, Babb J, Becske T, et al. Safety and efficacy of adjunctive balloon remodeling during endovascular treatment of intracranial aneurysms: a literature review. AJNR Am J Neuroradiol 2008;29: 1777–81.
13. Cohen JE, Melamed I, Itshayek E. X-microstenting and transmesh coiling in the management of wide-necked tent-like anterior communicating artery aneurysms. J Clin Neurosci 2013;21(4):664–7.
14. Huang QH, Wu YF, Shen J, et al. Endovascular treatment of acutely ruptured, wide-necked anterior communicating artery aneurysms using the Enterprise stent. J Clin Neurosci 2013;20(2):267–71.
15. Perlmutter D, Rhoton AL Jr. Microsurgical anatomy of the anterior cerebral-anterior communicating-recurrent artery complex. J Neurosurg 1976;45: 259–72.
16. Rhoton AL Jr, Perlmutter D. Microsurgical anatomy of anterior communicating artery aneurysms. Neurol Res 1980;2:217–51.
17. Rhoton AL Jr. The supratentorial arteries. Neurosurgery 2002;51:S53–120.
18. Cinnamon J, Zito J, Chalif DJ, et al. Aneurysm of the azygos pericallosal artery: diagnosis by MR imaging and MR angiography. AJNR Am J Neuroradiol 1992;13:280–2.
19. Gorczyca W, Mohr G. Microvascular anatomy of Heubner's recurrent artery. Neurol Res 1987;9: 259–64.
20. Maga P, Tomaszewski KA, Krzyżewski RM, et al. Branches and arterial supply of the recurrent artery of Heubner. Anat Sci Int 2013;88:223–9.
21. Alberts MJ. Results of a multicenter prospective randomized trial of carotid artery stenting vs. carotid endarterectomy. The Publications Committee of WALLSTENT [abstract]. Stroke 2001;32:325.
22. Nathal E, Yasui N, Sampei T, et al. Intraoperative anatomical studies in patients with aneurysms of the anterior communicating artery complex. J Neurosurg 1992;76:629–34.
23. Stehbens WE. Aneurysms and anatomical variation of cerebral arteries. Arch Pathol 1963;75:45–64.
24. Wilson G, Riggs HE, Rupp C. The pathologic anatomy of ruptured cerebral aneurysms. J Neurosurg 1954;11:128–34.
25. Itoyama Y, Fujioka S, Takaki S, et al. Occlusion of internal carotid artery and formation of anterior communicating artery aneurysm in cervicocephalic fibromuscular dysplasia–follow-up case report. Neurol Med Chir (Tokyo) 1994;34:547–50.
26. Inoue T, Tsutsumi K, Adachi S, et al. Clipping and superficial temporal artery-M2 bypass for unruptured anterior communicating artery aneurysm associated with atherosclerotic internal carotid artery occlusion: report of 2 cases. Surg Neurol 2007;68:226–31 [discussion: 232].
27. De Gast AN, van Rooij WJ, Sluzewski M. Fenestrations of the anterior communicating artery: incidence on 3D angiography and relationship to aneurysms. AJNR Am J Neuroradiol 2008;29:296–8.
28. Van Rooij SB, van Rooij WJ, Sluzewski M, et al. Fenestrations of intracranial arteries detected with 3D rotational angiography. AJNR Am J Neuroradiol 2009;30:1347–50.
29. Hunt WE, Hess RM. Surgical risk as related to time of intervention in the repair of intracranial aneurysms. J Neurosurg 1968;28:14–20.
30. McDougall CG, Spetzler RF, Zabramski JM, et al. The barrow ruptured aneurysm trial. J Neurosurg 2012;116:135–44.
31. Lownie SP, Drake CG, Peerless SJ, et al. Clinical presentation and management of giant anterior

communicating artery region aneurysms. J Neurosurg 2000;92:267–77.
32. Park JH, Park SK, Kim TH, et al. Anterior communicating artery aneurysm related to visual symptoms. J Korean Neurosurg Soc 2009;46:232–8.
33. Austin JR, Maceri DR. Anterior communicating artery aneurysm presenting as pulsatile tinnitus. ORL J Otorhinolaryngol Relat Spec 1993;55:54–7.
34. Shukla DP, Bhat DI, Devi BI. Anterior communicating artery aneurysm presenting with vision loss. J Neurosci Rural Pract 2013;4:305–7.
35. Dzhebrailbekov ES, Shishkina LV. The Korsakoff syndrome in a female patient operated on for an aneurysm of the anterior cerebral-anterior communicating arteries (a case report). Zh Vopr Neirokhir Im N N Burdenko 1996;(4):37–9 [in Russian].
36. Asari S, Satoh T, Sakurai M, et al. Delineation of unruptured cerebral aneurysms by computerized angiotomography. J Neurosurg 1982;57:527–34.
37. McKinney AM, Palmer CS, Truwit CL, et al. Detection of aneurysms by 64-section multidetector CT angiography in patients acutely suspected of having an intracranial aneurysm and comparison with digital subtraction and 3D rotational angiography. AJNR Am J Neuroradiol 2008;29:594–602.
38. Cirillo M, Scomazzoni F, Cirillo L, et al. Comparison of 3D TOF-MRA and 3D CE-MRA at 3T for imaging of intracranial aneurysms. Eur J Radiol 2013;82:e853–9.
39. Sailer AM, Wagemans BA, Nelemans PJ, et al. Diagnosing intracranial aneurysms with MR angiography: systematic review and meta-analysis. Stroke 2014;45(1):119–26.
40. Deutschmann HA, Augustin M, Simbrunner J, et al. Diagnostic accuracy of 3D time-of-flight MR angiography compared with digital subtraction angiography for follow-up of coiled intracranial aneurysms: influence of aneurysm size. AJNR Am J Neuroradiol 2007;28:628–34.
41. Romijn M, Gratama van Andel HA, van Walderveen MA, et al. Diagnostic accuracy of CT angiography with matched mask bone elimination for detection of intracranial aneurysms: comparison with digital subtraction angiography and 3D rotational angiography. AJNR Am J Neuroradiol 2008;29:134–9.
42. Agid R, Lee SK, Willinsky RA, et al. Acute subarachnoid hemorrhage: using 64-slice multidetector CT angiography to "triage" patients' treatment. Neuroradiology 2006;48:787–94.
43. Jane JA, Winn HR, Richardson AE. The natural history of intracranial aneurysms: rebleeding rates during the acute and long term period and implication for surgical management. Clin Neurosurg 1977;24:176–84.
44. Jane JA, Kassell NF, Torner JC, et al. The natural history of aneurysms and arteriovenous malformations. J Neurosurg 1985;62:321–3.
45. Molyneux AJ, Kerr RS, Birks J, et al. Risk of recurrent subarachnoid haemorrhage, death, or dependence and standardised mortality ratios after clipping or coiling of an intracranial aneurysm in the International Subarachnoid Aneurysm Trial (ISAT): long-term follow-up. Lancet Neurol 2009;8:427–33.
46. Schievink WI, Wijdicks EF, Piepgras DG, et al. The poor prognosis of ruptured intracranial aneurysms of the posterior circulation. J Neurosurg 1995;82:791–5.
47. Spetzler RF, McDougall CG, Albuquerque FC, et al. The barrow ruptured aneurysm trial: 3-year results. J Neurosurg 2013;119:146–57.
48. Unruptured intracranial aneurysms–risk of rupture and risks of surgical intervention. International Study of Unruptured Intracranial Aneurysms Investigators. N Engl J Med 1998;339:1725–33.
49. UCAS Japan Investigators, Morita A, Kirino T, et al. The natural course of unruptured cerebral aneurysms in a Japanese cohort. N Engl J Med 2012;366:2474–82.
50. Brizzi RE. 2 cases of congenital arteriovenous aneurysm of the brain treated by means of embolization with lipiodol-wax. Riv Neurobiol 1964;10:3–16 [in Italian].
51. Sashin D, Goldman RL, Zanetti P, et al. Electronic radiography in stereotaxic thrombosis of intracranial aneurysms and catheter embolization of cerebral arteriovenous malformations. Radiology 1972;105:359–63.
52. Guglielmi G, Viñuela F, Sepetka I, et al. Electrothrombosis of saccular aneurysms via endovascular approach. Part 1: electrochemical basis, technique, and experimental results. J Neurosurg 1991;75:1–7.
53. Guglielmi G, Viñuela F, Dion J, et al. Electrothrombosis of saccular aneurysms via endovascular approach. Part 2: preliminary clinical experience. J Neurosurg 1991;75:8–14.
54. Guglielmi G, Viñuela F, Duckwiler G, et al. Endovascular treatment of posterior circulation aneurysms by electrothrombosis using electrically detachable coils. J Neurosurg 1992;77:515–24.
55. Viñuela F, Duckwiler G, Mawad M. Guglielmi detachable coil embolization of acute intracranial aneurysm: perioperative anatomical and clinical outcome in 403 patients. J Neurosurg 1997;86:475–82.
56. Guglielmi G. The beginning and the evolution of the endovascular treatment of intracranial aneurysms: from the first catheterization of brain arteries to the new stents. J Neurointerv Surg 2009;1:53–5.
57. Ding YH, Lewis DA, Kadirvel R, et al. The Woven EndoBridge: a new aneurysm occlusion device. AJNR Am J Neuroradiol 2011;32:607–11.

58. Elias T, Ogungbo B, Connolly D, et al. Endovascular treatment of anterior communicating artery aneurysms: results of clinical and radiological outcome in Newcastle. Br J Neurosurg 2003;17: 278–86.
59. Proust F, Debono B, Hannequin D, et al. Treatment of anterior communicating artery aneurysms: complementary aspects of microsurgical and endovascular procedures. J Neurosurg 2003;99:3–14.
60. Birknes JK, Hwang SK, Pandey AS, et al. Feasibility and limitations of endovascular coil embolization of anterior communicating artery aneurysms: morphological considerations. Neurosurgery 2006;59: 43–52 [discussion: 43–52].
61. Guglielmi G, Viñuela F, Duckwiler G, et al. Endovascular treatment of 306 anterior communicating artery aneurysms: overall, perioperative results. J Neurosurg 2009;110:874–9.
62. Songsaeng D, Geibprasert S, Willinsky R, et al. Impact of anatomical variations of the circle of Willis on the incidence of aneurysms and their recurrence rate following endovascular treatment. Clin Radiol 2010;65:895–901.
63. Finitsis S, Anxionnat R, Lebedinsky A, et al. Endovascular treatment of ACom intracranial aneurysms. Report on series of 280 patients. Interv Neuroradiol 2010;16:7–16.
64. Raslan AM, Oztaskin M, Thompson EM, et al. Neuroform stent-assisted embolization of incidental anterior communicating artery aneurysms: long-term clinical and angiographic follow-up. Neurosurgery 2011;69:27–37 [discussion: 37].
65. Choi JH, Kang MJ, Huh JT. Influence of clinical and anatomic features on treatment decisions for anterior communicating artery aneurysms. J Korean Neurosurg Soc 2011;50:81–8.
66. Schuette AJ, Hui FK, Spiotta AM, et al. Endovascular therapy of very small aneurysms of the anterior communicating artery: five-fold increased incidence of rupture. Neurosurgery 2011;68:731–7 [discussion: 737].
67. Johnson AK, Munich SA, Heiferman DM, et al. Stent assisted embolization of 64 anterior communicating artery aneurysms. J Neurointerv Surg 2013;5(Suppl 3):iii62–5.
68. Gurbel PA, Antonino MJ, Tantry US. Recent developments in clopidogrel pharmacology and their relation to clinical outcomes. Expert Opin Drug Metab Toxicol 2009;5:989–1004.
69. Müller-Schunk S, Linn J, Peters N, et al. Monitoring of clopidogrel-related platelet inhibition: correlation of nonresponse with clinical outcome in supra-aortic stenting. AJNR Am J Neuroradiol 2008;29: 786–91.
70. Maruyama H, Takeda H, Dembo T, et al. Clopidogrel resistance and the effect of combination cilostazol in patients with ischemic stroke or carotid artery stenting using the VerifyNow P2Y12 Assay. Intern Med 2011;50:695–8.
71. Gaba RC, Ansari SA, Roy SS, et al. Embolization of intracranial aneurysms with hydrogel-coated coils versus inert platinum coils: effects on packing density, coil length and quantity, procedure performance, cost, length of hospital stay, and durability of therapy. Stroke 2006;37:1443–50.
72. Piotin M, Mandai S, Murphy KJ, et al. Dense packing of cerebral aneurysms: an in vitro study with detachable platinum coils. AJNR Am J Neuroradiol 2000;21:757–60.
73. Vanninen R, Koivisto T, Saari T, et al. Ruptured intracranial aneurysms: acute endovascular treatment with electrolytically detachable coils–a prospective randomized study. Radiology 1999;211: 325–36.
74. Raftopoulos C, Goffette P, Vaz G, et al. Surgical clipping may lead to better results than coil embolization: results from a series of 101 consecutive unruptured intracranial aneurysms. Neurosurgery 2003;52:1280–7 [discussion: 1287–90].
75. Horowitz M, Gupta R, Jovin T. The dual catheter technique for coiling of wide-necked cerebral aneurysms. An under-reported method. Interv Neuroradiol 2005;11:155–60.
76. Pan J, Xiao F, Szeder V, et al. Stent, balloon-assisted coiling and double microcatheter for treating wide-neck aneurysms in anterior cerebral circulation. Neurol Res 2013;35:1002–8.
77. Fang S, Brinjikji W, Murad MH, et al. Endovascular treatment of anterior communicating artery aneurysms: a systematic review and meta-analysis. AJNR Am J Neuroradiol 2013. [Epub ahead of print].
78. Leng B, Zheng Y, Ren J, et al. Endovascular treatment of intracranial aneurysms with detachable coils: correlation between aneurysm volume, packing, and angiographic recurrence. J Neurointerv Surg 2013. [Epub ahead of print].
79. Sluzewski M, van Rooij WJ, Beute GN, et al. Late rebleeding of ruptured intracranial aneurysms treated with detachable coils. AJNR Am J Neuroradiol 2005;26:2542–9.
80. Kang HS, Han MH, Kwon BJ, et al. Repeat endovascular treatment in post-embolization recurrent intracranial aneurysms. Neurosurgery 2006;58: 60–70 [discussion: 60–70].
81. Slob MJ, Sluzewski M, van Rooij WJ, et al. Additional coiling of previously coiled cerebral aneurysms: clinical and angiographic results. AJNR Am J Neuroradiol 2004;25:1373–6.
82. Dorfer C, Gruber A, Standhardt H, et al. Management of residual and recurrent aneurysms after initial endovascular treatment. Neurosurgery 2012;70:537–53 [discussion: 553–4].
83. Abdihalim M, Watanabe M, Chaudhry SA, et al. Are coil compaction and aneurysmal growth two

distinct etiologies leading to recurrence following endovascular treatment of intracranial aneurysm? J Neuroimaging 2013;24(2):171–5.
84. Levy DI, Ku A. Balloon-assisted coil placement in wide-necked aneurysms. Technical note. J Neurosurg 1997;86:724–7.
85. Akiba Y, Murayama Y, Viñuela F, et al. Balloon-assisted Guglielmi detachable coiling of wide-necked aneurysms: part I–experimental evaluation. Neurosurgery 1999;45:519–27 [discussion: 527–30].
86. Lefkowitz MA, Gobin YP, Akiba Y, et al. Ballonn-assisted Guglielmi detachable coiling of wide-necked aneurysma: part II–clinical results. Neurosurgery 1999;45:531–7 [discussion: 537–8].
87. Moret J, Cognard C, Weill A, et al. The "Remodelling Technique" in the treatment of wide neck intracranial aneurysms. Angiographic results and clinical follow-up in 56 cases. Interv Neuroradiol 1997;3:21–35.
88. Cottier JP, Pasco A, Gallas S, et al. Utility of balloon-assisted Guglielmi detachable coiling in the treatment of 49 cerebral aneurysms: a retrospective, multicenter study. AJNR Am J Neuroradiol 2001;22:345–51.
89. Chalouhi N, Jabbour P, Tjoumakaris S, et al. Single-center experience with balloon-assisted coil embolization of intracranial aneurysms: safety, efficacy and indications. Clin Neurol Neurosurg 2013;115: 607–13.
90. Cekirge HS, Yavuz K, Geyik S, et al. HyperForm balloon remodeling in the endovascular treatment of anterior cerebral, middle cerebral, and anterior communicating artery aneurysms: clinical and angiographic follow-up results in 800 consecutive patients. J Neurosurg 2011;114:944–53.
91. Santillan A, Gobin YP, Greenberg ED, et al. Intraprocedural aneurysmal rupture during coil embolization of brain aneurysms: role of balloon-assisted coiling. AJNR Am J Neuroradiol 2012;33:2017–21.
92. Sluzewski M, van Rooij WJ, Beute GN, et al. Balloon-assisted coil embolization of intracranial aneurysms: incidence, complications, and angiography results. J Neurosurg 2006;105:396–9.
93. Pierot L, Spelle L, Leclerc X, et al. Endovascular treatment of unruptured intracranial aneurysms: comparison of safety of remodeling technique and standard treatment with coils. Radiology 2009;251:846–55.
94. Pierot L, Cognard C, Anxionnat R, et al, CLARITY Investigators. Remodeling technique for endovascular treatment of ruptured intracranial aneurysms had a higher rate of adequate postoperative occlusion than did conventional coil embolization with comparable safety. Radiology 2011;258: 546–53.
95. Santillan A, Gobin YP, Mazura JC, et al. Balloon-assisted coil embolization of intracranial aneurysms is not associated with increased periprocedural complications. J Neurointerv Surg 2013;5(Suppl 3): iii56–61.
96. Mericle RA, Lanzino G, Wakhloo AK, et al. Stenting and secondary coiling of intracranial internal carotid artery aneurysm: technical case report. Neurosurgery 1998;43:1229–34.
97. Akgul E, Aksungur E, Balli T, et al. Y-stent-assisted coil embolization of wide-neck intracranial aneurysms. A single center experience. Interv Neuroradiol 2011;17:36–48.
98. Martínez-Galdámez M, Saura P, Saura J, et al. Y-stent-assisted coil embolization of anterior circulation aneurysms using two Solitaire AB devices: a single center experience. Interv Neuroradiol 2012; 18:158–63.
99. Zeleňák K, Zeleňáková J, DeRiggo J, et al. Flow changes after endovascular treatment of a wide-neck anterior communicating artery aneurysm by using X-configured kissing stents (cross-kissing stents) technique. Cardiovasc Intervent Radiol 2011;34:1308–11.
100. Saatci I, Geyik S, Yavuz K, et al. X-configured stent-assisted coiling in the endovascular treatment of complex anterior communicating artery aneurysms: a novel reconstructive technique. AJNR Am J Neuroradiol 2011;32:E113–7.
101. Lazzaro MA, Zaidat OO. X-configuration intersecting Enterprise stents for vascular remodeling and assisted coil embolization of a wide neck anterior communicating artery aneurysm. J Neurointerv Surg 2011;3:348–51.
102. Chalouhi N, Jabbour P, Singhal S, et al. Stent-assisted coiling of intracranial aneurysms: predictors of complications, recanalization, and outcome in 508 cases. Stroke 2013;44:1348–53.
103. Ismail Alhothi A, Qi T, Guo S, et al. Neuroform stent-assisted coil embolization: a new treatment strategy for complex intracranial aneurysms. Results of medium length follow-up. Neurol Neurochir Pol 2010;44:366–74.
104. Liang G, Gao X, Li Z, et al. Neuroform stent-assisted coiling of intracranial aneurysms: a 5 year single-center experience and follow-up. Neurol Res 2010;32:721–7.
105. Amenta PS, Dalyai RT, Kung D, et al. Stent-assisted coiling of wide-necked aneurysms in the setting of acute subarachnoid hemorrhage: experience in 65 patients. Neurosurgery 2012;70:1415–29 [discussion: 1429].
106. Becske T, Kallmes DF, Saatci I, et al. Pipeline for uncoilable or failed aneurysms: results from a multicenter clinical trial. Radiology 2013;267:858–68.
107. Chalouhi N, Tjoumakaris S, Starke RM, et al. Comparison of flow diversion and coiling in large unruptured intracranial saccular aneurysms. Stroke 2013;44:2150–4.

108. Rouchaud A, Saleme S, Gory B, et al. Endovascular exclusion of the anterior communicating artery with flow-diverter stents as an emergency treatment for blister-like intracranial aneurysms. A case report. Interv Neuroradiol 2013;19:471–8.
109. Lubicz B, Mine B, Collignon L, et al. WEB device for endovascular treatment of wide-neck bifurcation aneurysms. AJNR Am J Neuroradiol 2013;34: 1209–14.
110. Pierot L, Liebig T, Sychra V, et al. Intrasaccular flow-disruption treatment of intracranial aneurysms: preliminary results of a multicenter clinical study. AJNR Am J Neuroradiol 2012;33:1232–8.
111. Cho WS, Kim SS, Lee SJ, et al. The effectiveness of 3T time-of-flight magnetic resonance angiography for follow-up evaluations after the stent-assisted coil embolization of cerebral aneurysms. Acta Radiol 2013. [Epub ahead of print].

Middle Cerebral Artery Aneurysm Endovascular and Surgical Therapies

Comprehensive Literature Review and Local Experience

Osama O. Zaidat, MD, MS[a,b,c,*], Alicia C. Castonguay, PhD[a],
Mohamed S. Teleb, MD[a], Kaiz Asif, MD[a],
Ayman Gheith, MD[a], Chris Southwood, MD[a],
Glen Pollock, MD[a,c], John R. Lynch, MD[a,b,c]

KEYWORDS

• Middle cerebral artery • Aneurysm • Clipping • Coiling • Endovascular • Intracranial aneurysm

KEY POINTS

- The middle cerebral artery (MCA) is the most common location for cerebral aneurysms and is associated with a lower risk of rupture than aneurysms located in the anterior or posterior communicating arteries.
- There is no definitive evidence to support the superiority of clipping over coiling to treat middle cerebral artery aneurysm (MCAA) or vice versa.
- The current available data and review of the literature indicate that the feasibility of treating the MCAA with endovascular therapy (ET) as the first choice of treatment in cohorts of nonselected aneurysms exceeds 90%.
- No significant increase in the risk of rebleeding with endovascular approaches was shown, and there are no significant differences in the long-term morbidity and mortality (M&M) between the 2 treatments. However, the review of the literature indicates that treatment of MCAAs is also associated with low M&M rates with surgical clipping in unruptured aneurysms.
- Based on the literature, it seems that there is no significant difference between the 2 therapies, with only hypothetical advantages of one approach over the other. A randomized clinical trial comparing the 2 approaches in nonselected cases with long-term follow-up will shed light on which patients may benefit from one approach over another.

INTRODUCTION

Since the publication of the International Subarachnoid Aneurysm Trial (ISAT) and Barrow Ruptured Aneurysm Treatment (BRAT) randomized clinical trials, ET is the most frequently used approach for treating cerebral aneurysms.[1–5] Incremental improvements of interventional

Disclosures: None.
[a] Department of Neurology, SNN (Stroke, Neurocritical Care, and Neurointerventional) Research Center, Froedtert Hospital, Medical College of Wisconsin, 9200 West Wisconsin Avenue, Milwaukee, WI 53226, USA; [b] Department of Radiology, SNN (Stroke, Neurocritical Care, and Neurointerventional) Research Center, Froedtert Hospital, Medical College of Wisconsin, 9200 West Wisconsin Avenue, Milwaukee, WI 53226, USA; [c] Department of Neurosurgery, SNN (Stroke, Neurocritical Care, and Neurointerventional) Research Center, Froedtert Hospital, Medical College of Wisconsin, 9200 West Wisconsin Avenue, Milwaukee, WI 53226, USA
* Corresponding author. Froedtert Hospital, Medical College of Wisconsin, 9200 West Wisconsin Avenue, Milwaukee, WI 53226.
E-mail address: szaidat@mcw.edu

Neurosurg Clin N Am 25 (2014) 455–469
http://dx.doi.org/10.1016/j.nec.2014.04.005
1042-3680/14/$ – see front matter

techniques now permit treatment of more complex cerebral aneurysms endovascularly, resulting in a higher proportion of aneurysms being treated with ET than with open surgical techniques.[6] Despite the mounting evidence, the debate of coiling versus clipping continues to persist, most vigorously directed at the treatment of MCAAs. More emphasis is placed on choosing treatment based on clinical factors, complex anatomic and morphologic features (including age, location, size, projection, and relationship with branching vessels), and the potential of lifelong durability over the initial gain of coiling safety.

This ongoing controversy is well illustrated by the unresolved question regarding the best approach to treating MCAAs and the lack of consensus on which treatment provides balanced safety and long-term protection. It is assumed that the specific anatomic aneurysmal location of the MCA may be more suitable to open surgical therapy than to ET. Although the MCA is an appealing location for surgical treatment with a direct and feasible approach, there is potential difficulty in cases with early vasospasm, as well as potential additional morbidity of the open surgical approach, such as retraction injury and perioperative hematoma. These difficulties and complications may be avoided by an endovascular approach; however, no randomized controlled trial data currently exist to specifically guide MCAA treatment decisions.

The lack of consensus on best treatment practices may have originated from initial data on MCAA coiling outcomes collected during early-era ET when coiling techniques had limited feasibility in treating challenging complex-shaped aneurysms. The introduction of advanced microcatheter designs for superior aneurysm access, complex 3-dimensional coil designs coupled with neck-bridging microstents, and balloon-assisted coiling options that offer safer and more dense packing result in feasibility rates for ET that exceed 90%.[7–11] In a study of 300 MCAAs by Mortimer and colleagues,[11] the feasibility of MCAA coiling as a primary treatment was shown to be approximately 95.8%. In this monograph, we provide a comprehensive literature review of MCAA coiling and clipping, then present our initial experience of MCAA coiling of nonselective consecutive cases.

MCA EMBRYOLOGY AND ANATOMY

An understanding of MCA embryology, anatomy, and expected anomalies is imperative to best treatment approach planning. During the 8th to 12th week of gestation, the distal primitive internal carotid artery (ICA) and its anterior cerebral artery (ACA) divide into the anterior choroidal artery and numerous small arterial twigs. The latter develops into the future anterior and middle embryologic cerebral arteries. This rete coalesces into the main MCA trunk, and the remaining twigs are the future perforators. The MCA is thus a continuation of the ICA. Failure to coalesce can lead to accessory MCA and a dominant anterior temporal artery. These variations become important in the discussion of the accessory MCA types.

From microsurgical data, the MCA outer diameter is 3 ± 0.1 mm bilaterally with a length of 15 ± 1.1 mm in the right hemisphere and 15.7 ± 1.3 mm in the left hemisphere.[12] However, in an autopsy study of 610 MCAs, the horizontal segment length was 16 mm (range 5–30 mm), with a diameter of 3 to 5 mm.[13] The MCA main trunk horizontal segment is referred to as M1 (sphenoidal), followed by the M2 (insular), then M3 (opercular), and finally M4 (cortical) segments.[13,14]

The MCA horizontal segment branching patterns are bifurcation (78%–90% of cases), trifurcation (12%), and multiple branches (10%), with the subsequent branching being mainly bifurcated.[13,14] A true trifurcation may be confused with a dominant intermediate trunk with a gap between the latter and the bifurcation point. A dominant trunk was found to be close to the MCA division, masking as a true trifurcation in 15% of cases. In 55% of cases, it originates within a short distance of one of the MCA divisions, whereas in 30% of cases, it originates distal to the MCA divisions. The dominant intermediate trunk originated more commonly from the superior division. The more proximal the intermediate trunk is to the MCA division point, the larger its contribution to the cortical territories.[15] The intermediate trunk commonly supplies the parietal lobe. The superior trunk supplies the frontal convexity, and the inferior division supplies the temporal lobe in conjunction with the posterior cerebral artery and part of the parietal lobe, depending on the dominance of each division.

The anterior temporal artery is the first branch of the M1 segment and a common location of proximal M1 aneurysms, as was seen in 19 of the 23 specimens in one autopsy study and in all MCA samples in another study.[13,16] In addition, the perforators (Charcot striate arteries, varies from 6 to 20 perforators) are a common location for proximal M1 aneurysms.[13] The perforators can originate from the proximal M1 segment (51.1%), distal M1 segment and the first branching point (25.6%), or from one of the MCA/M2 branches distal to the first division (20.3%).[13]

Accessory MCA was found in 3% of the autopsies and 0.12% of the magnetic resonance angiographic (MRA) studies.[13,17] Failure of perforators off the ACA to coalesce and form a single MCA leads to MCA duplication with various dominance and origins leading to different types (Manelfe types I, II, and III). This duplication or accessory MCA commonly occurs unilaterally. However, when identified on one side, the likelihood of finding a mirror contralateral accessory MCA is 16.5%.[13] The accessory MCA arose from the ACA in 80% of cases (type 2 from proximal A1 segment of the ACA and type 3 from the distal A1 segment) and from the ICA in 20% of cases (type I) (**Fig. 1**).[13] Fenestration of the MCA is rarely encountered and was found in 3 of 3491 MRA studies or 0.09% of cases.[17]

EPIDEMIOLOGY AND RISK OF RUPTURE

Incidence, Multiplicity, and Location

The MCA is a common location of cerebral aneurysms and constitutes 14.4% to 43% of all diagnosed aneurysms.[1–4,18–24] A large series of 561 MCAAs from Finland showed that MCAAs may be found as single (60.6%), multiple (9.8%), or associated with aneurysms in other locations (19.6%).[19] Bilateral mirror aneurysms in the same location but on opposite sides were found in two-thirds of multiple MCAA cases.[19] The presence of proximal MCAA increased the occurrence of associated intracranial aneurysms by 2.6-fold.[19] The exact location of MCAA was evaluated by multiple investigators, with the most common site being the MCA bifurcation, followed by proximal M1, then distal MCA (**Fig. 2**).[19,25–28]

Familial Occurrence

In patients with subarachnoid hemorrhage (SAH), 10% of the aneurysms are familial.[29,30] However, familial association increases with MCAA multiplicity as it occurred in 11%, 14%, 20%, and 22% in single, multiple, pure bilateral, and pure bilateral at the bifurcation MCAs, respectively.[19]

Rupture Risk

The risk of future aneurysmal rupture and SAH seems to be less common when the aneurysms are encountered in the MCA territory versus other locations, such as anterior communicating and posterior communicating arteries, according to data from unruptured aneurysm trials. In the Unruptured Cerebral Aneurysm Study, the rate of rupture of MCAAs per year was 0.23 (0.09–0.54), 0.31 (0.10–0.96), 1.56 (0.74–3.26), 4.11 (2.22–7.66), and 16.87 (2.38–119.77) for aneurysm sizes of 3 to 4, 5 to 6, 7 to 9, 10 to 24, and greater than or equal to 25 mm, respectively.[21] In the International Study of Unruptured Intracranial Aneurysms 2, the annual rate of MCAA rupture was 0%, 1.5%, 2.6%, 14.5%, and 40% in less than 7 with no history of SAH, less than 7 with history of SAH, 7 to 12, 13 to 24, and greater than or equal to 25 mm MCAA.[22] In addition to the absolute aneurysm maximum size, other features may predict aneurysm rupture. For example, in a computerized tomographic angiography (CTA) serial imaging study of 151 patients with unruptured aneurysms, aneurysm size, interval growth, and multilobulation were the main predictors of rupture.[31]

PRESENTATION

MCAAs may be discovered incidentally or after rupture leading to SAH. In the Finnish consecutive MCAA series, patients presented with SAH in greater than 90% of the cases.[19] An associated hematoma of 2.5 cm or more was seen in 43% of MCAAs and was more common than in any

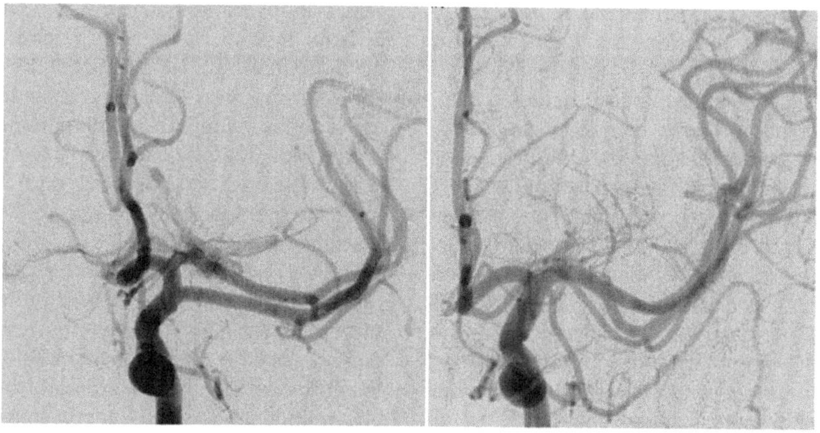

Fig. 1. Example of accessory middle cerebral artery, from the proximal A1 on the left side and from the distal A1 on the right side; also note on the right-hand side the origin of the anterior temporal artery off the distal ICA.

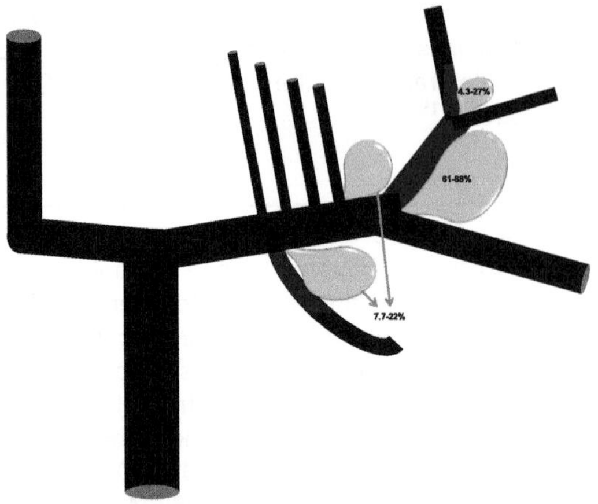

Fig. 2. Frequency of MCA aneurysm distribution across different location.

other aneurysm location (11%),[19] which may in part explain the higher grade of Hunt and Hess (H&H) at presentation with MCAA.[19] Intraventricular hemorrhage (IVH) was seen in 24% of MCA bifurcation aneurysms versus 19% and 11% in the proximal and distal locations, respectively. IVH was also seen less often with aneurysms at other sites.[19]

ANEURYSMAL FEATURES ASSOCIATED WITH OUTCOME

When assessing future rupture risk and planning the best treatment approach, morphologic features of MCAAs need to be evaluated and considered. MCAAs are typically classified into 3 types: proximal, bifurcation, and distal (see **Fig. 2**). As shown in **Fig. 2**, most MCAAs are located at the bifurcation (61%–88%), distal to the bifurcation (4.3%–27%), and proximally between the MCA origin and the bifurcation (7.7%–22%).[11,19,20,28,32–34] Proximal aneurysms are further classified into lenticulostriate (40%) or early M1 branch (60%) MCAAs.[32]

In addition to the classical locations identified earlier, other features of MCAAs may be examined to evaluate outcome after therapy, including side, size, multilobulation, dome to neck ratio, aneurysm size to parent vessel diameter ratio, incorporation of MCA lenticulostriate or distal branches, angulation of the branches, orientation and projection from the parent vessel, height from the origin of the ophthalmic artery, and distance between the ICA bifurcation and the aneurysm origin. We propose an angiographic classification of the bifurcation MCAAs for the purpose of predicting ET outcome and technical difficulty based on our experience of treating greater than 98% of all MCAAs presenting to our institution with ET (**Fig. 3**). Incorporated branches and acute angulations are 2 of the main limitations of ET. Our classification system may aid in predicting the acute branch angulations that would challenge adjunctive device use and incorporated branches that may also lead to technical difficulties (see **Fig. 3**).

For clipping, the distance between the MCA and aneurysm origin was found to be linked to increased perforator injury.[20,33] In a study of 91 clipping cases with an event rate of 15%, both the height (from the origin of the ophthalmic artery) and the distance (between the ICA bifurcation and the aneurysm origin) were significantly associated with perforator injuries.[35] In another study of 151 ruptured and unruptured MCAAs that underwent clipping, independent predictors for the risk of rupture intraoperatively and for postsurgical outcomes were the presence of SAH, location on the M2 segment, maximum length, and neck size.[34]

THERAPEUTIC APPROACHES

Middle Cerebral Artery Aneurysm Coiling Outcomes

There are multiple MCAA coiling series that show increased feasibility and improved procedural safety over time. However, most of these studies suffered from a lack of rigorous adjudication and randomization with an additional predilection for selection bias of treatment choice (based on institution preference and operator experience).

Feasibility and success rate

Although it has been argued that only a small proportion of the MCAAs are amenable to ET, recent large case series have shown that greater than 90% of the MCAAs are amenable to endovascular treatment. Mortimer and colleagues[11] reported a series of 295 consecutive patients with 300 MCAAs treated with ET from 1996 to 2012. The feasibility of primary coiling was 93%, with only 8 MCAAs treated by clipping based on anatomic consideration and an additional 13 due to failed ET attempts. In a similar nonselected 55 MCAA case series, when ET was implemented as the first-choice therapy, a feasibility rate of 91.7% was achieved.[28] Vendrell and colleagues[36] showed the feasibility of coiling MCAA as the first-choice therapy in 160 of 174 (92%) cases. In a study of 115 MCAAs treated during the early to middle era of ET (1990–2007), the feasibility rate of treating MCAAs was 93%; however, this study did not include consecutive MCAAs.[37] The high feasibility of ET as the first line of treatment was shown in a series of 154 aneurysms, 149 (96.5%) of which were treated successfully with coil embolization.[38]

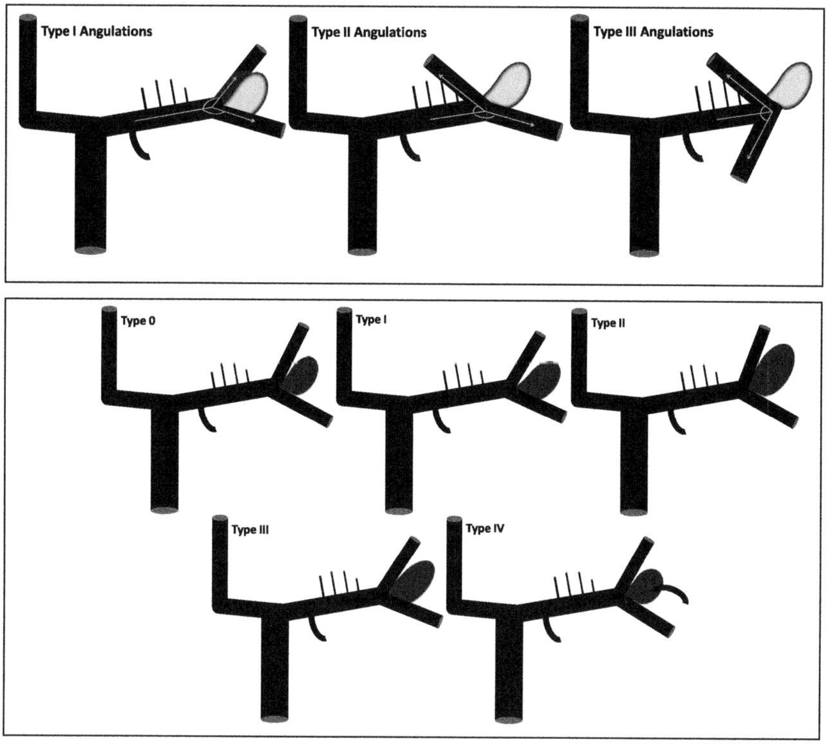

Fig. 3. Proposed classification for predicting outcomes of the branching angulations typing (*upper panel*): type I has both branching arteries at angles of greater than 90°, allowing for easy access for stent or balloon use if needed. Type II has 1 challenging angulation at less than 90° in 1 branch, and type III has both branches at less than 90°. Similar proposed classification of how many branches the aneurysm neck is incorporating (*lower panel*): type 0 no vessels are incorporated, type I and II involving inferior or superior division, type III incorporating 2 branches, and type IV when a branch is arising off the aneurysm dome, making it the most complex MCAA to treat.

In our local center experience, we treated 161 consecutive MCAAs during a 6-year period (2005–2011) with ET as the first-choice therapy. Our technical feasibility was 159 of 161 (98.8%) (2 cases were blister ruptured MCAAs of <1.5 mm). However, our adjunctive device utilization rate was 43%, which may have contributed to the high feasibility rate.[10]

Occlusion and retreatment rates

Across the literature, occlusion rates varied as did the definitions used to define occlusion grade. However, most reports defined occlusion rate as achieving complete embolization with no residual aneurysm or neck as opposed to residual dome filling. The range of recurrence rate requiring retreatment was 1.8% to 17.4%. The near-occlusion rate in the Mortimer and colleagues[11] series of 300 MCAAs was 91.4%, and the retreatment rate was 4.3%. In the Vendrell and colleagues[36] series of 174 MCAAs, the retreatment rate was 10.5% and the occlusion rate was 89.5%. In a prospective study of 131 MCAAs by Gory and colleagues,[39] the obliteration rate was 84.4% at 1.5-year follow-up, with a retreatment rate of 7.4%. Recurrence was predicted by aneurysm size (P = .02; odds ratio, 1.2; 95% confidence interval [CI], 1.02–1.4).[39] Quadros and colleagues[28] reported an obliteration rate of 95.3% with a retreatment rate of 1.8%. In a retrospective series of 152 consecutive MCAA patients (48% presenting with SAH), obliteration occurred in 83.3%, 79.5%, and 80.2% of aneurysms at 1, 3, and 5 years posttreatment.[40] The recurrence rate was 20% on the follow-up angiogram with half of these aneurysms (10%) retreated.[40] In the unruptured aneurysm series of 100 MCAAs treated by Vanzin and colleagues,[41] the recurrence rate requiring retreatment was reported as 9.8%. In another series of 76 unruptured MCAAs with a mean follow-up of 6 months, an 87% rate of complete obliteration was reported. Recurrence requiring retreatment was seen in 3 cases (4.3%).[42] Oishi and colleagues[43] reported a recanalization rate of 17.1% in a mixed group of both ruptured and unruptured MCAAs. In the Jin and colleagues[44] 103 MCAA series, from the 80 MCAAs that had follow-up (17.4%), a total of 14 recurrences were retreated with recoiling ($n = 12$) and clipping ($n = 2$) without complications. Predictors of recurrence were young age, rupture, and a wide aneurysm neck.[44] In a smaller report of 38 MCAAs, complete occlusion was achieved in 33 of 38 (87%) cases.[45] In our series of 161 nonselective MCAAs, the retreatment rate was 11%.[10]

Morbidity and mortality and rebleeding rate

The overall rate of M&M in ruptured MCAAs treated with ET was 16.8%, with a range (between 5.5% and 29.4%) that varies across the literature and over time (**Table 1**). Some literature reported only procedure-related complications, whereas others reported global outcome.

In one of the largest retrospective case series of 300 MCAAs with 80.7% presenting with SAH, the M&M rate was 7.8%[11]; in another 174 nonselective MCAAs (59.2% ruptured), the rate of M&M was 5.7%.[36] A large cohort (115 MCAAs; 42% ruptured) spanning the early and middle eras (between 1990 and 2007) of ET showed an overall M&M rate of 9.9%, with a rebleeding rate of less than 1% (1 in 115) in a giant partially treated MCAA.[37] In the Mortimer and colleagues[11] study, the rebleeding rate was 1%. M&M was seen in 7.9% (2% mortality) of the Quadros and colleagues[28] nonselective series (55.9% ruptured). In the Iijima and colleagues[38] series of 154 MCAAs (46.8% ruptured), the rate of symptomatic disability or death was 7% in ruptured aneurysms and 3% in unruptured aneurysms. In a prospective study of 131 nonselective MCAAs with ET as the first line of therapy, 32.4% presented as SAH and modified Rankin scale (mRS) of 2 or less was found in 93% of cases.[39] In the Bracard and colleagues[40] coiling series of 152 MCAAs, the overall procedure-related mortality rate was 0.7% and permanent morbidity was 2.6%. Early rebleeding occurred in 3 cases and was delayed in 1 case at a mean follow-up period of 4.3 years.[40]

In one series that examined the outcome in ruptured and unruptured aneurysms of 112 patients with 113 MCAAs treated with primary coiling from 2001 to 2007, the long-term outcome and M&M was 22.4% in those with SAH.[43] In the Jin and colleagues[44] series of 103 MCAAs, the M&M of ruptured aneurysms was 15.5%, whereas favorable outcome was noted in 72.4%. In 17 cases of ruptured MCAAs that were treated with endovascular coiling, M&M was seen in 5 of 17 (29.4%) cases, with no rebleeding on the long-term follow-up.[45] In 59 patients with 65 MCAAs, primary coiling was shown to be safe, with a bad outcome (mRS 4–6) in 7.7% of patients with H&H grades 1 to 3 and in 41.3% with H&H grades 4 and 5.[46] In our local experience, we treated 161 MCAAs during a 6-year period, 33% of which were ruptured and presented with SAH. The procedure-related M&M rate was 4% in this cohort of nonselected cases.[10]

Unruptured aneurysm coiling outcome

ET in unruptured aneurysms demonstrated lower M&M rates than ruptured aneurysms, with range between 0% and 5.9% (mean of 2.4%) (see **Table 1**). In a single-center experience with 100 unruptured MCAAs in 84 patients treated with coil embolization, the reported M&M rate was 2.4% (0% mortality).[41] In a retrospective case series of 70 patients with 76 unruptured MCAAs, no permanent morbidity was reported, with only 1 patient (1 in 70, 1.4%) who died of SAH within 9 hours of performing coiling.[42] In another series with both ruptured and unruptured aneurysms of 112 patients with 113 MCAAs, treated with primary coiling, the M&M rate was 2.2% in those with unruptured aneurysms.[43] In a case series of unruptured MCAAs, 1 in 17 (5.9%) had moderate disability and 0% mortality with no rebleeding with long-term follow-up.[45] In a case series of 103 MCAAs by Jin and colleagues,[44] the M&M rate was 0% for 42 of 103 unruptured MCAAs, with no rebleeding or new disability during a 29.5-month follow-up period, with 40 of 42 patients maintaining follow-up.

In summary, several smaller studies have shown similar results with M&M rates ranging from 0% to 10% and comparable retreatment rates (see **Table 1**).[47–49] Moreover, in a systematic review of 12 studies of endovascular MCAA coiling, the death and permanent morbidity rate was 5.1% for unruptured aneurysm and 6% for ruptured aneurysm, with an 82.4% rate of complete obliteration.[50]

MCA Clipping

Similar to the coiling data, the clipping and surgical data for the MCAAs are mostly limited to self-reported case series and retrospective studies that lack independent adjudication or randomization.

Morbidity and mortality in ruptured MCAA

The range of M&M from surgical therapy with ruptured aneurysms is difficult to accurately estimate given the natural history of SAH versus surgical morbidity specific to clipping (see **Table 1**).

In a study of 543 patients with 632 MCAAs who underwent clipping, 282 (51.9%) had ruptured MCAAs. Treatment approach was clipping (88.6%), thrombectomy/clip reconstruction (6.2%), and bypass/aneurysm occlusion (3.3%). Complete obliteration was achieved in 98.3% of cases. The overall rate of poor outcome (mRS 3–6) was seen in 29.8% of ruptured aneurysms inclusive of a mortality rate of 9.6%. Predictors of worse outcomes were rupture (*P* = .04), poor grade (*P* = .001), giant size (*P* = .03), and hemicraniectomy ($P \leq .001$).[51]

In another large series of 561 MCAAs from the Finnish study, a total of 496 (88.4%) patients were treated with surgical approaches.[19] A significant proportion of patients were not treated with surgery in this series (11.6%) because of rebleeding, technical reasons, patient choice, old age, or poor grade. The overall poor outcome rate was close to the ISAT trial results at 32.6% and was almost equal across the MCAA locations (34%, 32%, and 30% for proximal, bifurcation, and distal MCAAs). Surgical outcome was associated with aneurysm size in this series (29%, 33%, 31%, and 43% in very small, small, large, and giant aneurysms, respectively). Moreover, those pointing laterally in both anteroposterior and lateral projections were associated with worse surgical outcome than those pointing inferiorly on both projections. In addition, patients with multiple MCAAs had a 37% rate of poor outcome versus 39% in those with multiple intracranial aneurysms and 1 MCAA.[19] In another retrospective analysis of data from a single-center case series of 151 consecutive MCAAs treated with clipping between 2001 and 2006, 20% of the ruptured aneurysms had poor outcome (mRS 3–6).[52] In 1984, Suzuki and colleagues[53] reported on their single-center experience of 413 MCAAs whereby 265 of them were single aneurysms that were treated with a surgical approach. The single MCAAs had an overall M&M incidence at 6 months of 13.4% inclusive of a 5.1% mortality rate. However, patients treated earlier in this center's practice had poorer outcome (20%) than patients treated later (5.6%).

Morbidity and mortality in the unruptured MCAAs

The M&M rate of surgical therapy in unruptured MCAAs, based on available case series data, ranges from 0% to 8% (mean 3.2%) (see **Table 1**). In the Rodríguez-Hernández and colleagues[51] study of 543 patients with 632 MCAAs, 261 (48.1%) had unruptured aneurysms. Poor outcome (mRS 3–6) was demonstrated in 8%, inclusive of a mortality rate of 1.5%. In van Dijk and colleagues[52] series, 28 patients had unruptured MCAAs treated with clipping and 0% had long-term M&M. In another study of 263 patients (339 unruptured MCAAs) who underwent surgical clipping, the overall M&M rate was 5% (95% CI, 2.9%–8.3%). Patients younger than 60 years with an aneurysm 12 mm or less had the lowest complication rate of 0.6% (95% CI, 0%–3.8%) versus 22.2% (95% CI, 8.5%–45.8%) for those 60 years or older with an aneurysm greater than 12 mm in size.[54] In a retrospective single-center series of 201 unruptured MCAAs treated with a surgical approach, the overall total procedural complication rate was 2.5%. However, the permanent morbidity rate was only 0.6%, with size being the most predictive of outcome.[55] Unruptured MCAA surgical therapy was also studied in 125 patients (143; <10 mm aneurysms) treated from January 2007 to December 2010. An M&M rate of 2.4% (3 of 125) (intracranial hemorrhage [ICH], meningitis, and wound infection) was found in this study; however, the investigators reported that all patients had good clinical outcomes during follow-up (mRS 0–1). Imaging follow-up was mixed with CTA and conventional catheter angiography, which showed complete occlusion in 137 of 143 (95.8%) aneurysms and residual neck or residual aneurysm in 6 of 143 (4.4%).[56] Predictors of poor outcome from clipping of 91 unruptured MCAAs included higher distance between the MCAA and ophthalmic artery origin and shorter distance between the MCA origin and the bifurcation. In the same series, a total of 14 of 91 (15%) new infarctions were found on postoperative imaging, of which 4 of 91 (4.4%) led to permanent deficit.[35] Finally, in a single-center small series of 24 unruptured MCAAs that used imaging guidance navigation to perform craniotomy and clipping, no complications were reported.[57]

Clipping Versus Coiling Data

At present, no randomized controlled trial data comparing coiling to clipping in a pure cohort of MCAAs exist in the literature. However, in the prospective and randomized BRAT trial, patients with ruptured anterior circulation aneurysms who were assigned to coiling versus clipping at 3 years demonstrated an mRS greater than 2 in 21 of 89 (23.4%) in the coiling group versus 66 of 215 (30.7%) in the clipping group (*P* = .21). Assuming that most anterior circulation aneurysms were MCAAs, one may then hypothesize a numerically lower likelihood of poor outcome with coiling. However, because the BRAT trial is a single-center small sample size study with surgeons that had extensive coiling and clipping experience, the results may not be generalizable.[4]

There are several retrospective studies with the following limitations: small sample size, imbalanced groups, single center, and self-adjudication. In the ISAT trial, ruptured MCAA subgroup analysis showed a poor outcome rate of 46 of 162 (28.4%) in the coiling arm versus 39 of 139 (28.1%) in the clipping arm, with no

Table 1
Result from studies of outcomes from coiling and clipping of MCAAs

	Author, Year	*N*	SAH (%)	Population	Dead I	Poor I	Total M&M I	Dead R	Poor R	Total MM R	Outcome
Coil	Mortimer et al,[11] 2014	295	80.7	Retrospective analysis of prospective data	1.9	0	1.9	13.6	7	20.6	Obliteration rate, 91.4%. Retreatment rate, 4.3%. Coiling with hematoma, good outcome in 40%. Feasibility rate of MCAAs coiling is 95.8%
	Quadros et al,[28] 2007	55	60	Retrospective: 55/59 MCAAs	0	4.5	4.5	3	6.1	9.1	Multidisciplinary team referred 76.6% for coiling, obliteration rate, 95.3%; retreatment, 1.8%
	Doerfler et al,[45] 2006	36	50	Retrospective: 36/38	0	5.6	5.6	5.9	23.5	29.4	Retreatment, 7.9% Feasibility, 86.8%
	Bracard et al,[40] 2010	140	48	Retrospective, single center	0	1.5	1.5	9.6	9.6	19.2	Obliteration rate, 83.3%. Rebleed occurred in 1 patient (4.3 y follow-up)
	Gory et al,[39] 2014	120	34.2	Prospective nonselective	2.5	4.8	7.3	4.9	2.4	6.3	Retreatment rate, 7.6%
	Jin et al,[44] 2013	100	58	Retrospective: 100/103	0	0	0	12.1	15.5	27.6	Feasibility rate, 99%. Retreatment: 12 with recoiling and 2 with clipping
	Vendrell et al,[36] 2009	153	59.2	Retrospective: single center 153/174	0	9.8	9.8	2.2	3.3	5.5	Feasibility 160/174 (92%). Recurrence in 10.5%
	Suzuki et al,[37] 2009	115	42	Retrospective, single center	0	1.5	1.5	4.2	16.7	20.9	Rebleeding in 1/115 cases in partially treated aneurysm 0.09%. Recanalization, 10.5%.
	Oishi et al,[43] 2009	112	53.6	Retrospective, single center	0	2.2	2.2	5	17.4	22.4	Long-term recanalization in 17.1% Feasibility, 91.1%
	Kim et al,[42] 2011	70	0	Retrospective, single center	1.4	0	1.4	NA	NA	NA	Retreatment, 4.3%. Rebleeding rate, 0% over 25 mo follow-up
	Iijima et al,[38] 2005	142	46.8	Retrospective, single center	1	3	4	6	1	7	Retreatment, 10% Coiling was feasible in 96.5%

CLIP	Rodríguez-Hernández et al,[51] 2013	543	51.9	Retrospective	1.5	6.5	8	9.6	20.2	29.8	Improved or unchanged postsurgery was 86.9% in ruptured and 92.7% unruptured MCAAs
	Rinne et al,[19] 1996	561	100	Finnish study of consecutive cases	NA	NA	NA	13	25.6	32.6	Overall poor outcome was 32.6% vs 25% in the rest of anterior circulation
	Suzuki et al,[53] 1984	413	100	Retrospective, single center	NA	NA	NA	4.2	18.5	22.6	Early cases poor outcome, 20% vs 5.6% in the later cases
	Morgan et al,[54] 2010	263	0	Retrospective, single center, incidental: 263/339 MCAAs	0.4	4.6	5	NA	NA	NA	<60 y of age and ≤12 mm size had M&M of 0.6% (95% CI, 0%–3.8%) vs 22.2% (95% CI, 8.5%–45.8%) for those ≥60 y of age and >12 mm in size
	Moroi et al,[55] 2005	201	0	Retrospective, single center, unruptured	0	2.4	2.5	NA	NA	NA	Total permanent and temporary deficit was 5/201 (2.5%) with no mortality
	Choi et al,[56] 2012	125	0	Retrospective, single center	0	2.4	2.4	NA	NA	NA	Occlusion rate, 95.8%. Events: ICH, meningitis, wound infection
	van Dijk et al,[52] 2011	105	73.3	Retrospective, single center	NA	NA	NA	NA	NA	20	Rebleeding 1/77 of cases (1.3%) Occlusion rate, 89%
	Yeon et al,[35] 2011	91	0	Retrospective, single center	0	4.4	4.4	NA	NA	NA	Imaging infarction in 14/91 (15%). Permanent in 4.4%
	Zhu et al,[33] 2013	58	46.6	Retrospective, single center	NA	NA	NA	NA	NA	NA	Poor or death 11.9% (6.8% death). Retreatment, 1.7%; residual neck, 19%
	Son et al,[57] 2007	24	0	Retrospective, single center	0	0	0	NA	NA	NA	
	Park et al,[20] 2008	23	82.6	Retrospective	0	25	25	30.5	5.3	36.8	Permanent deficit 3/23 (13.04%) MCAA at frontal branch in 78.3%, and lenticulostriate in 13%

Abbreviations: I, Incidental or unruptured aneurysms; *N*, sample size; NA, not applicable; R, ruptured aneurysms.

statistical difference and a risk ratio of 1.01 (95% CI, 0.71–1.45).[2]

In a retrospective single-center study of 84 patients (90 MCAAs), 50 (20% SAH) patients were treated with ET compared with 34 (26.5% SAH) treated with surgical clipping. Six-month poor outcome (defined as an mRS 3–6) was 10% in the endovascular group versus 5.9% in the clipping group (*P* = .5). The complete obliteration rate was 86% versus 95%, respectively.[58]

In a single-center study comparing 30 MCAAs treated with coiling versus 78 clipped aneurysms during the same period, coiling was implemented for difficult clipping cases, whereas clipping was the first-choice therapy. The most common reason for performing coiling instead of clipping was a short M1 length in 17 of 30 patients (56.7%). Complete obliteration of the aneurysm was achieved in 28 of 30 (93%) patients who were treated with coiling and in 72 of 78 (92%) patients who were treated with clipping, with no difference in the M&M rates (3.3% vs 2.6%, respectively).[59]

Another single-center retrospective case series compared clipping with coiling in patients with ruptured MCAAs and demonstrated poor outcome (mRS 3–6) rates of 45% in 163 clipping cases versus 45% in 21 coiling cases. In unruptured MCAAs, only 4% in the clipping group versus 5% in the coiling group had a poor outcome.[60]

Finally, the risk of epilepsy after aneurysmal SAH was significantly higher in patients with MCAA treated with clipping as compared with those treated with coiling. In the coiling group, the risk for epilepsy at 1 year was 6.5% versus 11.5% for the clipping group.[61] **Table 2** summarizes some of the available comparative study results of the 2 treatment approaches.

Special Situations

There are certain features of MCAAs such as associated hematoma, complex shape, and location that may make treatment a challenge. Here, we briefly present some of these particularly challenging situations.

MCAA with cerebral hemorrhage and mass effect

ICH associated with ruptured MCAA poses a challenge and historically resulted in a bias toward hematoma evacuation and clipping in the same session. However, this approach may actually result in an increased risk of intraoperative aneurysm rupture due to detamponading, whereas the hematoma may make access to the aneurysm neck more complex.[62] Alternatively, performing coiling before evacuation may provide protection against detamponading. In a series of 300 MCAAs treated with coiling, 20 patients had associated

Table 2
Results from studies comparing clipping with coiling of MCAAs

Study	Study Design	Sample Size	Clipping (%)	Coiling (%)	Results
ISAT investigators	2005: SAH study, prospective, RCT Outcome: mRS >2	139 clipping vs 162 coiling	28.1	28.4	Risk ratio: 1.01 (95% CI, 0.71–1.45)
Güresir et al	2011: Retrospective, single center SAH outcome: mRS >2 long term	163 SAH clip vs 21 SAH coil	45	45	NS
	2011: Unruptured Outcome: mRS >2 long term	108 unruptured clip vs 38 unruptured coil	5	5	NS
Kim et al	2013: Retrospective, single center Mainly unruptured Permanent disability	30 coiling vs 78 clipping	2.6	3.3	NS
	Postoperative events		6.4	3.3	NS
	Obliteration rate		92	93	NS
Diaz et al	2012: Retrospective Both SAH and unruptured single-center study Outcomes: 6 mo mRS >2	50 (59.5%) coiling with 10/50 ruptured vs 34 (40.5%) clipping, 9/34 ruptured	5.9	10	0.5
	Obliteration rate		95	86	0.2

Abbreviation: RCT, randomized clinical trial.

ICH and/or mass effect where 40% had a good clinical outcome.[11] In another series of 30 patients with MCAA and ICH implementing a similar strategy of coiling followed by evacuation, 56.7% had a favorable Glasgow Outcome Scale of 4 and 5 at a mean follow-up of 18 months.[63]

Fusiform and blow out cerebral MCAAs

The percentage of aneurysms that are fusiform is small at 0.6% versus 3% in other locations.[19] The morphologic appearance of the MCAA offers potential for a combined approach of bypass procedure and coiling, open surgical clipping, or modified reconstructive surgery depending on the aneurysmal anatomy. In a series of 9 patients with large complex and fusiform aneurysms who underwent bypass surgery followed by clipping or trapping, 6 patients had long-term good outcomes and 3 patients had significant disability or death.[64] However, a similar approach may be applied with endovascular coiling and occlusion after bypass instead of the clip for trapping. In a 9-case series of giant/fusiform aneurysms, 3 cases were treated with coiling and 6 were treated with combination of Superficial temporal artery (STA)-MCA/occipital-MCA bypass surgery, which was performed first, followed by aneurysm coil embolization and occlusion. Only 1 in 9 patients had minor neurologic disability.[65]

Advances in ET may increase the proportion of aneurysms amenable to newer techniques that allow a reconstructive approach. Flow-diverting devices such as Pipeline Embolization Device (PED) (Covidien, Irvine, CA, USA) may also offer potential future ET for complex MCAAs without bypass procedures. Using PED to treat 10 complex MCAAs, 7 of which were fusiform, morbidity was seen in 3 of 10 (30%) cases with no mortality. Long-term occlusion was achieved in 7 of 9 (77.8%) cases.[66] In addition, one case report using the LEO stent (Balt, Montmorency, France) showed progressive thrombosis of the MCA fusiform aneurysm to complete reconstruction of the arterial lumen with no recurrence.[67]

M1 segment aneurysms

A small proportion (16%) of MCAAs is located in the proximal segment.[19,27] Zhou and colleagues[68] examined 29 MCAAs (both ruptured and unruptured) involving the M1 segment that were treated mainly with primary coiling, stent-assisted coiling (1 of 3), and with balloon assistance (1 case) and found a periprocedural neurologic deterioration rate of 2 of 29 (6.9%). In a larger series of endovascular coiling involving 59 patients (61 M1 aneurysms, 43 involving the superior wall and 17 the inferior wall), no permanent disability or mortality was reported, with 1 delayed transient neurologic deficit. Long-term complete occlusion or residual neck was attained in 87% of patients with a 4.3% major recurrence rate.[69]

Clipping outcome was reported in several studies, with one of these studies examining the outcome in 23 patients with 25 M1 aneurysms (SAH in 19 of 25).[20] Eighteen of the aneurysms involved early frontal branches and 3 involved the lenticulostriate arteries. Fixed severe disability was seen in 3 of 23 (13%) patients.[20]

Adjunctive devices

Adjunctive devices such as stents and balloons improve the ability to treat wide-neck and complex-shaped aneurysms.[10,36] In our initial series spanning 2005 to 2011 with 161 MCAAs, stent-assisted coiling was used in 34% of the cases and balloon remodeling in 9%, for a total of 43%. The use of adjunctive devices allowed us to achieve an endovascular feasibility rate of 98.2% as the first choice in our nonselective cohort.[10] In a prospective registry looking at outcomes and its predictors in 120 patients with 131 MCAAs treated with endovascular coiling nonselectively (34.2% presented with SAH), 33 (25.2%) were treated with coiling, 79 (60.3%) with balloon-assisted coiling, and 19 (14.5%) with stent-assisted coiling. The 1-month permanent morbidity (mRS$\leq$2) and mortality rates were 3.3%. No significant difference was found between endovascular techniques.[70]

In 23 patients with unruptured MCAAs treated with stent-assisted coiling using Neuroform (Stryker, Fremont, CA, USA) stents, a success rate was seen in 22 of 23 (96%) patients. There were no mortalities or morbidities. The aneurysm occlusion rate was 83%, with a 17% recurrence rate and only 1 in 18 (6%) of the cases with follow-up required retreatment. No bleeding or neurologic events were seen with median follow-up of 1 year.[71]

In addition, stent-assisted coiling was used in 16 patients harboring 16 MCAAs. Seventeen stents were deployed in this series: 12 Neuroform, 4 LEO, and 1 Enterprise (Codman, MA, USA). Of the 13 aneurysms treated with stent-assisted coil embolization, 10 (77%) had complete aneurysm occlusion or residual neck, whereas residual aneurysm was present in 3. Procedure-related morbidity occurred in 1 of 16 patients with no permanent deficit. There was no rebleeding or other adverse neurologic events at the mean follow-up of 20.1 months.[72] The Y-stent technique can be implemented to span the aneurysm neck and protect the superior and inferior divisions using most of the aneurysm stents available on the market with good results.[73] **Fig. 4** illustrates the use of

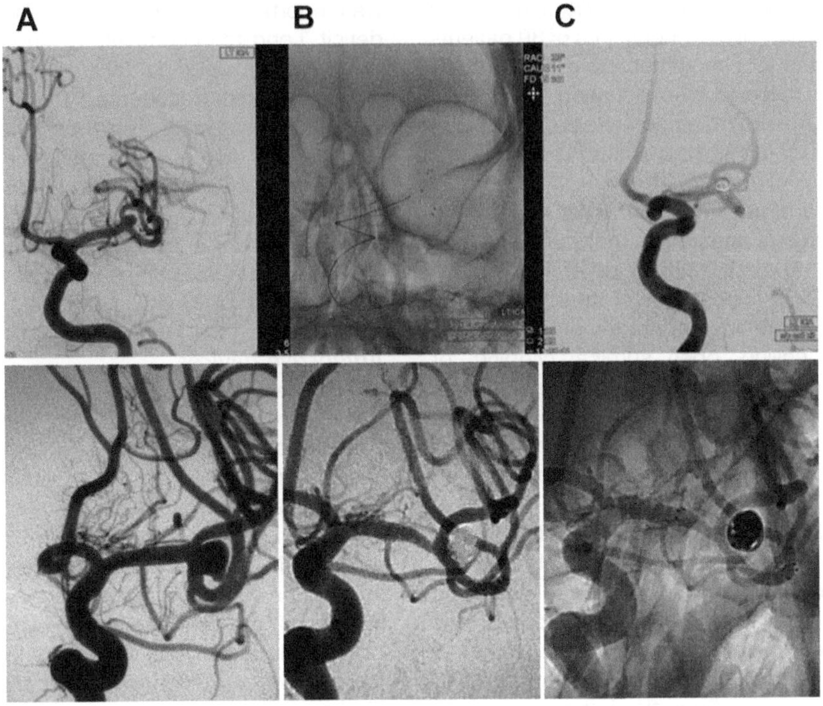

Fig. 4. Two cases of MCAAs treated with stent assistance (Y-stent upper case, and single stent into the inferior division, the lower case) and Penumbra 400 coils. Upper panel demonstrates an MCA bifurcation aneurysm, before (*A*) and after (*C*) angiograms of a Y configuration stent-assisted MCA aneurysm coiling. (*B*) The figure displays the native image after stent deployment. Notice the angulations of the 2 branches making stent deployment less challenging. Case 2 is depicted in the lower panel with precoiling angiogram and 6-month follow-up angiogram with single stent showing complete and persistent obliteration of the MCA bifurcation aneurysm. The native image on the left-hand side shows complete endothelialization at the aneurysm neck.

Y-stents in one of the cases and single stent in another case.

Future Directions

ET continues to improve and newer devices and techniques are specifically trying address the shortcomings of the current technology. In addition to potential improvements to flow diverters that make them more feasible and safe to treat MCAAs, promising new devices for the MCAAs are currently being evaluated in humans, including Web (Sequent medical, Aliso Viejo, CA, USA), Luna AES (Nfocus Neuromedical, Palo Alto, CA, USA), and pCONus (Phenox GmbH, Bochum, Germany). The pCONus stent-based platform device has distal ends that open like a blossoming flower inside the proximal end of the aneurysm and is available currently in Europe.[74] In addition, primary coiling with compaction resistance coils may reduce the likelihood of recurrence. Finally, **Fig. 4** shows an example of 2 cases we treated in our institution using the Y-stent technique with Penumbra-400 coils (Penumbra Inc, Alameda, CA, USA).

SUMMARY

The MCA is the most common location for cerebral aneurysms and is associated with a lower risk of rupture than aneurysms located in the anterior or posterior communicating arteries. There is no definitive evidence to support the superiority of clipping over coiling to treat MCAA or vice versa. The current available data and review of the literature indicate that the feasibility of treating the MCAA with ET as the first choice of treatment in cohorts of nonselected aneurysms exceeds 90%. No significant increase in the risk of rebleeding with endovascular approaches was shown and there are no significant differences in the long-term M&M between the 2 treatments. However, the review of the literature indicates that treatment of MCAAs is also associated with low M&M rates with surgical clipping in unruptured aneurysms. Based on the literature, it seems that there is no significant difference between the 2, therapies with only hypothetical advantages of one approach over another. A randomized clinical trial comparing the 2 approaches in nonselected cases with long-term follow-up will shed light on which patients may benefit from one approach over another.

REFERENCES

1. Molyneux AJ, Kerr RS, Stratton I, et al. International Subarachnoid Aneurysm Trial (ISAT) of neurosurgical clipping versus endovascular coiling in 2143 patients with ruptured intracranial aneurysms: a randomised trial. Lancet 2002;360:1267–74.
2. Molyneux AJ, Kerr RS, Yu LM, et al. International Subarachnoid Aneurysm Trial (ISAT) of neurosurgical clipping versus endovascular coiling in 2143 patients with ruptured intracranial aneurysms: a randomised comparison of effects on survival, dependency, seizures, rebleeding, subgroups, and aneurysm occlusion. Lancet 2005;366:809–17.
3. McDougall CG, Spetzler RF, Zabramski JM, et al. The barrow ruptured aneurysm trial. J Neurosurg 2012;116(1):135–44.
4. Spetzler RF, McDougall CG, Albuquerque FC, et al. The barrow ruptured aneurysm trial: 3-year results. J Neurosurg 2013;119(1):146–57.
5. Lanzino G, Murad MH, d'Urso PI, et al. Coil embolization versus clipping for ruptured intracranial aneurysms: a meta-analysis of prospective controlled published studies. AJNR Am J Neuroradiol 2013; 34(9):1764–8.
6. Brinjikji W, Lanzino G, Rabinstein AA, et al. Age-related trends in the treatment and outcomes of ruptured cerebral aneurysms: a study of the nationwide inpatient sample 2001-2009. AJNR Am J Neuroradiol 2013;34(5):1022–7.
7. Regli L, Uske A, de Tribolet N. Endovascular coil placement compared with surgical clipping for the treatment of unruptured middle cerebral artery aneurysms: a consecutive series. J Neurosurg 1999;90:1025–30.
8. Regli L, Dehdashti AR, Uske A, et al. Endovascular coiling compared with surgical clipping for the treatment of unruptured middle cerebral artery aneurysms: an update. Acta Neurochir Suppl 2002; 82:41–6.
9. Lozano AM, Lázaro RC, Andrés JM. Endovascular treatment of cerebral aneurysms: review of a ten year experience. Neurologia 2009;24(9):797–803.
10. Pandya D, Lazzaro M, Fitzsimmons BF, et al. Endovascular treatment of middle cerebral artery aneurysm: single center case series. Neurology 2012; 78. P05.251.
11. Mortimer AM, Bradley MD, Mews P, et al. Endovascular treatment of 300 consecutive middle cerebral artery aneurysms: clinical and radiologic outcomes. AJNR Am J Neuroradiol 2014;35(4):706–14.
12. Umansky F, Juarez SM, Dujovny M, et al. Microsurgical anatomy of the proximal segments of the middle cerebral artery. J Neurosurg 1984;61(3): 458–67.
13. Jain KK. Some observations on the anatomy of the middle cerebral artery. Can J Surg 1964;7(2): 134–9.
14. Gibo H, Carver CC, Rhoton AL Jr, et al. Microsurgical anatomy of the middle cerebral artery. J Neurosurg 1981;54(2):151–69.
15. Kahilogullari G, Ugur HC, Comert A, et al. The branching pattern of the middle cerebral artery: is the intermediate trunk real or not? An anatomical study correlating with simple angiography. J Neurosurg 2012;116(5):1024 34.
16. Delong WB. Anatomy of the middle cerebral artery: the temporal branches. Stroke 1973;4:412–8.
17. Uchino A, Saito N, Okada Y, et al. Duplicate origin and fenestration of the middle cerebral artery on MR angiography. Surg Radiol Anat 2012;34(5): 401–4.
18. Zaidat OO, Kalia JS, Batista LM, et al. For Endovascular Coiling of Small Aneurysm multicenter study group (ECOSA study). Safety and feasibility of elective endovascular coiling of very small (2-7 mm) Unruptured Cerebral Aneurysms (ECOSA Study): a multicenter experience analysis. Stroke 2010; 41(4):E242.
19. Rinne J, Hernesniemi J, Niskanen M, et al. Analysis of 561 patients with 690 middle cerebral artery aneurysms: anatomic and clinical features as correlated to management outcome. Neurosurgery 1996;38:2–11.
20. Park DH, Kang SH, Lee JB, et al. Angiographic features, surgical management and outcomes of proximal middle cerebral artery aneurysms. Clin Neurol Neurosurg 2008;110(6):544–51.
21. UCAS Japan Investigators, Morita A, Kirino T, et al. The natural course of unruptured cerebral aneurysms in a Japanese cohort. N Engl J Med 2012; 366(26):2474–82.
22. Wiebers DO, Whisnant JP, Huston J 3rd, et al, International Study of Unruptured Intracranial Aneurysms Investigators. Unruptured intracranial aneurysms: natural history, clinical outcome, and risks of surgical and endovascular treatment. Lancet 2003;362(9378):103–10.
23. Pierot L, Spelle L, Vitry F, ATENA Investigators. Immediate clinical outcome of patients harboring unruptured intracranial aneurysms treated by endovascular approach: results of the ATENA study. Stroke 2008;39(9):2497–504.
24. Unruptured intracranial aneurysms — risk of rupture and risks of surgical intervention. The international study of unruptured intracranial aneurysms investigators. N Engl J Med 1998;339: 1725–33.
25. Dashti R, Hernesniemi J, Niemelä M, et al. Microneurosurgical management of distal middle

cerebral artery aneurysms. Surg Neurol 2007; 67(6):553–63.
26. Dashti R, Hernesniemi J, Niemelä M, et al. Microneurosurgical management of middle cerebral artery bifurcation aneurysms. Surg Neurol 2007; 67(5):441–56.
27. Dashti R, Rinne J, Hernesniemi J, et al. Microneurosurgical management of proximal middle cerebral artery aneurysms. Surg Neurol 2007;67(1):6–14.
28. Quadros RS, Gallas S, Noudel R, et al. Endovascular treatment of middle cerebral artery aneurysms as first option: a single center experience of 92 aneurysms. AJNR Am J Neuroradiol 2007;28(8):1567–72.
29. Ronkainen A, Niskanen M, Piironen R, et al. Familial subarachnoid hemorrhage. Outcome study. Stroke 1999;30(5):1099–102.
30. Ronkainen A, Hernesniemi J, Ryynanen M. Familial subarachnoid hemorrhage in East Finland 1977-1990. Neurosurgery 1993;33:787–97.
31. Mehan WA Jr, Romero JM, Hirsch JA, et al. Unruptured intracranial aneurysms conservatively followed with serial CT angiography: could morphology and growth predict rupture? J Neurointerv Surg 2013. http://dx.doi.org/10.1136/neurintsurg-2013-010944.
32. Elsharkawy A, Lehečka M, Niemelä M, et al. A new, more accurate classification of middle cerebral artery aneurysms: computed tomography angiographic study of 1,009 consecutive cases with 1,309 middle cerebral artery aneurysms. Neurosurgery 2013;73(1):94–102 [discussion: 102].
33. Zhu W, Liu P, Tian Y, et al. Complex middle cerebral artery aneurysms: a new classification based on the angioarchitecture and surgical strategies. Acta Neurochir (Wien) 2013;155(8):1481–91.
34. Schebesch KM, Proescholdt M, Steib K, et al. Morphology of middle cerebral artery aneurysms: impact on surgical strategy and on postoperative outcome. ISRN Stroke 2013;2013:7. http://dx.doi.org/10.1155/2013/838292. Article ID 838292.
35. Yeon JY, Kim JS, Hong SC. Angiographic characteristics of unruptured middle cerebral artery aneurysms predicting perforator injuries. Br J Neurosurg 2011;25(4):497–502.
36. Vendrell JF, Menjot N, Costalat V, et al. Endovascular treatment of 174 middle cerebral artery aneurysms: clinical outcome and radiologic results at long-term follow-up. Radiology 2009;253(1):191–8.
37. Suzuki S, Tateshima S, Jahan R, et al. Endovascular treatment of middle cerebral artery aneurysms with detachable coils: angiographic and clinical outcomes in 115 consecutive patients. Neurosurgery 2009;64(5):876–88 [discussion: 888–9].
38. Iijima A, Piotin M, Mounayer C, et al. Endovascular treatment with coils of 149 middle cerebral artery berry aneurysms. Radiology 2005;237:611–9.
39. Gory B, Rouchaud A, Saleme S, et al. Endovascular treatment of middle cerebral artery aneurysms for 120 nonselected patients: a prospective cohort study. AJNR Am J Neuroradiol 2014;35(4):715–20.
40. Bracard S, Abdel-Kerim A, Thuillier L, et al. Endovascular coil occlusion of 152 middle cerebral artery aneurysms: initial and midterm angiographic and clinical results. J Neurosurg 2010;112(4): 703–8.
41. Vanzin JR, Mounayer C, Piotin M, et al. Endovascular treatment of unruptured middle cerebral artery aneurysms. J Neuroradiol 2005;32(2):97–108.
42. Kim BM, Kim DI, Park SI, et al. Coil embolization of unruptured middle cerebral artery aneurysms. Neurosurgery 2011;68(2):346–53 [discussion: 353–4].
43. Oishi H, Yoshida K, Shimizu T, et al. Endovascular treatment with bare platinum coils for middle cerebral artery aneurysms. Neurol Med Chir (Tokyo) 2009;49(7):287–93.
44. Jin SC, Kwon OK, Oh CW, et al. Simple coiling using single or multiple catheters without balloons or stents in middle cerebral artery bifurcation aneurysms. Neuroradiology 2013;55(3):321–6.
45. Doerfler A, Wanke I, Goericke SL, et al. Endovascular treatment of middle cerebral artery aneurysms with electrolytically detachable coils. AJNR Am J Neuroradiol 2006;27:513–20.
46. Hirota N, Musacchio M, Cardoso M, et al. Angiographic and clinical results after endovascular treatment for middle cerebral artery berry aneurysms. Neuroradiol J 2007;20(1):89–101.
47. Abla AA, Jahshan S, Kan P, et al. Results of endovascular treatment of middle cerebral artery aneurysms after first giving consideration to clipping. Acta Neurochir (Wien) 2013;155(4):559–68. http://dx.doi.org/10.1007/s00701-012-1594-8.
48. Horowitz M, Gupta R, Gologorsky Y, et al. Clinical and anatomic outcomes after endovascular coiling of middle cerebral artery aneurysms: report on 30 treated aneurysms and review of the literature. Surg Neurol 2006;66(2):167–71 [discussion: 171].
49. Lubicz B, Graca J, Levivier M, et al. Endovascular treatment of middle cerebral artery aneurysms. Neurocrit Care 2006;5:93–101.
50. Brinjikji W, Lanzino G, Cloft HJ, et al. Endovascular treatment of middle cerebral artery aneurysms: a systematic review and single-center series. Neurosurgery 2011;68(2):397–402 [discussion: 402].
51. Rodríguez-Hernández A, Sughrue ME, Akhavan S, et al. Current management of middle cerebral artery aneurysms: surgical results with a "clip first" policy. Neurosurgery 2013;72(3):415–27.
52. van Dijk JM, Groen RJ, Ter Laan M, et al. Surgical clipping as the preferred treatment for aneurysms of the middle cerebral artery. Acta Neurochir (Wien) 2011;153(11):2111–7.
53. Suzuki J, Yoshimoto T, Kayama T. Surgical treatment of middle cerebral artery aneurysms. J Neurosurg 1984;61:17–23.

54. Morgan MK, Mahattanakul W, Davidson A, et al. Outcome for middle cerebral artery aneurysm surgery. Neurosurgery 2010;67(3):755–61 [discussion: 761].
55. Moroi J, Hadeishi H, Suzuki A, et al. Morbidity and mortality from surgical treatment of unruptured cerebral aneurysms at Research Institute for Brain and Blood Vessels-Akita. Neurosurgery 2005; 56(2):224–31 [discussion: 224–31].
56. Choi SW, Ahn JS, Park JC, et al. Surgical treatment of unruptured intracranial middle cerebral artery aneurysms: angiographic and clinical outcomes in 143 aneurysms. J Cerebrovasc Endovasc Neurosurg 2012;14(4):289–94.
57. Son YJ, Han DH, Kim JE. Image-guided surgery for treatment of unruptured middle cerebral artery aneurysms. Neurosurgery 2007;61(5 Suppl 2):266–71 [discussion: 271–2].
58. Diaz OM, Rangel-Castilla L, Barber S, et al. Middle cerebral artery aneurysms: a single-center series comparing endovascular and surgical treatment. World Neurosurg 2014;81(2):322–9. http://dx.doi.org/10.1016/j.wneu.2012.12.011. pii: S1878-8750(12)01443-X.
59. Kim KH, Cha KC, Kim JS, et al. Endovascular coiling of middle cerebral artery aneurysms as an alternative to surgical clipping. J Clin Neurosci 2013;20(4):520–2.
60. Güresir E, Schuss P, Berkefeld J, et al. Treatment results for complex middle cerebral artery aneurysms. A prospective single-center series. Acta Neurochir (Wien) 2011;153(6):1247–52.
61. Hart Y, Sneade M, Birks J, et al. Epilepsy after subarachnoid hemorrhage: the frequency of seizures after clip occlusion or coil embolization of a ruptured cerebral aneurysm: results from the International Subarachnoid Aneurysm Trial. Neurosurgery 2011;115:1159–68.
62. Houkin K, Kuroda S, Takahashi A, et al. Intra-operative premature rupture of the cerebral aneurysms. Analysis of the causes and management. Acta Neurochir (Wien) 1999;141:1255–63.
63. Tawk RG, Pandey A, Levy E, et al. Coiling of ruptured aneurysms followed by evacuation of hematoma. World Neurosurg 2010;74:626–31.
64. Seo BR, Kim TS, Joo SP, et al. Surgical strategies using cerebral revascularization in complex middle cerebral artery aneurysms. Clin Neurol Neurosurg 2009;111(8):670–5.
65. Shi ZS, Ziegler J, Duckwiler GR, et al. Management of giant middle cerebral artery aneurysms with incorporated branches: partial endovascular coiling or combined extracranial-intracranial bypass–a team approach. Neurosurgery 2009;65(Suppl 6): 121–9 [discussion: 129–31].
66. Zanaty M, Chalouhi N, Tjoumakaris SI, et al. Flow diversion for complex middle cerebral artery aneurysms. Neuroradiology 2014. [Epub ahead of print].
67. Pumar JM, Lete I, Pardo MI, et al. LEO stent monotherapy for the endovascular reconstruction of fusiform aneurysms of the middle cerebral artery. AJNR Am J Neuroradiol 2008;29:1775–6.
68. Zhou Y, Yang PF, Fang YB, et al. Endovascular treatment for saccular aneurysms of the proximal (M1) segment of the middle cerebral artery. Acta Neurochir (Wien) 2012;154(10):1835–43.
69. Cho YD, Lee WJ, Kim KM, et al. Endovascular coil embolization of middle cerebral artery aneurysms of the proximal (M1) segment. Neuroradiology 2013;55(9):1097–102.
70. Vendrell JF, Costalat V, Brunel H, et al. Stent-assisted coiling of complex middle cerebral artery aneurysms: initial and midterm results. AJNR Am J Neuroradiol 2011;32:259–63.
71. Fields JD, Brambrink L, Dogan A, et al. Stent assisted coil embolization of unruptured middle cerebral artery aneurysms. J Neurointerv Surg 2013;5(1): 15–9.
72. Yang P, Liu J, Huang Q, et al. Endovascular treatment of wide-neck middle cerebral artery aneurysms with stents: a review of 16 cases. AJNR Am J Neuroradiol 2010;31(5):940–6.
73. Sani S, Lopes DK. Treatment of a middle cerebral artery bifurcation aneurysm using a double neuroform stent "Y" configuration and coil embolization: technical case report. Neurosurgery 2005;57:E209.
74. Mpotsaris A, Henkes H, Weber W. Waffle Y technique: pCONus for tandem bifurcation aneurysms of the middle cerebral artery. J Neurointerv Surg 2013:1–3.

Vertebrobasilar Fusiform Aneurysms

Joseph C. Serrone, MD[a], Yair M. Gozal, MD, PhD[a], Aaron W. Grossman, MD, PhD[a], Norberto Andaluz, MD[b], Todd Abruzzo, MD[b,c], Mario Zuccarello, MD[b], Andrew Ringer, MD[b,*]

KEYWORDS

• Aneurysm • Vertebrobasilar • Vertebral • Fusiform • Dolichoectatic

KEY POINTS

- Vertebrobasilar aneurysms present most commonly with brainstem ischemic stroke or compressive symptoms of the brainstem, cerebellum, or cranial nerves.
- The natural history of patients with fusiform vertebrobasilar aneurysms presenting with ischemic stroke or compressive symptoms is for the presenting signs and symptoms to steadily progress.
- Flow reduction or flow reversal is the most time-tested management strategy for fusiform vertebrobasilar aneurysms presenting with compressive symptoms, but this treatment relies largely on the presence of adequate collateralization through the posterior communicating arteries.
- Mixed results have been reported with the use of flow diversion for fusiform vertebrobasilar aneurysms, and their use should be reserved for patients with compressive symptoms and poor collateralization through the posterior communicating arteries.
- Patients with vertebrobasilar aneurysms presenting with ischemic stroke and no compressive symptoms are best managed with anticoagulation.

INTRODUCTION

Vertebrobasilar fusiform aneurysms are among the most daunting lesions treated by cerebrovascular surgeons. Many names have been linked to these lesions, including giant serpentine aneurysm, giant fusiform aneurysm, S aneurysm, megadolichobasilar artery, dolichoectacic artery, fusiform aneurysm, and transitional aneurysm. Perhaps the most universal definition of these lesions is aneurysms with separate inflow and outflow ostia. The earliest descriptions of fusiform aneurysms of the vertebrobasilar arterial system were most consistent with a dolichoectatic basilar artery. There is no arteriography available for most cases, and most patients presented with cranial neuropathies.[1]

A fusiform aneurysm of the basilar artery was first described by Wells in 1922[2] on surgical exploration in a patient with paresis of cranial nerves 6 to 8 and obstructive hydrocephalus. Dr Walter Dandy[3] operated on a series of 10 patients with trigeminal neuralgia and described a so-called S aneurysm. Greitz and Lofstedt[4] in 1954 reported 5 cases of ectasia of the basilar artery. The patients of their series were more consistent with compressive or ischemic presentations that are associated with fusiform aneurysms. Reports since this time have drastically expanded our understanding of these lesions. In this article, fusiform vertebrobasilar aneurysms are reviewed, including incidence, presentation, natural history, pathophysiology, and treatment, with a suggested algorithm for treatment based on review of the literature. Dissecting aneurysms, which have a distinct behavior of presenting with subarachnoid

Disclosures: None.
[a] Department of Neurosurgery, UC College of Medicine, Cincinnati, OH, USA; [b] Comprehensive Stroke Center, UC Neuroscience Institute, Cincinnati, OH, USA; [c] Mayfield Clinic, Cincinnati, OH, USA
* Corresponding author. 260 Stetson Street, Suite 2200, Cincinnati, OH 45267.
E-mail address: aringer@mayfieldclinic.com

Neurosurg Clin N Am 25 (2014) 471–484
http://dx.doi.org/10.1016/j.nec.2014.04.006
1042-3680/14/$ – see front matter

hemorrhage (SAH) followed by frequent early rebleeding, are not discussed.[5–9]

INCIDENCE

The incidence of fusiform aneurysms of the vertebrobasilar system is low. Dolichoectasia of any intracranial artery in the general population is estimated at less than 0.05%.[10] In cases of vertebral angiography, the incidence ranges from 17 of 10,000 (0.17%) for all indications to 132 of 2265 (5.8%) in cases of stroke.[11,12] Another series of 387 patients undergoing computed tomography (CT) or magnetic resonance (MR) angiography (MRA) for stroke showed 10 patients (2.6%) with vertebrobasilar dolichoectasia.[13] Autopsy series also show a wide range, but remain low in incidence, ranging from 6 of 5762 (0.10%) in a series from 1914 to 1956 at Columbia University[14] to 5 of 7500 (0.07%) in a VA hospital series.[15] One clinical series of treated posterior circulation aneurysms[16] classified 4 of 528 (0.76%) aneurysms as fusiform vertebrobasilar aneurysms.

The discrepancy in incidence in these studies is likely related to a combination of the loose definitions of these lesions and subselection. In addition, the incidence may increase in high-risk populations. Yu and colleagues[11] found a strong correlation with hypertension (64%) and tobacco smoking (74%) with intracranial arterial ectasia. In addition, Mitsias and Levine[17] described a high incidence in Fabry disease, with symptomatic disease of a dilated vertebrobasilar system found in 60% of heterozygotes and 67% of homozygotes. Conversely, vertebrobasilar aneurysms have been reported in children but are rare.[18–20] In 3000 postmortem brain examinations in children, Housepian and Pool[14] found no case of any intracranial aneurysm.

PRESENTATION

Because of the low incidence of these lesions and the relative paucity of reported cases, initial reports focused primarily on the striking pathologic features and rarely provided adequate clinical details.[1] However, a review of published series and case reports shows some common features. Unlike saccular aneurysms, vertebrobasilar fusiform aneurysms show a significant male predominance, accounting for greater than 70% of the 408 reported cases (**Tables 1** and **2**). Although affected patients ranged from age 5 years to 87 years, the average reported age at diagnosis was ~60 years, significantly older than that typically presenting with saccular aneurysms.[21] Although not often reported, commonly encountered comorbidities include hypertension (31%–69%), diabetes mellitus (10%–15%), hyperlipidemia (40%), coronary artery disease (23%–28%), and smoking (50%).[21,28,31] Data regarding connective tissue disorders were almost universally absent, an oddity given the mechanisms underlying vessel ectasia and the known importance of family history in the risk of aneurysm formation.[39,40] This subject was addressed only in the well-studied Mayo Clinic cohort, in whom 4% were found to have a known connective tissue disorder, including Fabry disease and autosomal-dominant polycystic kidney disease.[21,41,42]

In addition to the small subset of patients in whom vertebrobasilar fusiform aneurysms were incidentally diagnosed, the presenting symptoms in most patients are related to 3 basic mechanisms: mass effect, ischemia, or aneurysmal rupture. Mass effect, which was observed in 43% of patients (see **Table 1**), occurred when the ectatic vessel compressed surrounding tissues, including the brainstem and cerebellum, resulting in numerous cranial nerve palsies or in noncommunicating hydrocephalus, and typically developed over years.[1,28] In our experience, even although the clinical course is characteristically slowly progressive, it is often punctuated by stuttering episodes of abrupt exacerbation, typically as an early manifestation but also as a late preterminal manifestation. These episodes often correspond to intramural hemorrhage or microdissection evident on brain MR imaging (MRI) studies (**Fig. 1**).

When discussing cranial neuropathies caused by vertebrobasilar fusiform aneurysms, the most common cranial nerves involved are V to VIII.[21] Nishizaki and colleagues,[25] for example, reported dysfunction affecting the facial nerve in 4 of 6 patients, whereas in Herpers and colleagues' study,[26] hemifacial spasm accounted for 22% of patients presenting with compressive cause. Similarly, trigeminal neuralgia and abducens nerve palsy were frequently implicated as clinical correlates of brainstem compression.[1,26–29] Defects involving other cranial nerves, including cranial nerves IX, X, and XII, were more rarely described.[25,33] Although varying by aneurysm location, obstructive hydrocephalus was consistently reported as a sequela of brainstem compression.[21,23,28] In many of these patients, headache was a principal presenting symptom.[28]

Perhaps the most common presentation of patients with vertebrobasilar fusiform aneurysms involves ischemic stroke symptoms. Accounting for ~44% of patients (see **Table 1**), this subgroup comprises clinical syndromes ranging from transient ischemic attacks (TIAs) to catastrophic pontine ischemia consistent with a locked-in

Table 1
Summary of the principal clinical presentation in studies of vertebrobasilar fusiform aneurysms

Author, Year	Number of Patients	Male (n) (%)	Mass Effect	Ischemic Event	SAH	Notable
Flemming et al,[21] 2005	159	118 (74)	35	44	5	63 (incidental)
Drake & Peerless,[22] 1997	61	30 (49)	35	15	NR	11 (headache)
Coert et al,[23] 2007	39	NR	8	5	26	
Milandre et al,[24] 1991	23	16 (76)	13	9	1	
Nishizaki et al,[25] 1986	23	19 (82)	6	11	2	2 (incidental); 1 (cerebellar intracranial hemorrhage)
Herpers et al,[26] 1983	22	11 (50)	9	9	1	2 (incidental); 1 (dementia)
Anson et al,[27] 1996	20	17 (85)	10	5	4	
Echiverri et al,[28] 1989	13	11 (85)	4	9	1	
Boeri & Passerini,[1] 1964	10	7 (70)	8	NR	2	
Kalani et al,[29] 2013	7	6 (86)	6	1	0	
Pessin et al,[30] 1989	7	5 (71)	0	7	0	
Giang et al,[31] 1988	6	5 (83)	3	2	0	1 (incidental)
Meckel et al,[32] 2013	5	4 (80)	3	2	0	
Nakatomi,[39] 2000	4	3 (75)	3	1	0	
Sluzewski et al,[33] 2001	3	3 (100)	1	1	1	
Wenderoth et al,[34] 2003	2	2 (100)	0	1	1	
Binning et al,[35] 2011	1	1 (100)	1	0	0	
Cohen,[74] 2012	1	1 (100)	0	1	0	
Greenberg,[93] 2007	1	1 (100)	0	0	1	
Islak et al,[36] 2002	1	0 (0)	0	0	1	

Abbreviation: NR, not reported.

syndrome.[27] In the Mayo Clinic cohort, Flemming and colleagues[21] further delineated the distribution of infarction in these patients, showing a preference for the pons (50%), lateral medulla (9%), cerebellar hemispheres (7%), midbrain/thalamus (4.5%), and occipital lobes (4.5%). TIAs comprised 25% of clinical presentations in the population of patients with ischemia. In the cohort described by Echiverri and colleagues,[28] ischemic insult most often affected the pons (33%) and thalamus (11%), whereas 55% of patients experienced TIAs alone. Similarly, in a review of 23 dolichoectatic vertebrobasilar aneurysms, Nishizaki and colleagues[25] identified ischemia to the pons (30%) and temporal lobe (9%). Cerebral lacunar infarcts accounted for 17% of patients in this series, whereas TIAs and vertebrobasilar insufficiency occurred in 22% of patients. Pessin and colleagues[30] found that 43% of patients presented with extensive ischemic insult to the pons. The remaining patients in this series initially suffered TIAs (57%) and subsequently progressed to develop formal ischemic lesions.

Unlike giant saccular aneurysms, aneurysmal rupture is, perhaps, the least common diagnostic phenotype of vertebrobasilar fusiform aneurysms.[43] Invariably developing sudden headache with or without focal neurologic signs, only ~13% of all patients (see **Table 1**) presented with corresponding SAH.[21] Most of these patients were described in a study on the treatment of vertebrobasilar aneurysms at Stanford University.[23] In this report, only 39% of 26 patients with ruptured fusiform aneurysms had good neurologic status (Hunt and Hess grade 1–2). Conversely, 61% of patients presented with a pretreatment Hunt and Hess grade of 3 to 4. In all, aneurysmal rupture comprised 67% of their study population. In contrast, only 23% of patients in Anson and colleague' study[27] and 3% of described cases in Flemming and colleagues' study[21] presented with SAH. All 5 patients with SAH in Flemming and colleagues' study[21] were of a poor clinical grade.

NATURAL HISTORY

The natural history of vertebrobasilar fusiform aneurysms is dependent on the presenting signs and symptoms. Flemming and colleagues[21] reported the most complete longitudinal evaluation

Table 2
Surgical/endovascular series with ≥5 patients

Author, Year	Years Treated	n	Location	Aneurysm Type	Treatment (%)	Good Outcome by Location (%)[a]
Drake & Peerless,[22] 1997	1965–1992	61	Basilar (37) VBJ (10) Vertebral (14)	Fusiform	Flow reduction (18) Flow reversal (64) Trapping (10) Wrap/explore (7) Clip reconstruction (2)	Basilar (73) VBJ (60) Vertebral (64)
Coert et al,[23] 2007	1991–2005	39	Basilar/VBJ (18) Vertebral/PICA (21)	Fusiform/dolichoectatic	Surgery (26) Embolization (67) Surgery and embolization (8)	Basilar/VBJ (39) Vertebral/PICA (62)
Anson et al,[27] 1996	1986–1994	19	Basilar (8) VBJ (5) Vertebral (6)	Fusiform (13) Dolichoectatic (6)	Heterogeneous[b]	Basilar (28) VBJ (80) Vertebral (83)
Leibowitz et al,[37] 2003	1997–2000	10	Basilar (1) VBJ (5) Vertebral (4)	Fusiform	Endovascular balloon or coil occlusion	Basilar/VBJ (16)[c] Vertebral (25)[d]
Aymard et al,[38] 1991	NR	9	Basilar (3) VBJ (3) Vertebral (3)	Fusiform	Endovascular balloon occlusion	Basilar (33) VBJ (100) Vertebral (67)

Abbreviations: GOS, glasgow outcome score; NR, not reported; PICA, posterior inferior cerebellar artery; VBJ, vertebrobasilar junction.
[a] mRS ≤2, GOS ≥4, or reported good or normal.
[b] Combinations of thrombectomy with aneurysmorrhaphy, proximal or distal occlusion, bypasses, anticoagulation, clip reconstruction, trapping.
[c] Continued aneurysm filling in all cases; 67% died.
[d] All completely occluded, 100% improved mRS from presentation.

of fusiform vertebrobasilar aneurysms over a 12-year period, yielding 159 cases with 719 patient-years of follow-up. Dissecting vertebrobasilar aneurysms were excluded from this analysis.[41,42] These lesions were defined as having a vessel caliber 1.5 times normal without an identifiable neck as previously defined by Huber.[44] These investigators proposed a radiographic classification of vertebrobasilar fusiform aneurysms, including fusiform = aneurysmal dilation of the involved segment; dolichoectactic = uniform dilation of the involved segment; transitional = uniform dilation of the involved segment with superimposed aneurysmal dilation.

In the classification scheme by Flemming and colleagues,[21] 57% of patients had a dolichoectatic artery, 25% had a transitional aneurysm, and 18% had a fusiform aneurysm. Of patients in this series, 20.8% had an indeterminate type. The transitional-type or fusiform-type aneurysms were more likely to be symptomatic than dolichoectactic aneurysms. In this series, predictors for mortality after adjustment for age were transitional type (hazard ratio [HR] = 3.56), fusiform type (HR = 7.7), and basilar involvement (HR = 8.77). Conversely, dolichoectatic aneurysms appeared more benign. Of patients presenting asymptomatically, 66% had a dolichoectatic-type aneurysm. Asymptomatic patients did not often become symptomatic, developing stroke caused by the aneurysm in 7.8% of cases, mass effect caused by aneurysm in 3.1% of cases, and hemorrhage in 1.6%. In their description of nonatheromatous fusiform cerebral aneurysms, Mizutani and colleagues[7] reported the natural history of 6 vertebrobasilar dolichoectatic lesions (Mizutani type 2). Similar to the findings by Flemming and colleagues,[21] all dolichoectatic vertebrobasilar aneurysms reported by Mizutani and colleagues[7] were incidentally discovered with no significant neurologic sequelae in 2 to 5 years of follow-up. Both Mizutani and colleagues and Flemming and colleagues reported no cases of transformation of a dolichoectactic aneurysm to a fusiform aneurysm.

Ischemic Stroke

Flemming and colleagues[21] found that the ischemic stroke risk of these lesions after their diagnosis was higher than the hemorrhagic risk. The rate of any cerebral infarction after diagnosis at 1-year, 5-year, and 10-year follow-up was 6.1,

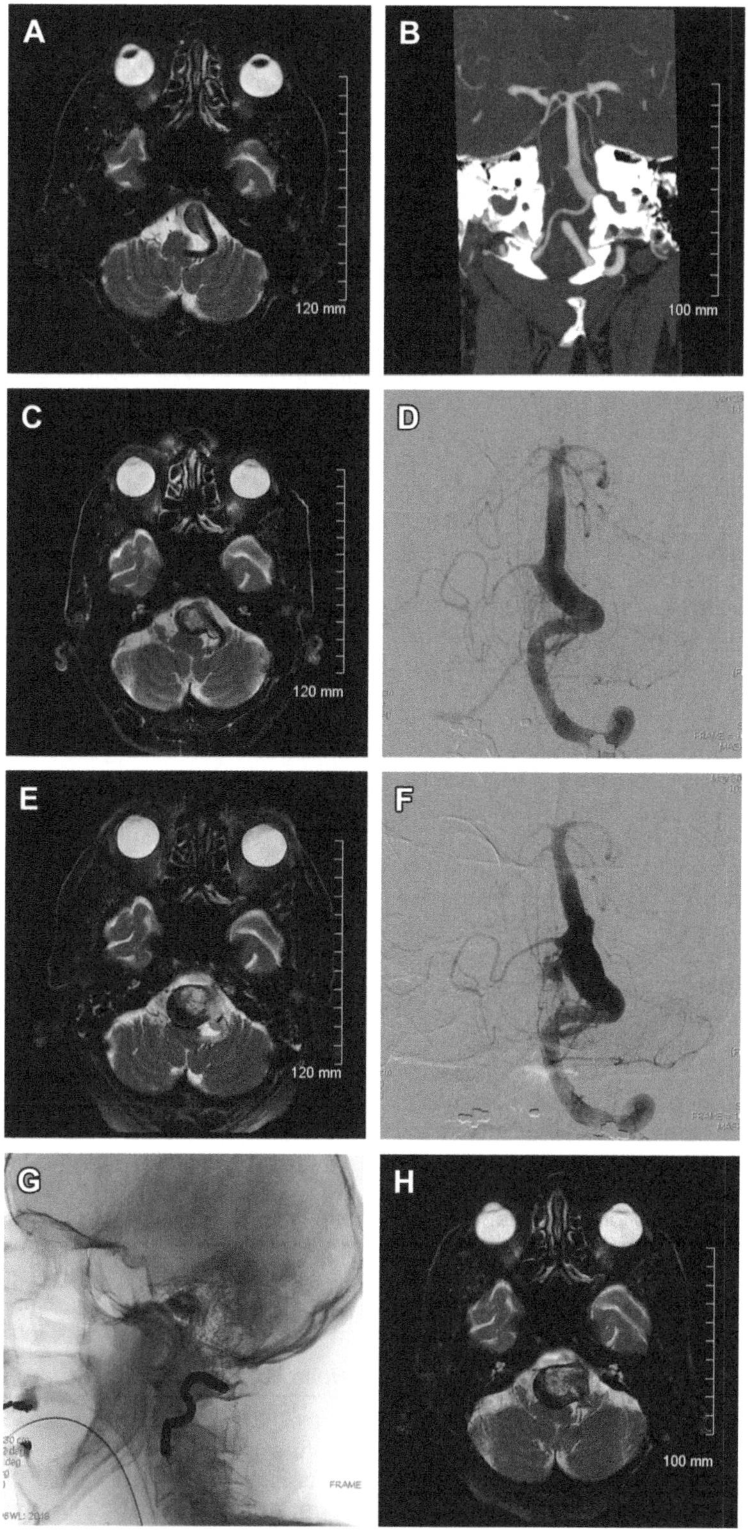

Fig. 1. Evolution of more than 5 years of a fusiform vertebrobasilar aneurysm in a 69-year-old man. Axial MRI and CT angiography or digital subtraction angiography in February, 2008 (*A*, *B*), January, 2012 (*C*, *D*), and May, 2013 (*E*, *F*) shows interval enlargement of a fusiform vertebrobasilar aneurysm with progressive brainstem compression. Despite endovascular coil occlusion of the left vertebral artery in May, 2013 (*G*), subtle continued expansion of the aneurysm was noted on follow-up MRI in August, 2013 (*H*).

17.3, and 25.4%, respectively. The rate of cerebral infarction related to the aneurysm at 1-year, 5-year, and 10-year follow-up was 2.7%, 11.3%, and 15.9%, respectively. For patients presenting with stroke, the risk of a recurrent ischemic stroke was 6.7%/y at a median time of 1.73 years. Risk factors for stroke in the Mayo Clinic cohort included patients who were initially symptomatic, previous history of ischemia caused by the aneurysm, and a transitional type of aneurysm with HRs of 16.2, 3.88, and 3.3, respectively. The median survival in their cohort was 7.8 years, with death caused by stroke occurring in more than one-third of cases (the most common cause). Recurrent stroke was less common in anticoagulated patients and more common in patients treated with antiplatelets. Recurrent stroke was not affected by thrombus presence, enlargement over time, size, hypertension, hyperlipidemia, or gender.[21]

The risk of recurrent stroke was also seen in the series of dolichoectatic vertebrobasilar arteries reported by Milandre and colleagues.[24] Of 21 patients presenting with stroke or compressive signs and symptoms, 8 (38%) had an ischemic event after presentation, and this was more common in patients initially presenting with stroke. Ince and colleagues[13] evaluated all patients with stroke presenting to the Mayo Clinic from 1985 to 1989 and found that dolichoectasia of any distribution had a relative risk of 2.4 for recurrent stroke compared with patients without dolichoectasia. The 2 patient groups had no difference in age, gender, or medical comorbidities. Eighty-three percent of these patients at least had some involvement of the vertebrobasilar system.

In a report of 23 cases with dolichoectatic basilar arteries defined as the basilar bifurcation at least 21 mm above the dorsum sellae, Nishizaki and colleagues[25] managed 19 cases conservatively. These investigators did not discern between dolichoectatic-type or fusiform-type aneurysms. Two of the 7 patients presenting with pontine infarction died of medical complications. The other 5 patients were treated conservatively, with stable signs and symptoms at follow-up. The natural history after the ictus described in this smaller series is seemingly more benign than that described by Flemming and colleagues.[21]

Compressive Symptoms

In the series by Flemming and colleagues,[21] 35 patients (22% of the cohort) presented with symptoms caused by compression. Compressive symptoms included brainstem compression, hydrocephalus, or cranial neuropathies. Of these 35 patients, 77% had mild or no disability at presentation. At 1 year, only 46% had mild or no disability, 25% moderate, and 25% severe disability or were dead. At 5 years, only 18% remained with mild or no disability, and 50% of the patients had severe disability or death. In addition, 12 patients in the cohort (7.5%) who did not initially present with compressive symptoms developed compressive symptoms.

Compressive symptoms correlate with growth of the aneurysm. Fifty-two of 159 patients in the Mayo Clinic cohort had serial imaging. Twenty-five patients (48%) had radiographic documentation of aneurysm growth with cross-sectional enlargement of 1.3 mm per year. Lesion growth was statistically associated with symptomatic compression at initial diagnosis, a transitional or fusiform type of aneurysm, and a larger diameter at diagnosis (15 vs 8 mm). These investigators also found more intramural hemorrhage in the enlarging aneurysms by T1 MRI compared with aneurysms that did not enlarge, but this was not statistically significant. The 5-year mortality of growing aneurysms was 56.5% versus 3.7% for aneurysms that were not growing.[42]

Nishizaki and colleagues[25] followed 7 patients with compressive symptoms. These symptoms included 4 brainstem compression symptoms, 1 vertigo, 1 dysarthria and cerebellar compression, and 1 with cranial nerve 9–12 palsy. The patient with cerebellar compression and vertigo improved with medical therapy. The remaining patients remained stable in their signs and symptoms. Mizutani and colleagues[7] reported the natural history of 8 Mizutani type 3 vertebrobasilar aneurysms (consistent with a fusiform or translational aneurysm defined by Flemming and colleagues), with follow-up ranging from 1 to 5 years. All patients initially presented with brainstem compression. Six aneurysms (75%) grew over the follow-up period. This finding is consistent with a 71% growth rate of fusiform and transitional aneurysms seen by Flemming and colleagues.[21] One patient (18%) died of progressive brainstem compression.[7]

Hemorrhage

In the 12-year Mayo Clinic experience, the annual rupture risk was 0.9% for all fusiform vertebrobasilar aneurysms. The annual risk was 2.3% for fusiform and transitional aneurysms but only 0.4% for dolichoectatic aneurysms. This risk was increased with aneurysm enlargement (4 of 6 ruptures had documented growth). Flemming and colleagues[41] also quoted the risk of rupture being increased with aneurysm diameter, because all cases that ruptured with imaging were greater than 10 mm, whereas only 34% of unruptured cases were greater than 10 mm. The exception to this theory was very large aneurysms (30–40 mm), which always had thrombus and never presented with rupture. Of the 8 patients with fusiform basilar aneurysms followed by Mizutani and colleagues[7] for 1 to 5 years, 3 patients (38%) had fatal SAH.

Fusiform cerebral aneurysms have a not insignificant hemorrhage rate of 2.3% per year. The natural history of unruptured symptomatic lesions is for the presenting symptoms to continue to worsen, whether this is compressive or ischemic in nature. However, recurrent ischemic events may be reduced with anticoagulation more than with antiplatelet therapy. The natural history for asymptomatic dolichoectatic lesions, conversely, is relatively benign.

PATHOLOGY

Formation

The pathophysiology of aneurysm formation in the vertebrobasilar system may be unique, considering that this is the only location in the human body in which 2 arteries merge into a larger artery. However, some well-known pathophysiology concepts of aneurysms at arterial bifurcations overlap. The initiation of saccular cerebral aneurysms is through loss of the internal elastic lamina, which allows dilation of the vessel.[45] Meng and colleagues[46] reported the classic histologic changes of aneurysm formation (ie, fragmentation of internal elastic lamina and tunica media thinning) in areas of high wall shear stress and high wall shear stress spatial gradients.[45] Identical histologic changes have been seen in histologic specimens of fusiform vertebrobasilar aneurysms. In postmortem examination of 2 patients with basilar ectasia, Hegedus[47] described disruption of the internal elastic lamina and loss of reticular fibers in the tunica media without evidence of atherosclerosis.

Postmortem specimens from 8 of 16 cases of fusiform aneurysms (2 posterior circulation) analyzed by Nakatomi and colleagues[39] described 4 distinct histologic features. These investigators found (1) fragmentation of the internal elastic lamina with intimal hyperplasia, (2) neoangiogenesis within the thickened intima, (3) intramural hemorrhage and intraluminal thrombus, and (4) vessel formation with intramural thrombus. Based on these observations, the investigators suggested that the inciting event of internal elastic lamina fragmentation leads to intima hyperplasia, neovascularization of the intima, bleeding from these intimal vessels causes intramural hemorrhage and vascularization of the thrombus, with further bleeding and growth of the aneurysm wall. Intimal neoangiogenesis was seen only in aneurysms larger than 12 mm, and intramural hemorrhage was seen only in aneurysms larger than 28 mm.

Fusiform Vertebrobasilar Aneurysms: the Controversial Role of Atherosclerosis

Some of the earliest reports indicated arteriosclerosis as the likely culprit of fusiform aneurysm formation.[3,4,14,15] This theory has been refuted by subsequent reports.[7,48,49] This discrepancy may be explained by the fact that many of the early reports described arteriosclerosis on gross examination but made no other mention of histologic features regarding the intima or internal elastic membrane. In a detailed histologic examination of 18 intracranial elongated/distended arteries, Sacks and Lindenburg[48] reported an absence of arteriosclerotic plaques. These investigators found multiple gaps in the internal elastic membrane, thinning of the tunica media with replacement by hypertrophic connective tissue that extended through internal elastic lamina defect, resulting in intraluminal plaquelike bulges. These lesions were perhaps mistaken by previous investigators for arteriosclerotic disease. In autopsy examination of 4 fusiform basilar arteries, Hulten-Gyllensten and colleagues[50] observed fragmentation of the internal elastic membrane without atherosclerosis in 3 of 4 cases. In the large series of 120 patients with fusiform aneurysms published by Drake and Peerless,[22] only 6 of these aneurysms were attributed to arteriosclerosis.

There is undoubtedly some degree of atherosclerosis in patients with fusiform vertebrobasilar aneurysms, especially in older patients, but this is not likely the primary mechanism for their development or growth. Atherosclerosis develops in regions of low shear stress (<5 dyn/cm^2) through mechanisms of decreased endothelial nitric oxide synthase, which leads to endothelial dysfunction, increased reactive oxygen species, increased leukocyte adhesion, increased lipoprotein permeability, and inflammation with subsequent atheroma formation.[51–53] It has been hypothesized that this sequence of events could occur at the inner curvature of a dolichoectactic basilar artery,[54] and this likely does occur, as reported in autopsy findings by Nijensohn and colleagues[55] in 23 fusiform basilar aneurysms and 27 saccular basilar aneurysms from 1952 to 1972. Atherosclerosis was identified in less than half of fusiform aneurysms (10 of 23) compared with no saccular aneurysms. Although the occurrence of atherosclerosis in this series may be a secondary factor caused by long segments of low wall shear stress, diminished mural elasticity and intramural inflammation associated with atherosclerosis may contribute to the maladaptive expansive remodeling and aneurysmal dilatation.

Aneurysm Growth

After fusiform aneurysm formation, these aneurysms begin an aggressive course of growth and worsening signs and symptoms.[7,21,41,42] When discussing growth of fusiform aneurysms, it is important to distinguish between (1) growth of the aneurysm lumen and (2) growth of the wall. The mechanism of the former may be related to low wall shear stress. Low wall shear stress causing luminal growth has been evaluated using computational fluid dynamic simulations from MRA. In 7 aneurysms without intramural thrombus that had morphologies unsuitable for clipping or coiling, Boussel and colleagues[56] correlated wall shear stress with radial displacement of the aneurysm wall as an indirect marker of aneurysm growth. These investigators reported that more radial displacement occurs at areas of low wall shear stress. Areas of low wall shear stress are prone to endothelial dysfunction (reduced vasodilatory substances, increased vasosconstrictive substances, increased endothelial permeability, and increased endothelial expression of leukocyte adhesion molecules and prothrombotic surface molecules). Endothelial dysfunction leads to mural thrombus formation, transendothelial migration of leukocytes and metalloproteinase-mediated cavitation of the extracellular matrix.[52,57–61] Any of these factors may contribute to aneurysm growth. So, whereas the initial formation of cerebral aneurysms occurs in areas of high wall shear stress, luminal growth occurs in areas of low shear stress.

The mechanism of growth of a fusiform vertebrobasilar aneurysm wall is different. In analyzing 8 postmortem specimens, Nakatomi and colleagues concluded that mural hemorrhage led to growth of the wall of the aneurysm, which also correlated with signs and symptoms. Histologically, these investigators identified intimal hyperplasia with neovascularization, mural hemorrhage, neovascularization into the mural thrombus, and evidence of recurrent mural hemorrhages. In studying MRIs from the same cases series, Nakatomi and colleagues[39] found that 8 of 9 symptomatic cases had both contrast enhancement of the aneurysm wall and intramural hemorrhage, whereas 6 of the 7 asymptomatic cases had neither of these features. Similarly, Schubiger and colleagues[62] reported imaging and intraoperative findings in 4 cases of growing giant intracranial aneurysms (1 posterior circulation). These investigators found peripheral enhancement of these lesions, which correlated with new hemorrhage intraoperatively. These investigators hypothesized that neovascularization and recurrent hemorrhage may cause enlargement of these lesions, much like the process that occurs with chronic subdural hematomas.

Microdissections may also contribute to growth of the aneurysm wall. In an attempt to classify aneurysms, Mizutani and colleagues[7] described 4 types of aneurysms. Fusiform vertebrobasilar aneurysms were identified as type 3 aneurysms. All type 3 aneurysms occurred in the basilar artery and angiographically had irregular lumens. Histologically, intimal dissection points with laminated thrombus as well as a fragmented internal elastic lamina were observed. Intimal disruptions were also grossly seen in the 2 cases examined by Anson and colleagues.[27] Chronic microdissections may allow another mechanism for intramural hematoma expansion.

TREATMENT

Surgical/Endovascular Flow Reduction/ Reversal

The treatment of vertebrobasilar fusiform aneurysms began in the 1960s with the surgical treatment that has been best described by Dr Charles Drake.[22,43,63] The surgical treatment involved either flow reduction if the patient did not have sufficient posterior circulation collaterals, flow reversal if the patient had adequate collaterals, or trapping with mural hematoma decompression for lesions presenting with acute mass effect.

In Drake and colleagues' series, multiple factors likely determined which treatment to perform, and these may have included the patient's clinical status, presentation, ability to tolerate vessel occlusion, or the status of collaterals. Patients who underwent flow reduction, usually by single vertebral artery occlusion or tourniquet-induced stenosis, had an excellent/good outcome in 63% of cases. Patients undergoing flow reversal by complete proximal flow arrest, usually by bilateral vertebral or basilar occlusion, had a 74% chance of excellent/good outcome. Also, 14 patients underwent trapping of the aneurysm with thrombectomy, achieving good outcomes in 71% of patients.[63] Drake and Peerless[22] found that the risk of thromboembolic events with Hunterian ligation increases with the increase in the length of involved vessel. Drake and colleagues reported that although rarely encountered, the management of atherosclerotic aneurysms inevitably led to brainstem stroke, despite adequate collateralization. These investigators recommend medical management with antihypertensives and antiplatelets as first-line treatment.

To evaluate the efficacy of Hunterian ligation for any posterior circulation aneurysm, including saccular aneurysms, Steinberg and colleagues retrospectively reviewed 201 cases in the series by Drake. Of these 201 cases, 118 occurred at the vertebral artery, vertebrobasilar junction (VBJ), or basilar trunk and 34 were classified as fusiform morphology. Therefore most of these lesions were complex saccular aneurysms not amenable to clip ligation. Similar to when evaluating only fusiform aneurysm, 61% of patients had improvement after Hunterian ligation. This has been the finding in other surgical series as well.[64]

Although the series reported by Steinberg and colleagues[63] does not completely consist of fusiform aneurysms, a pertinent finding related to treating these lesions emerged from these data. The tolerance to Hunterian ligation of the lower basilar artery was predicted by the size of the posterior communicating arteries (PCoAs). Patients with at least 1 large PCoA (>1 mm) had a 6.7% incidence of brainstem ischemia versus 43% in patients with 2 small PCoAs (<1 mm). In addition, the long-term outcome in patients with at least 1 large PCoA was excellent in 83% versus only 57% in patients with 2 small PCoAs. Drake had the practice of clipping the basilar artery without tourniquet test occlusion as long as 1 large PCoA was present.[65]

If poor collaterals exist, then cerebral bypass before vessel occlusion is usually required. Kalani and colleagues[29] reported 11 cases of vertebrobasilar aneurysms managed with flow reversal or reduction by surgical or endovascular means after superficial temporal artery bypass to the superior cerebellar or posterior cerebral artery. Patients in this series had a preoperative modified Rankin score (mRS) of 2.1 and postoperative mRS of 3.45 with a 45% mortality within 1 month of surgery. However, the 6 long-term survivors had an mRS of 2.5. Given the severe signs and symptoms of these patients with a poor natural history, the investigators still advocated treatment.

In the modern era, vessel sacrifice can be achieved by endovascular means as well. In their study of endovascular treatment of basilar trunk aneurysms, Uda and colleagues[66] reported the use of unilateral or bilateral vertebral occlusion in the treatment of 5 basilar/vertebrobasilar aneurysms. Three patients presented with SAH and 2 patients presented with mass effect. Complete occlusion was achieved in 2 patients, a neck remnant in 1 patient, and incomplete in 2 patients. Four of 5 patients achieved good or excellent outcomes.

Leibowitz and colleagues[37] looked at their results of parent vessel occlusion by endovascular techniques in 13 cases, 10 of which were fusiform vertebrobasilar aneurysms. Flow reduction by dominant vertebral artery occlusion was attempted in 6 patients with VBJ or basilar fusiform. Four of the 6 patients with palliative flow reduction died, 1 patient worsened to an mRS of 4, and 1 patient remained stable with an mRS of 1. However, patients with vertebral fusiform aneurysms that could be angiographically cured with vertebral artery occlusion did well. Four of 4 patients receiving this treatment improved from an average preoperative mRS of 4 to a postoperative mRS of 2.5. Although patients who could be cured angiographically did better, these patients also had simpler disease, which could be angiographically cured with unilateral vertebral artery sacrifice. The finding of better outcomes with complete proximal flow arrest was also seen in Steinberg and colleagues' series,[63] in which 45% of patients with incompletely thrombosed aneurysms had neurologic complications compared with 4% of patients with complete thrombosis.

Aymard and colleagues[38] treated 10 patients who had fusiform aneurysms of the vertebral artery, VBJ, or basilar artery. These investigators started with endovascular balloon occlusion of 1 vertebral artery. If the aneurysm did not regress at follow-up, the contralateral vertebral was sacrificed with a balloon. These investigators used balloon test occlusion with Xenon CT before vessel sacrifice. Eight of 10 patients (80%) with fusiform aneurysms had angiographic cure, and 90% had improvement or normalization of their clinical examination. One patient worsened after occlusion of the vertebral artery distal to posterior inferior cerebellar artery. Unilateral vertebral occlusion was used in every case of a fusiform aneurysm, with excellent results, which contradicts the findings of Leibowitz and colleagues.[37] However, a principle of proximal vessel occlusion for treatment of aneurysms is shown in the series by Aymard and colleagues,[38] in which only 2 of 7 basilar terminus lesions resolved with vertebral artery ligation. This finding may indicate that the efficacy of proximal vessel occlusion correlates with the proximity of the occlusion point to the vascular lesion.

Sluzewski and colleagues[33] reported 6 cases of basilar fusiform aneurysms treated with bilateral vertebral balloon occlusion. Three patients presenting in good condition did well and 3 patients presenting in poor condition did poorly. Two patients in this series required bypass for either clinical failure of balloon test occlusion or identification of small PCoAs. Wenderoth and colleagues[34] reported basilar artery sacrifice by coil embolization of 3 giant fusiform basilar aneurysms. All patients tolerated this procedure, with complete occlusion of their lesion and no neurologic complications. This finding leads many physicians to conclude that a fusiform and partially thrombosed basilar artery is likely defunctionalized with collaterals supplying the brainstem and cerebellum, thus allowing sacrifice of the vessel.

Stent/Coil

Stent-assisted coiling for fusiform vertebrobasilar aneurysms preserves the native basilar artery and may be considered in patients with poor collaterals who would not tolerate vessel sacrifice. The use of stent coiling of fusiform aneurysms with preservation of perforating side branches was shown to be effective in a swine model by Massoud and colleagues.[67] Higashida and colleagues[68] were the first to report stent and coil reconstruction of a fusiform basilar artery. Lanzino and colleagues[69] reported their experience in stenting with or without coil in wide-necked aneurysms. Two patients in this report had stenting with coiling of the basilar trunk fusiform aneurysms. These patients had incomplete follow-up at the time of the publication but had acceptable initial radiographic and clinical results. Other investigators have reported similar findings.[66] The literature is scarce for reports of this technique, but it can be a consideration if a constructive technique is required.

Flow Diversion

The initial treatment of anterior circulation cerebral aneurysms with flow-diverting stents has been positive, with a high occlusion rate of complex lesions.[70] This treatment strategy as a constructive approach (opposed to the destructive approach of vessel sacrifice) for vertebrobasilar fusiform aneurysms is attractive, especially in cases with small PCoAs that preclude vertebral artery sacrifice. Before dedicated intracranial flow-diverting stents, case reports of cardiac stents for treatment of vertebrobasilar fusiform aneurysms had promising results.[36,71] Also before dedicated cerebral flow-diverting stents, several investigators reported overlapping multiple high-porosity stents to create a lower-porosity construct, with good results in case reports.[32,72,73]

Meckel and colleagues[32] reported their experience with flow-diverting stents in 10 patients with complex vertebrobasilar aneurysms. Flow diverters were primarily used as adjunctive devices, with 9 of 10 patients having contralateral vertebral artery sacrifice and 5 of 10 patients having additional coil embolization. Good outcomes (mRS 0–2) were seen 6 patients (60%), and 4 patients died (40%). Many other case reports of flow-diverting stents for fusiform posterior circulation aneurysms have been published, with good outcomes.[35,74–76] However, the use of flow diverters in the posterior circulation should be approached with caution, because some physicians have noted high complication rates and poor long-term outcomes.[77] Continued analysis of flow diverters for select fusiform vertebrobasilar aneurysms is required before a strong recommendation on their routine use for this disease can be made.

Medical Therapy

The treatment options have acceptable results in properly selected patients, but these treatments are by no means benign. In addition, because patients with fusiform vertebrobasilar aneurysms are often older than patients with berry aneurysms, many patients cannot undergo extensive surgical procedures. Specifically, with growing fusiform aneurysms with mural thrombosis causing brainstem compression, there may be a role for medical therapy.

Vascular inflammation and adaptive remodeling processes rely extensively on matrix metalloproteinase (MMP) activity. Nonspecific MMP inhibitors including doxycycline and roxithromycin have been shown to decrease the growth rate of aortic aneurysms in clinical trials.[78,79] Compared with berry aneurysms, aortic aneurysms have been characterized as more biologically unstable, with a greater dependence on mural thrombus, atherosclerosis, and related mural inflammation for growth and rupture.[80] In this regard, fusiform cerebral aneurysms and dolichoectatic cerebral aneurysms behave more like aortic aneurysms and may show a similar favorable response to MMP-directed therapies.[39,81,82]

Other therapies have been evaluated for the treatment of aortic aneurysms, but the transition of these therapies to vertebrobasilar fusiform disease has not been explored. Clinical trials of statin therapy in patients with aortic aneurysms have attempted to exploit the ability of these agents to reduce vascular inflammation by reducing circulating levels of atherogenic lipoproteins and blocking the effects of reactive oxygen species on the vascular wall. These trials have not shown that statins beneficially alter aortic aneurysm histology or growth rates.[83,84] Hemodynamic modulating drug interventions, including β-adrenergic receptor

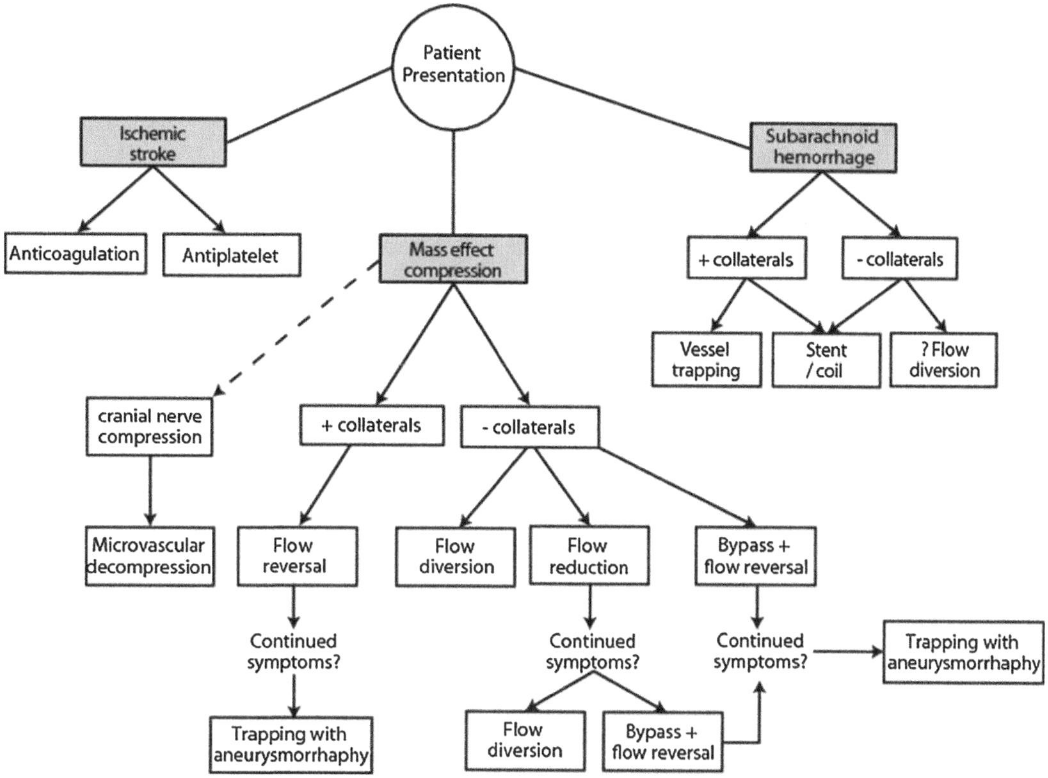

Fig. 2. Suggested treatment algorithm for fusiform vertebrobasilar aneurysms based on presentation.

blockers and angiotensin receptor blockers, have successfully reduced rates of aortic dilatation and dissection in patients with Marfan syndrome.[85–87] However, similar benefits have not been observed in the case of nonsyndromic abdominal aortic aneurysms.[88] Future research should report the use of these medications when following or treating patients with fusiform vertebrobasilar aneurysms.

As shown by examination of postmortem specimens of fusiform vertebrobasilar aneurysms, the mechanism of growth in these lesions is related to neoangiogenesis in the thickened intima and mural thrombus with subsequent hemorrhage.[39] Antiangiogenic drug interventions, such as bevacizumab, rapamycin, thalidomide, and celebrex, have enabled stabilization of abnormal vasculature in other diseases and may have a future role in treatment of fusiform vertebrobasilar aneurysms with mural neoangiogenesis.[89–92] There are no reports of use of MMP or antiangiogenic agents in fusiform cerebral aneurysms; however, these therapies should be considered for neurologically worsening patients when surgical and interventional options are not feasible or show limited efficacy.

For patients presenting with ischemic symptoms, anticoagulation is a reasonable option. Drake noted that older patients whose aneurysms were more likely to be attributed to atherosclerosis did not tolerate flow reduction methods. He recommended medical therapy as first-line treatment in this population. The literature on anticoagulation for this indication is scarce. In patients with fusiform vertebrobasilar aneurysms presenting with stroke, Echiverri and colleagues[28] reported no recurrent ischemic symptoms in 7 of 7 patients treated with warfarin, whereas 4 of 9 patients treated with aspirin had a recurrent stroke. Newer anticoagulation agents or dual antiplatelet regimens (eg, clopidogrel and aspirin) could also be considered.

Based on the reviewed literature, we propose an algorithm for symptomatic patients with fusiform vertebrobasilar aneurysms based on presentation (**Fig. 2**).

REFERENCES

1. Boeri R, Passerini A. The megadolichobasilar anomaly. J Neurol Sci 1964;11:475–84.
2. Wells HG. Intracranial aneurysms of the vertebral artery. Arch Neurol Psychiatry 1922;1:311.
3. Dandy WE. Intracranial arterial aneurysms. Ithaca (NY): Comstock; 1944.

4. Greitz T, Lofstedt S. The relationship between the third ventricle and the basilar artery. Acta Radiol 1954;42(2):85–100.
5. Pozzati E, Andreoli A, Limoni P, et al. Dissecting aneurysms of the vertebrobasilar system: study of 16 cases. Surg Neurol 1994;41(2):119–24.
6. Yoshimoto Y, Hoya K, Tanaka Y, et al. Basilar artery dissection. J Neurosurg 2005;102:476–81.
7. Mizutani T, Miki Y, Kojima H. Proposed classification of nonatherosclerotic cerebral fusiform and dissecting aneurysms. Neurosurgery 1999;45(2):253.
8. Rabinov JD, Hellinger FR, Morris PP, et al. Endovascular management of vertebrobasilar dissecting aneurysms. AJNR Am J Neuroradiol 2003;24: 1421–8.
9. Kocaeli H, Chaalala C, Andaluz N, et al. Spontaneous intradural vertebral artery dissection: a single-center experience and review of the literature. Skull Base 2009;19(3):209–18.
10. Casas PI, Abruzzi M, Lehkuniec E, et al. Dolichoectatic intracranial arteries. Advances in images and therapeutics. Medicina (B Aires) 1995;55(1):59–68.
11. Yu YL, Moseley IF, Pullicino P, et al. The clinical picture of ectasia of the intracerebral arteries. J Neurol Neurosurg Psychiatry 1982;45:29–36.
12. Resta M, Gentile MA, Di Cuonzo F, et al. Clinical-angiographic correlations in 132 patients with megadolichovertebrobasilar anomaly. Neuroradiology 1998;26:213–6.
13. Ince B, Petty GW, Brown RD Jr, et al. Dolichoectasia of the intracranial arteries in patients with first ischemic stroke: a population-based study. Neurology 1998;50(6):1694–8.
14. Housepian EM, Pool JL. A systematic analysis of intracranial aneurysms from the autopsy file of the Presbyterian Hospital, 1914 to 1956. J Neuropathol Exp Neurol 1958;17:409–23.
15. Hayes WT, Bernhardt H, Young JM. Fusiform arteriosclerotic aneurysm of the basilar artery. Five cases including two ruptures. Vasc Surg 1967;1: 171–8.
16. Pia HW. Classification of vertebro-basilar aneurysms. Acta Neurochir 1979;47:3–30.
17. Mitsias P, Levine SR. Cerebrovascular complications of Fabry's disease. Ann Neurol 1996;40(1):8–17.
18. Holmin S, Ozanne A, Zhao WY, et al. Association of cervical internal carotid artery aneurysm with ipsilateral vertebrobasilar aneurysm in two children: a segmental entity? Childs Nerv Syst 2007;23:791–8.
19. Massimi L, Moret J, Tamburrini G, et al. Dissecting giant vertebra-basilar aneurysms. Childs Nerv Syst 2003;19:204–10.
20. Gandolfo C. Giant vertebrobasilar aneurysm in a child: a challenging management. Neuroradiology 2012;54(5):505–6.
21. Flemming KD, Wiebers DO, Brown RD, et al. The natural history of radiographically defined vertebrobasilar fusiform intracranial aneurysm. Cerebrovasc Dis 2005;20:270–9.
22. Drake CG, Peerless SJ. Giant fusiform intracranial aneurysms: review of 120 patients treated surgically from 1965 to 1992. J Neurosurg 1997;87: 141–62.
23. Coert BA, Chang SD, Do HM. Surgical and endovascular management of symptomatic posterior circulation fusiform aneurysms. J Neurosurg 2007;106:855–65.
24. Milandre L, Bonnefoi B, Pestre P, et al. Vertebrobasilar arterial dolichoectasia. Complications and prognosis. Rev Neurol (Paris) 1991;147(11):714–22.
25. Nishizaki T, Tamaki N, Takeda N, et al. Dolichoectatic basilar artery: a review of 23 cases. Stroke 1986;17:1277–81.
26. Herpers M, Lodder J, Janevski B, et al. The symptomatology of megadolicho basilar artery. Clin Neurol Neurosurg 1983;85(4):203–12.
27. Anson JA, Lawton MT, Spetzler RF. Characteristics and surgical treatment of dolichoectatic and fusiform aneurysms. J Neurosurg 1996;84:185–93.
28. Echiverri HC, Rubino FA, Gupta SR, et al. Fusiform aneurysm of the vertebrobasilar arterial system. Stroke 1989;20:1741–7.
29. Kalani MY, Zabramski JM, Nakaji P, et al. Bypass and flow reduction for complex basilar and vertebrobasilar junction aneurysms. Neurosurgery 2013;72(4):763–76.
30. Pessin MS, Chimovitz MI, Levine SR, et al. Stroke in patients with fusiform vertebrobasilar aneurysms. Neurology 1989;39:16–21.
31. Giang DW, Perlin SJ, Monajati A, et al. Vertebrobasilar dolichoectasia: assessment using MR. Neuroradiology 1988;30(6):518–23.
32. Meckel S, McAuliffe W, Fiorella D, et al. Endovascular treatment of complex aneurysms at the vertebrobasilar junction with flow-diverting stents: initial experience. Neurosurgery 2013;73(3):386–94.
33. Sluzewski M, Brilstra EH, van Rooij WJ, et al. Bilateral vertebral artery balloon occlusion for giant vertebrobasilar aneurysms. Neuroradiology 2001;43: 336–41.
34. Wenderoth JD, Khangure MS, Phatouros CC, et al. Basilar trunk occlusion during endovascular treatment of giant and fusiform aneurysms of the basilar artery. AJNR Am J Neuroradiol 2003;24(6):1226–9.
35. Binning MJ, Natarajan SK, Bulsara KR, et al. SILK flow-diverting device for intracranial aneurysms. World Neurosurg 2011;76(5):477.e1–6.
36. Islak C, Kocer N, Albayram S. Bare stent-graft technique: a new method of endoluminal vascular reconstruction for the treatment of giant and fusiform aneurysms. AJNR Am J Neuroradiol 2002; 23:1589–95.
37. Leibowitz R, Do HM, Marcellus ML, et al. Parent vessel occlusion for vertebrobasilar fusiform and

dissecting aneurysms. AJNR Am J Neuroradiol 2003;24:902–7.
38. Aymard A, Gobin YP, Hodes JE, et al. Endovascular occlusion of vertebral arteries in the treatment of unclippable vertebrobasilar aneurysms. J Neurosurg 1991;74:393–8.
39. Nakatomi H, Segawa H, Kurata A, et al. Clinicopathological study of intracranial fusiform and dolichoectatic aneurysms: insight on the mechanism of growth. Stroke 2000;31(4):896–900.
40. Kissela BM, Sauerbeck L, Woo D, et al. Subarachnoid hemorrhage: a preventable disease with a heritable component. Stroke 2002;33(5):1321–6.
41. Flemming KD, Wiebers DO, Brown RD, et al. Prospective risk of hemorrhage in patients with vertebrobasilar fusiform intracranial aneurysm. J Neurosurg 2004;101:82–7.
42. Mangrum WI, Huston J, Link MJ, et al. Enlarging vertebrobasilar fusiform intracranial aneurysms: frequency, predictors, and clinical outcome of growth. J Nurs Scholarsh 2005;102:72–9.
43. Drake CG. Giant intracranial aneurysms: experience with surgical treatment in 174 patients. Clin Neurosurg 1979;26:12–95.
44. Huber P. Cerebral angiography. New York: Thieme; 1982.
45. Krex D, Schackert HK, Schackert G. Genesis of cerebral aneurysms–an update. Acta Neurochir 2001; 143:429–49.
46. Meng H, Wang Z, Hoi Y, et al. Complex hemodynamics at the apex of an arterial bifurcation induces vascular remodeling resembling cerebral aneurysm initiation. Stroke 2007;38:1924–31.
47. Hegedus K. Ectasia of the basilar artery with special reference to possible pathogenesis. Surg Neurol 1985;24:463–9.
48. Sacks JG, Lindenburg R. Dolicho-ectatic intracranial arteries: symptomatology and pathogenesis of arterial elongation and distention. Johns Hopkins Med J 1969;125(2):95–106.
49. Shokunbi MT, Vinters HV, Kaufmann JC. Fusiform intracranial aneurysms. Clinicopathologic features. Surg Neurol 1988;29(4):263–70.
50. Hulten-Gyllensten IL, Lofstedt S, von Reis G. Observations on generalized arteriectasis. Acta Med Scand 1959;163(2):125–30.
51. Cunningham KS, Gotlieb AI. The role of shear stress in the pathogenesis of atherosclerosis. Lab Invest 2005;85(1):9–23.
52. Malek AM, Alper SL, Izumo S. Hemodynamic shear stress and its role in atherosclerosis. JAMA 1999; 282:2035–42.
53. Caro CG, Fitz-Gerald JM, Schroter RC. Atheroma and arterial wall shear: observation, correlation and proposal of a shear dependent mass transfer mechanism for atherogenesis. Proc R Soc Lond B Biol Sci 1971;177:109–59.
54. Kim C, Sohn JH, Choi HC. Vertebrobasilar angulation and its association with sudden sensorineural hearing loss. Med Hypotheses 2012;79(2):202–3.
55. Nijensohn DE, Saez RJ, Feagan TJ. Clinical significance of basilar artery aneurysms. Neurology 1974;24(4):301–5.
56. Boussel L, Rayz V, McCulloch C, et al. Aneurysm growth occurs at region of low wall shear stress: patient-specific correlation of hemodynamics and growth in a longitudinal study. Stroke 2008;39: 2997–3002.
57. Kaiser D, Freyberg MA, Friedl P. Lack of hemodynamic forces triggers apoptosis in vascular endothelial cells. Biochem Biophys Res Commun 1997;231:586–90.
58. Rieder MJ, Carmona R, Krieger JE, et al. Suppression of angiotensin-converting enzyme expression and activity by shear stress. Circ Res 1997;80: 312–9.
59. Korenaga R, Ando J, Kosaki K, et al. Negative transcriptional regulation of the vcam-1 gene by fluid shear stress in murine endothelial cells. Am J Physiol 1997;273:C1506–15.
60. Rubanyi GM, Romero JC, Vanhoutte PM. Flow-induced release of endothelium-derived relaxing factor. Am J Physiol 1986;250:H1145–9.
61. Nagahiro S, Takada A, Goto S, et al. Thrombosed growing giant aneurysms of the vertebral artery: growth mechanism and management. J Neurosurg 1995;82(5):796–801.
62. Schubiger O, Valavanis A, Wichmann W. Growth-mechanism of giant intracranial aneurysms; demonstration by CT and MR imaging. Neuroradiology 1987;29:266–71.
63. Steinberg GK, Drake CG, Peerless SJ. Deliberate basilar or vertebral artery occlusion in the treatment of intracranial aneurysms. J Neurosurg 1993;79:161–73.
64. Kellner CP, Haque RM, Meyers PM, et al. Complex basilar artery aneurysms treated using surgical basilar occlusion: a modern case series. Clinical article. J Neurosurg 2011;115(2):319–27.
65. Pelz DM, Vinuela F, Fox AJ, et al. Vertebrobasilar occlusion therapy of giant aneurysms. Significance of angiographic morphology of the posterior communicating arteries. J Neurosurg 1984;60:560–5.
66. Uda K, Murayama Y, Gobin P, et al. Endovascular treatment of basilar artery trunk aneurysms with Guglielmi detachable coils: clinical experience with 41 aneurysms in 39 patients. J Neurosurg 2001;95:624–32.
67. Massoud TF, Turjman F, Ji C, et al. Endovascular treatment of fusiform aneurysms with stents and coils: technical feasibility in a swine model. AJNR Am J Neuroradiol 1995;16:1953–63.
68. Higashida RT, Smith W, Gress D, et al. Intravascular stent and endovascular coil placement for a

ruptured fusiform aneurysm of the basilar artery. Case report and review of the literature. J Neurosurg 1997;87(6):944–9.
69. Lanzino G, Wakhloo AK, Fessler RD, et al. Efficacy and current limitations of intravascular stents for intracranial internal carotid, vertebral, and basilar artery aneurysms. J Neurosurg 1999;91:538–46.
70. Nelson PK, Lylyk P, Szikora I, et al. The pipeline embolization device for the intracranial treatment of aneurysms trial. AJNR Am J Neuroradiol 2011; 32(1):34–40.
71. Lylyk P, Cohen JE, Ceratto R, et al. Endovascular reconstruction of intracranial arteries by stent placement and combined techniques. J Neurosurg 2002; 97:1306–13.
72. Ansari SA, Lassig JP, Nicol E, et al. Thrombosis of a fusiform intracranial aneurysm induced by overlapping neuroform stents: case report. Neurosurgery 2007;60:E950–1.
73. Crowley RW, Evans AJ, Kassell NF, et al. Endovascular treatment of a fusiform basilar artery aneurysm using multiple "in-stent stents". Technical note. J Neurosurg Pediatr 2009;3:496–500.
74. Cohen JE, Gomori JM, Moscovici S, et al. Successful endovascular treatment of a growing megadolichoectasic vertebrobasilar artery aneurysm by flow diversion using the "diverter-in-stent" technique. J Clin Neurosci 2012;19(1):166–70.
75. Fiorella D, Woo HH, Albuquerque FC, et al. Definitive reconstruction of circumferential, fusiform intracranial aneurysms with the pipeline embolization device. Neurosurgery 2008;62:1115–21.
76. Tan LA, Moftakhar R, Lopes DK. Treatment of a ruptured vertebrobasilar fusiform aneurysm using pipeline embolization device. J Cerebrovasc Endovasc Neurosurg 2013;15(1):30–3.
77. Siddiqui AH, Abla AA, Kan P, et al. Panacea or problem: flow diverters in the treatment of symptomatic large or giant fusiform vertebrobasilar aneurysms. J Neurosurg 2012;116(6):1258–66.
78. Mosorin M, Juvonen J, Biancari F, et al. Use of doxycycline to decrease the growth rate of abdominal aortic aneurysms: a randomized, double-blind, placebo-controlled pilot study. J Vasc Surg 2001; 34:606–10.
79. Vammen S, Lindholt JS, Ostergaard L, et al. Randomized double-blind controlled trial of roxithromycin for prevention of abdominal aortic aneurysm expansion. Br J Surg 2001;88:1066–72.
80. Humphrey JD, Taylor CA. Intracranial and abdominal aortic aneurysms: similarities, differences, and need for a new class of computational models. Annu Rev Biomed Eng 2008;10:221–46.
81. Lou M, Caplan LR. Vertebrobasilar dilatative arteriopathy (dolichoectasia). Ann N Y Acad Sci 2010;1184:121–33.
82. Passero SG, Rossi S. Natural history of vertebrobasilar dolichoectasia. Neurology 2008;70:66–72.
83. Hurks R, Hoefer IE, Vink A, et al. Different effects of commonly prescribed statins on abdominal aortic aneurysm wall biology. Eur J Vasc Endovasc Surg 2010;39(5):569–76.
84. Ferguson CD, Clancy P, Bourke B, et al. Association of statin prescription with small abdominal aortic aneurysm progression. Am Heart J 2010; 159(2):307–13.
85. Shores J, Berger KR, Murphy EA, et al. Progression of aortic dilation and the benefit of long-term β-adrenergic blockade in Marfan's syndrome. N Engl J Med 1994;330:1335–41.
86. Keane MG, Pyeritz RE. Medical management of the Marfan syndrome. Circulation 2008;117:2802–13.
87. Brooke BS, Habashi JP, Judge DP, et al. Angiotensin II blockade and aortic-root dilation in Marfan's syndrome. N Engl J Med 2008;358:2787–95.
88. Propranolol Aneurysm Trial Investigators. Propranolol for small abdominal aortic aneurysms: results of a randomized trial. J Vasc Surg 2002;35(1):72–9.
89. Brinkerhoff BT, Poetker DM, Choong NW. Long-term therapy with bevacizumab in hereditary hemorrhagic telangectasia. N Engl J Med 2011;364(7): 688–9.
90. Hammill AM, Wentzel M, Gupta A, et al. Sirolimus for the treatment of complicated vascular anomalies in children. Pediatr Blood Cancer 2011;57(6): 1018–24.
91. Iacobas I, Burrows PE, Adams DM, et al. Oral rapamycin in the treatment of patients with hamartoma syndromes and PTEN mutation. Pediatr Blood Cancer 2011;57(2):321–3.
92. Klement G, Cervi D, Orbach D, et al. PTEN associated lesions regress in response to the anti-angiogenic therapy with thalidomide/Celebrex. Presented at the 17th International Workshop on Vascular Anomalies. Boston, June 21–24, 2008.
93. Greenberg E, Katz JM, Janardhan V, et al. Treatment of giant vertebrobasilar artery aneurysm using stent grafts. J Neurosurg 2007;107:165–8.

Endovascular Treatment of Basilar Aneurysms

Evan S. Marlin, MD, Daniel S. Ikeda, MD, Andrew Shaw, MD, Ciarán J. Powers, MD, PhD, Eric Sauvageau, MD*

KEYWORDS

- Basilar apex aneurysm • PCA aneurysm • SCA aneurysm • AICA aneurysm • Stent-assisted coil
- Balloon remodeling

KEY POINTS

- Posterior circulation aneurysms constitute 15% of intracranial aneurysms. Between 50% and 80% of these are located at the basilar artery apex.
- Most basilar apex aneurysms are wide-necked and require specialized techniques for treatment to ensure patency of the parent vessel and successful lesion embolization.
- Treated basilar artery aneurysms should be followed closely to monitor for delayed recanalization.
- In addition to basilar apex aneurysms, aneurysms of the basilar artery may involve the posterior cerebral artery, superior cerebellar artery, and the anterior inferior cerebellar artery.

INTRODUCTION

Intracranial aneurysms are found in approximately 3% to 5% of the population, with an annual rate of rupture of approximately 10 per 100,000. Of these, posterior circulation aneurysms constitute approximately 15% of all intracranial aneurysms.[1,2] The most common posterior circulation aneurysm location is the basilar artery (BA) apex. Basilar apex aneurysms constitute 50% to 80% of posterior circulation aneurysms.[3] Other locations of BA aneurysms include the basilar trunk and the junctions of the posterior cerebral arteries (PCAs), superior cerebellar arteries (SCAs), and anterior inferior cerebellar arteries (AICAs).

Traditional microsurgical approaches for the treatment of posterior circulation aneurysms often require significant brain retraction and temporary arterial occlusion that may result in significant morbidity and mortality. Specifically, third nerve palsies, perforator injury, and retraction injury are the most common.[4,5] Therefore, endovascular therapy has evolved to become a mainstay in treating these lesions.

BASILAR ARTERY ANATOMY

The basilar artery forms from the convergence of both vertebral arteries at the level of the pons. The BA continues to travel ventral to the pons until its termination and bifurcation into the posterior cerebral arteries in the interpeduncular cistern. During its ascent it provides numerous perforating branches to the pons and midbrain, including multiple median, circumferential, and lateral pontine branches. It emanates 3 major paired arteries: the AICAs proximally, the SCAs just proximal to its terminal bifurcation, and the PCAs as terminal branches. The posterior inferior cerebellar arteries (PICAs) most commonly arise from the vertebral artery. The AICAs and SCAs form an extensive and redundant collateral arterial system supplying the rest of the cerebellum.

In addition to the BA's close association with the brainstem, its branches have intimate relationships with several cranial nerves. The third cranial nerve exits the mesencephalon immediately inferior to the PCA and superior to the SCA. Lateral to this is the trochlear nerve before piercing the tentorial

Disclosures: None.
Department of Neurosurgery, The Ohio State University Wexner Medical Center, 410 West 10th Avenue, N-1004 Doan Hall, Columbus, OH 43210, USA
* Corresponding author.
E-mail address: ericsauvageau@hotmail.com

Neurosurg Clin N Am 25 (2014) 485–495
http://dx.doi.org/10.1016/j.nec.2014.04.007
1042-3680/14/$ – see front matter

dura. The SCA has a close relationship with the trigeminal nerve, and the distal AICA has a close relationship with the vestibulocochlear nerve.

Regarding endovascular treatment, the straight course of the BA and the position of apex aneurysms make them favorable to endovascular navigation and catheterization. The position of the BA does not influence the endovascular approach as it does with open vascular cases. In addition, important perforators arise from the neck and not the dome of the apex aneurysms, making endovascular approaches ideal. Approximately 60% of basilar apex aneurysms are wide-necked and may involve the PCA origins, making these more challenging to treat.[6] Various methods have evolved to keep these critical vessels patent.

CLINICAL PRESENTATION AND DIAGNOSIS

A large number of posterior circulation aneurysms are found incidentally on workup of unrelated symptoms. Nonruptured aneurysms may present secondary to mass effect and cranial nerve palsies. Infrequently, thrombosed and giant basilar aneurysms may present with hydrocephalus and a third ventricular mass.[7] Because of the low incidence of posterior circulation aneurysms, their natural history is not well understood. However, the International Study of Unruptured Intracranial Aneurysms investigation revealed that unruptured posterior circulation aneurysms have a 2.6% to 50.0% chance of rupture over a 5-year period, depending on their size.[1,8] Posterior circulation, and especially basilar apex aneurysms, in patients with a prior history of subarachnoid hemorrhage predict a poor outcome. This risk of rupture and poor outcome argues for aggressive treatment of these lesions, especially when the aneurysm is greater than 7 mm and life expectancy is greater than 5 years.

On rupture, presentation and prognosis are typically more severe than those of anterior circulation aneurysms, with survival rates as low as 32% within the first 48 hours of rupture and 11% at 30 days despite treatment.[9] The dismal prognosis is related to the BA's relationship to the brainstem and hemorrhage into the forth ventricle. Obstructive hydrocephalus secondary to rupture is particularly common among ruptured BA aneurysms.

ENDOVASCULAR CONSIDERATIONS

History

Endovascular surgery of the posterior circulation was primarily developed for the treatment of nonoperative aneurysms. Treatment most commonly involved Hunterian proximal arterial occlusion of the parent artery with detachable balloons.[10,11] The advent of detachable coils in 1992 by Guglielmi began a revolution in the treatment of aneurysms. Detachable coils were originally used only for aneurysms thought to be too difficult to clip or in patients with poor prognosis.[12] Therefore, many early series reveal frequent use with posterior circulation aneurysms.[12–15] In fact, a 1997 series of 403 intracranial aneurysms found that 57% of those treated were in the posterior circulation.[15] With the use of coiling, acutely ruptured aneurysms can be treated to significantly reduce the risk of rehemorrhage, allow aggressive therapy for the prevention of delayed cerebral ischemia, and prevent vasospasm.[3]

General Techniques and Principles

Several basic principles and steps help ensure safe interventional procedures. Interventional procedures are usually completed under general endotracheal anesthesia. All sheaths, guides, and microcatheters are continually flushed with heparinized saline. Generally, the procedure begins with a micropuncture needle, which is ultimately upsized to a 6F short sheath unless femoral access is tortuous and a long sheath is required. Once access is obtained, 70 U/kg of heparin is administered intravenously for an activated clotting time (ACT) goal of 250 seconds. Activated clotting time point of care testing is used through the duration of the procedure to ensure adequate heparinization. Meticulous attention of heparinization and ACT checks can prevent disastrous thromboembolic complications. Protamine must be immediately available in case of intraoperative rupture. Appropriate guide and selector catheters are used to select the vessel of interest. Once selected and treatment projections are chosen, 10 mg of intra-arterial verapamil are given to prevent catheter-induced vasospasm. The guide catheter is then brought to the V2 or V3 segment of the vertebral artery as it allows. Straight microcatheters are suitable for most aneurysms; however, this is even more assured for basilar apex aneurysms, in which the trajectory is straight. After treatment, a final ACT is measured and more heparin is given as needed. For aneurysms requiring stenting or with significant coil mass exposed at the neck, a heparin infusion at 8 U/kg/hr is often used overnight to prevent delayed thromboembolic complications. If delayed thromboembolism occurs, an abciximab infusion is initiated for 24 hours and the daily clopidogrel dose is increased. A postoperative systolic blood pressure goal of less than 160 mm Hg is strictly enforced.

Basilar Apex Aneurysms

Basilar apex aneurysms are the most common posterior circulation and BA aneurysm (**Fig. 1**). They compose approximately 50% of all posterior circulation aneurysms and 5% of all intracranial aneurysms. These aneurysms most commonly follow Rhoton's third law of aneurysms and point superiorly in the direction blood would have flowed if not for the artery's termination as the posterior cerebral arteries.[16] The anatomy of the BA and basilar apex aneurysms make these ideal for endovascular technology. These anatomies dictate the treatment and ultimate outcome. They may incorporate the posterior cerebral arteries, complicating treatment, and high flow can lead to long-term coil compaction, necessitating re-treatment.

Narrow-necked aneurysms can be primarily coiled; however, up to 60% of basilar apex aneurysms are wide-necked (>4 mm). Therefore, a variety of techniques have developed to prevent coil prolapse into the BA lumen or occlusion of the PCAs. The most common techniques include balloon remodeling, stent-assisted coiling, and multiple microcatheter techniques.

Balloon remodeling involves using a nondetachable balloon to segregate the aneurysm neck from the parent vessel during occlusion. After aneurysm catheterization, the balloon is inflated across the aneurysm neck, allowing coil deployment and preventing prolapse. The balloon should go across the aneurysm neck into the dominant P1 to protect the vessel. Highly formable balloons, such as the HyperForm (Covidien, Plymouth, MN, USA) or TransForm (Stryker, Kalamazoo, MI, USA), can be inflated and formed to protect bilateral P1 segments and the aneurysm neck. Deflation before coil detachment helps ensure prolapse will not occur. Large framing coils will further help prevent prolapse, whereas the balloon prevents coil loops from prolapsing during deployment. Intermittent balloon inflation can be performed throughout coiling. In a small series of 52 aneurysms, this technique allowed for complete occlusion in 40

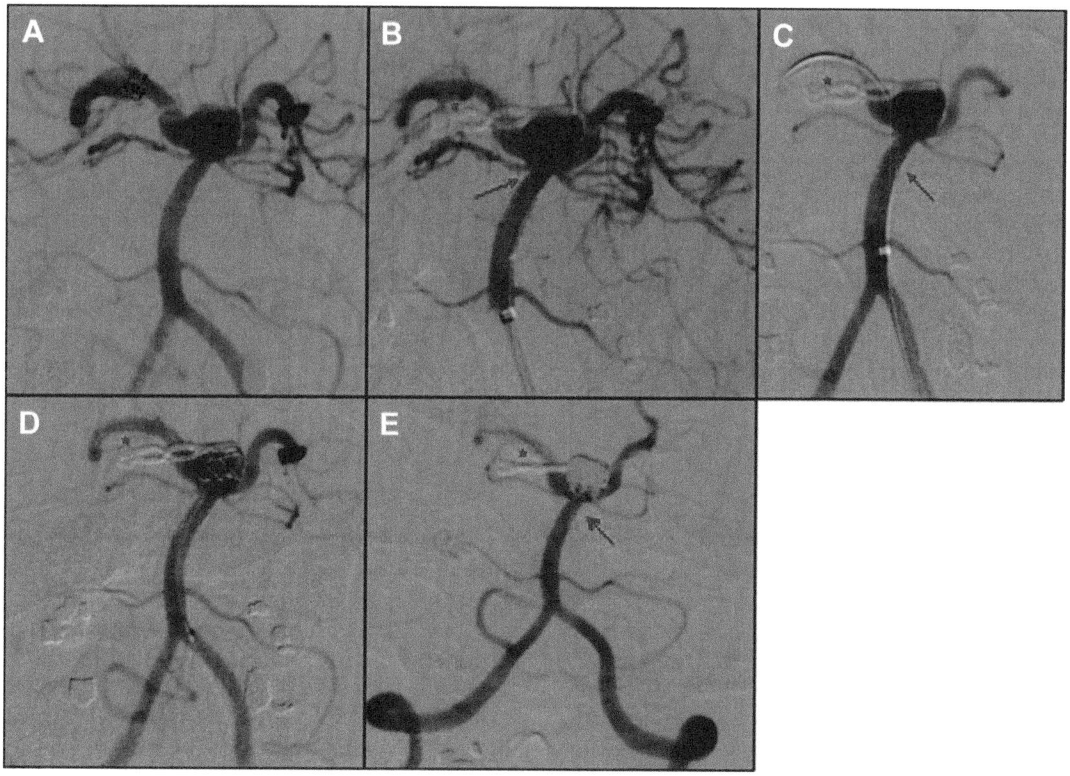

Fig. 1. A 57-year-old woman status post clipping of ruptured basilar apex aneurysm at age 20 years who presented after a reportedly negative diagnostic cerebral angiogram 2 years prior with new headaches and was found to have a recurrent 9 × 14 mm recurrent basilar apex aneurysm. (*A*) A wide-neck basilar apex aneurysm involving bilateral PCAs. Prior clip indicated by asterisk. (*B, C*) Left and right PCAs catheterized and Y stent protection of aneurysm neck. Arrow marks proximal tines of stents. (*D*) Microcatheterization of aneurysm through the Y stent and deployment of framing coil. (*E*) Final angiographic images revealing minimal residual neck and patency of bilateral PCAs. Proximal tines of stents are marked by the arrow.

patients (77%), subtotal in 9 (17%), and incomplete occlusion in 3 (6%).[17] Balloon remodeling is particularly beneficial in acutely ruptured aneurysms when stenting and dual antiplatelet therapy is less than optimal. It does, however, involve temporary flow arrest and no guarantee of coil stability after balloon deflation.

The use of dual balloon remodeling has been described but is infrequently required, because newer balloons are now highly formable. This technique involves balloons in each PCA that are intermittently inflated during embolization. Unfortunately, this technique frequently requires bilateral femoral access and is associated with a higher risk of thromboembolic complications.[18,19]

Stent-assisted coiling can also be used to prevent coil prolapse into the BA and obstruction of the PCAs (see **Fig. 1**). The stent configuration depends on the aneurysm's neck incorporation of the P1 segments. If a single P1 is incorporated at the base, frequently a single stent is required. However, if the neck is broad enough, stenting with a Y-configuration may be required, which involves 2 stents arising from the top portion of the BA into each P1 segment. Afterward, the microcatheter can be guided into the aneurysm and coiled (ie, the "coil through" technique). Alternatively, the microcatheter can be "jailed" into the aneurysm dome before embolization. A multicenter study of 45 aneurysms at 7 institutions were treated with Y stenting with good results: 92% of patients had Raymond I or II occlusion, 83% of Raymond III occluded aneurysms had better occlusion grade on delayed angiographic imaging, and 10% of patients recanalized, requiring repeat procedures.[20] Thromboembolic complications were lower in this series, and typically range from 4% to 8% in multiple series. In-stent stenosis was infrequent and asymptomatic in all patients.[20]

Unfortunately, placement of stents necessitates the need for dual antiplatelet therapy, which is less appealing after acute subarachnoid hemorrhage. The need for aggressive medical therapy and external ventricular drainage, and the possible future need for ventriculoperitoneal shunting for ruptured aneurysms, is associated with increased risk for hemorrhage during dual antiplatelet therapy.[21,22] In these cases that may require stent-assisted coiling, the authors attempt to secure the dome to prevent acute rehemorrhage, knowing that re-treatment will be required in a delayed fashion.

For elective aneurysm treatment, patients are treated with aspirin and clopidogrel for a minimum of 7 days before the procedure. Immediately post-procedure, all patients are kept on low-rate heparin infusions (8 U/kg/hr) overnight to prevent delayed presentation of thromboembolic events. Dual antiplatelet therapy is continued for a minimum of 6 weeks, after which the patient will remain on aspirin. Up to 47% of patients may be clopidogrel-nonresponders and should be evaluated preoperatively if possible to reduce thromboembolic complications. The authors favor the use of open-cell stents (NeuroForm stent systems, Stryker) as opposed to closed-cell stents because of the decreased risk of kinking and the possibility of poor vessel apposition requiring in-stent angioplasty after delivery. However, clinically there seems to be little difference in outcome between these stent types.[20]

Another technique that allows for the treatment of wide-necked aneurysm is the dual microcatheter technique.[23,24] This technique avoids the need for balloon remodeling when the risk of temporary occlusion is too high or in acutely ruptured aneurysms in which avoidance of stent-assisted coiling is preferred. This technique involves the use of 2 microcatheters within the aneurysm dome. The first catheter deploys a framing coil without detaching it. The second catheter is then used to deploy a second framing coil. The successive deployment of 2 coils helps interlock their position and provide coil stability in the aneurysm dome to prevent prolapse. They can subsequently be detached and coiling can continue, with filling coils alternating between both microcatheters. Tandem coil placement can also be performed with dual microcatheter access; through alternately partially deploying a coil from each of the microcatheters, a complex coil mass can be formed and prevent prolapse. When using this technique, special attention to microcatheter removal at the end of coiling is critical to prevent shifting of the coil mass.

Finally, less common practices for the treatment of basilar apex aneurysms include transcirculation techniques via a posterior communicating artery and use of flow diversion technology. Transcirculation approaches require guide catheters in the internal carotid artery to access a large posterior communicating artery and in a vertebral artery to access the basilar apex aneurysm.[25] As such, there is an increased risk of thromboembolic complications. Several case reports discuss the use of flow-diverting stents, such as the Pipeline Embolization Device (PED; Micro Therapeutics Inc, Irvine, CA, USA).[25] The use of this technology requires the use of dual antiplatelet therapy and may place small pontine perforator branches at risk. The long-term outcomes of PEDs for the treatment of BA aneurysms are not well-known, currently limiting this application.

Basilar Trunk Aneurysms

Basilar trunk aneurysms constitute fewer than 1% of intracranial aneurysms and approximately 8% of vertebrobasilar artery aneurysms.[26] Dissecting aneurysms of the basilar trunk are more common than saccular aneurysms. Saccular aneurysms of the basilar trunk most commonly occur in the distal third of the BA and often are categorized with AICA aneurysms. In a series of 8 saccular basilar trunk aneurysms, 7 presented with a subarachnoid hemorrhage. All 8 were treated with primary coiling with complete or near-complete occlusion; 1 patient died secondary to vasospasm, and 2 patients ultimately required additional treatments for coil compaction.[26]

Dissecting and fusiform BA trunk aneurysms are associated with a high rate of morbidity and mortality. They can lead to progressive brainstem compression and subarachnoid hemorrhage, with 2-year survival rates as low as 20%.[27,28] These lesions often require vessel remodeling and a combination of stenting and stent-assisted coiling. The use of flow diversion embolization has been reported with varying success; however, this should be used with caution, because the long-term risks of perforating arteries or subsequent basilar artery thrombosis are not well-known.[27,29]

PCA Aneurysms

Posterior cerebral artery aneurysms are uncommon and constitute approximately 1% of all intracranial aneurysms. Typically they are large and a mixture of saccular and fusiform in nature, involving the P1 or P2 segment, often at the junction of P2 and the posterior communicating artery (**Fig. 2**).[30] Most frequently, these aneurysms present with subarachnoid hemorrhage, visual deficits, or third nerve dysfunction. In a small series by Ciceri and colleagues,[31] 66% of PCA aneurysms were treated without parent vessel occlusion, with an associated 10% morbidity. The remaining third required parent vessel sacrifice. One of these cases presented with memory loss from a giant P3 aneurysm compressing the hippocampus. Vessel preservation must be attempted when treating P1 segment aneurysms, because this segment provides end-artery thalamoperforators and possibly the artery of Percheron. In another small series of 10 P2 aneurysms, distal vessel occlusion was found to be tolerated. This finding is thought to be caused by the hemodynamic balance between anterior and posterior choroidal arteries, pericallosal arteries, and middle cerebral artery branches with distal PCA branches.[32]

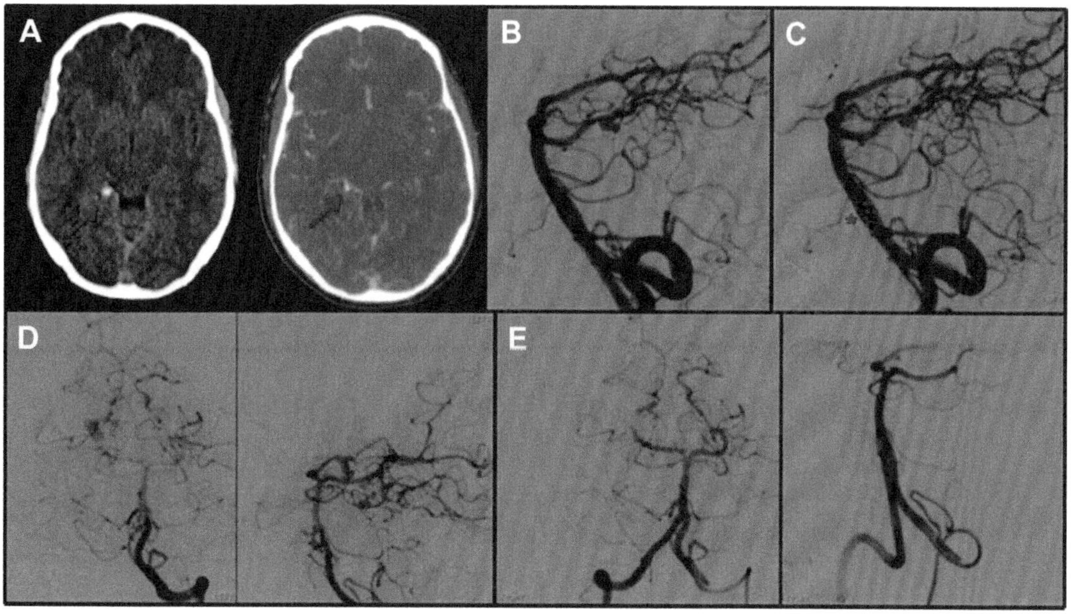

Fig. 2. A 43-year-old man presenting with a Hunt and Hess grade 2, Fisher grade 2 subarachnoid hemorrhage. (*A*) Computed tomography and computed tomography angiography reveal the site of hemorrhage. (*B*) Lateral mid-arterial injection digital subtraction angiography reveals a fusiform right P2 aneurysm. (*C*) Using a dual microcatheter technique, the aneurysm dome and extrusion was coiled. Asterisk reveals 2 microcatheters in the BA. (*D*) Short-term follow-up after discharge reveals an interval increase in fusiform aneurysm with coil compaction. (*E*) Stent-assisted coiling of aneurysm with complete occlusion.

SCA Aneurysms

Superior cerebellar artery aneurysms arise between the origin of the SCA and PCA (**Fig. 3**). They are amenable to endovascular treatment with low morbidity. Most commonly they require balloon remodeling to protect the SCA ostium and BA lumen. Large necks may preclude complete embolization. Although few case series are published, Haw and colleagues[33] present a series of 12 SCA aneurysms in 11 patients, 7 of which presented with subarachnoid hemorrhage. In this series, half of the aneurysms were completely excluded from circulation and half had only minimal residual at the neck because of SCA incorporation. One SCA stroke occurred, and overall good clinical outcomes were seen in 10 of the 11 patients. Uda and colleagues[34] presented similar results in a series of basilar trunk aneurysms in which 13 were SCA aneurysms; 10 of these patients had excellent outcomes without further recurrence or rehemorrhage at follow-up. Distal SCA aneurysms may be associated with arteriovenous malformations or trauma and can be treated with parent vessel sacrifice because of robust collateral circulation from the AICA and PICA.

AICA Aneurysms

Anterior inferior cerebellar artery aneurysms are also rare aneurysms and compose approximately 1% of intracranial aneurysms (**Fig. 4**).[35,36] AICA aneurysms typically present with either subarachnoid hemorrhage or brainstem compression. Additionally, distal or meatal segment AICA aneurysms can present with hearing disruption from compression of the vestibulocochlear nerve (see **Fig. 4**).[37] Surgical access is difficult because of the close relationship to the pons and middle cerebellar peduncle; there are also close relationships to cranial nerves VI through VIII.[38] Proximal AICA aneurysms may be amenable to endovascular occlusion; however, distal AICA aneurysms often require vessel sacrifice. The degree of tolerance to vessel occlusion is thought to be related to the comparative size of the PICA and SCA, such that occlusion is better tolerated with robust collateral PICAs and SCAs.

COMPLICATIONS AND CONCERNS

Procedural Morbidity and Mortality

The lack of clinical equipoise for posterior circulation aneurysms did not allow adequate comparison of the morbidity and mortality of open microsurgical treatment and endovascular modalities in the International Subarachnoid Aneurysm Trial.[39,40] However, retrospective analysis and case series have shown that coil embolization can be effective in completely excluding, and very effective in partially excluding, the basilar apex aneurysms from circulation. Periprocedural complications are low. The most common complications of BA aneurysm treatment include failure to treat, periprocedural rupture, coil malposition, thrombosis, and embolic events. Henkes and colleagues,[3] in a review of 6 basilar apex aneurysm coiling series found a procedural morbidity of 6.6% and mortality of 1.3%. In his own series of 316 aneurysms, morbidity was 5.4% and the mortality rate was 2.2%. Vasospasm complicated 22% of ruptured aneurysms.[3]

Lozier and colleagues[6] reviewed 12 single-institution case series for a total of 495 posterior circulation aneurysms; 82% of these were categorized as basilar apex aneurysms and 81% were either unruptured or in good clinical condition.

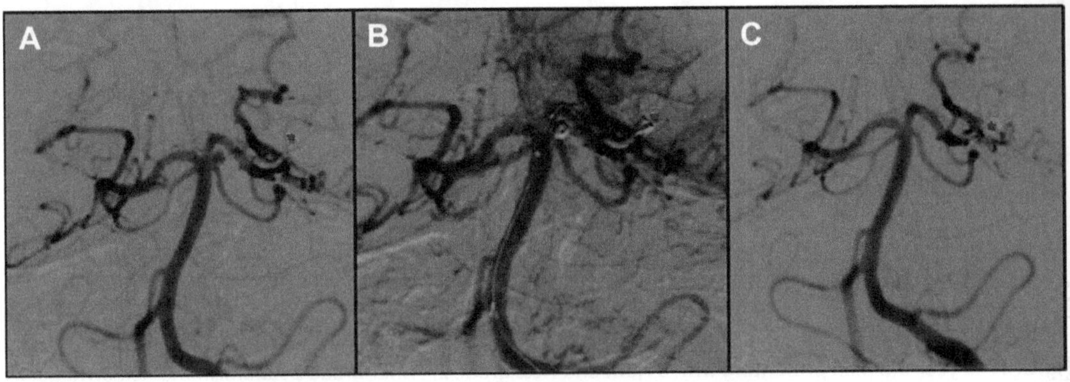

Fig. 3. A 58-year-old woman with a previously symptomatic clipped posterior communicating artery aneurysm who presented with an incidental left 4-mm SCA aneurysm. Given her prior history of symptomatic aneurysm, treatment was pursued. (*A*) Mid-arterial anteroposterior projection revealing saccular SCA aneurysm. Clip from the prior craniotomy is evident and marked by the asterisk. (*B*) Balloon remodeling and coiling of aneurysm. (*C*) Complete embolization of SCA aneurysm.

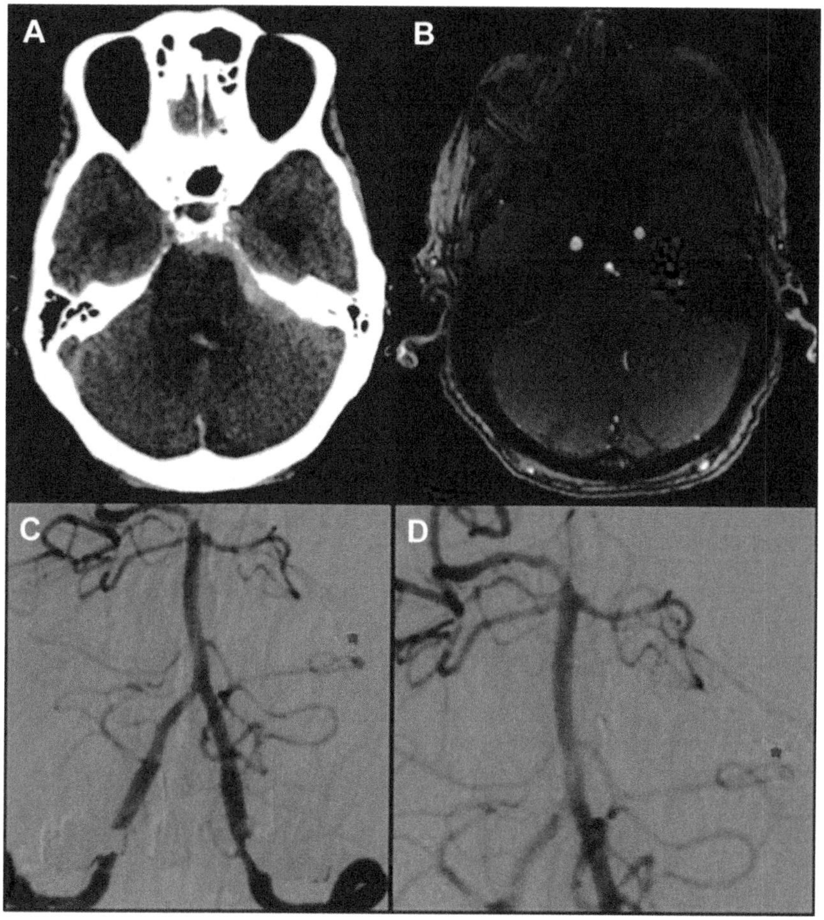

Fig. 4. A 91-year-old woman with multiple medical comorbidities presents after several weeks of left hearing disturbances and acute headache with Hunt and Hess grade 3, Fisher grade 3 subarachnoid hemorrhage. (*A*) Noncontrast head computed tomography revealing subarachnoid hemorrhage in the prepontine cistern and cerebellopontine angle. (*B*) Magnetic resonance angiogram revealing distal AICA aneurysm, marked by the asterisk. (*C*) After extensive discussion with the family regarding the patient's poor prognosis aggressive medical care was requested. Diagnostic cerebral angiogram revealed a distal AICA aneurysm in the meatal segment of the AICA. (*D*) Coil embolization of the aneurysm with distal AICA patency. Three days postcoiling, the patient had new facial droop and complete hearing loss, indicating possible distal vessel thrombosis and stroke.

Overall procedural complication and morbidity rates were 12.5% and 5.1%, respectively. Coil was deployed in 97.6% of treated aneurysms, and 91.0% of aneurysms were treated with complete or near-complete occlusion.

Coil Compaction and Aneurysm Recanalization

The morphology and anatomic location of basilar apex aneurysm increase the risk of coil compaction. Models have shown that complete coil obliteration of an aneurysm only fills 30% of the aneurysm with coil mass.[41,42] For most aneurysms, 90% to 100% occlusion should protect from hemorrhage by excluding the aneurysm fundus from circulation. Partial occlusion of 50% to 90% is helpful in acutely ruptured aneurysms by covering the site of rupture with coil mass. Less than 50% occlusion is likely to be ineffective in providing protection from rerupture.[2]

Aneurysms with smaller necks are easier to achieve complete occlusion.[34] Wider-necked aneurysms (>4 mm) are at high risk for recanalization and should be followed closely. This risk is most likely related to flow dynamics and stress, which can lead to coil compaction. Rates of early recanalization can be substantial in wide-necked or partially treated aneurysms.[3,6,12,13]

Coil compaction and aneurysm recanalization were seen in 24% of treated aneurysms in the series by Henkes and colleagues.[3] The degree of occlusion and packing density are the greatest predictors of future aneurysm recanalization. Retreatment was pursued in 15% of those with 90% to 100% occlusion. Of those, 83% were successfully retreated and had an overall good clinical outcome. Procedural morbidity of a second treatment was 4%.[3] In the series of basilar apex aneurysms by Lozier and colleagues,[6] recanalization rates were estimated at 10% for completely occluded aneurysms, 37% for near occlusion, and 60% if incompletely occluded.[6]

CLINICAL OUTCOMES

Posterior circulation aneurysms are poorly represented in trials comparing clipping and coiling; however, this evidence favors coiling over clipping for reducing morbidity. In a meta-analysis of clipping versus coiling of ruptured aneurysms, poor outcome was seen in 31.1% of clipped aneurysms as opposed to 23.4% of coiled aneurysms, whereas the rehemorrhage rate was 1.2% versus 2.3%, respectively. For coiled aneurysms, the rehemorrhage rate was related to degree of occlusion.[4]

Aneurysm necks greater than 4 mm are more difficult to completely occlude because of coil migration and prolapse into the parent vessel.[39] Complete occlusion rate varies in literature from 21% to 84%.[3,12,43–45] The series by Henkes and colleagues[3] achieved complete occlusion in 61% coiled aneurysms. Rerupture in 11 patients for a rate of 1.3% in completely occluded aneurysms and 2.1% in partially occluded aneurysms. Complete occlusion was durable in 78.0% of patients at first follow-up.[3] Increased risk of recanalization with wide necks was seen. Lozier and colleagues[6] found a rerupture risk equal to 0.7% per year, with a return to independent function in 85.0% of patients and an overall follow-up mortality rate of 9.8% in their cohort.[6]

In a series of 33 basilar apex aneurysms by McDougall and colleagues,[13] immediate angiographic occlusion was achieved in 21.2% of patients and greater than 90% occlusion in 51.5%. Twenty of these aneurysms were wide-necked and 23 presented with subarachnoid hemorrhage. At follow-up angiography, 21.0% of the aneurysms were completely occluded and 63.2% were occluded greater than 90% but less than 100%. A single patient experienced recurrent hemorrhage at 6-month follow-up.

Other small series reflect similar results. Bavinzski and colleagues[12] reported on a group of 45 coiled basilar apex aneurysms, of which 75% presented with subarachnoid hemorrhage. Of these, 73% were categorized as excellent outcomes. Complete occlusion occurred in 67% of patients and greater than 90% (but <100%) occlusion was seen in 20%. These results were durable at follow-up, with 12 patients displaying angiographic coil compaction, 8 of whom underwent re-treatment. Recanalization occurred in 57% of wide-necked aneurysms and 8% of narrow-necked aneurysms. Rehemorrhage occurred in one previously ruptured aneurysm and none of the unruptured aneurysms. Raymond and colleagues[14] treated 31 basilar apex aneurysms with coiling, with a 94% success rate. Seven recurrences occurred within 42 months, 5 of which required re-treatment. No rehemorrhage events were documented at the conclusion of the study.

Regarding functional outcomes, the rate of independence in the series by Henkes and colleagues[3] was 82.0%.[2] The series by Lozier and colleagues[6] showed similar results, with 84.0% of coiled basilar apex aneurysms being independent, 6.8% dependent, and 9.5% dead. When divided into treated ruptured and nonruptured aneurysms, 80.2% of patients with ruptured aneurysms were independent and 90.6% of those with unruptured aneurysms were independent at last follow-up.[6]

FOLLOW-UP CONSIDERATIONS

Although no consensus exists regarding follow-up of treated aneurysms, close follow-up is recommended, particularly for wide-necked basilar apex aneurysms.

All patients receive a formal diagnostic cerebral angiogram (DCA) at 6 months to document complete occlusion or early recanalization. For ruptured aneurysms, noninvasive diagnostic imaging is then obtained 1 year later, then annually for 2 years, and then once every 2 to 5 years. For nonruptured aneurysms, noninvasive imaging is obtained after 1 year. If no recurrence is seen, patients are typically discharged, with follow-up as needed. If recanalization or coil compaction is seen at follow-up, re-treatment or close follow-up is required. Re-treatment is especially important in wide-necked ruptured aneurysms that were not stent-coiled at the time of rupture, which prevented sufficient packing density within the aneurysm. This practice is consistent with the recommendations of the American Heart Association.[46]

The authors prefer magnetic resonance angiography with contrast as the noninvasive study to limit coil- and stent-related artifacts seen on computed tomography (CT). They also find that the gadolinium-enhanced study improves visualization of flow-through stents.

Regarding antiplatelet therapy, patients that undergo stenting remain on dual antiplatelet therapy for a minimum of 3 months. After 3 months, if the patient is asymptomatic and without any thromboembolic complications, clopidogrel is held and full-dose aspirin is continued. Full-dose aspirin is transitioned to 81 mg indefinitely at 6 months if occlusion remains complete.

Delayed Thromboembolism

To prevent delayed thromboembolism, a combination of antiplatelet therapy is used. In acutely ruptured aneurysms with wide necks and an exposed coil mass, aspirin is started after a stable head CT on the day of treatment. Stenting in these patients is avoided to prevent the need for dual antiplatelet therapy.

Dual antiplatelet therapy is used in all patients undergoing stenting. Some patients are unresponsive to clopidogrel inhibition and are at greater risk for a periprocedural ischemic stroke, because the target moiety of platelets, $P2Y_{12}$, has been shown to have a variable response to clopidogrel.[47,48] The real-time evaluation of platelet inhibition with the VerifyNow $P2Y_{12}$ assay (Accumetrics, San Diego, CA, USA) is a measure some interventionists use to guide therapy.[49] However, no standard of care has been established regarding the medication regimen to be used in patients who experience no response to standard clopidogrel inhibition. At the authors' institution, the daily dose of clopidogrel is typically doubled to 150 mg in divided doses, whereas other investigators have advocated adding cilostazol or ticlopidine to standard clopidogrel therapy.[50]

SUMMARY

Basilar artery aneurysms constitute a small percentage of intracranial aneurysms; however, they are a diverse group, requiring many different treatment techniques for unruptured and ruptured aneurysms. Basilar apex aneurysms are the most common type and are frequently wide-necked, necessitating stent-assisted coiling or balloon remodeling. The prevention of delayed thromboembolic complications with dual antiplatelet therapy in patients with stents is critical. After treatment, basilar aneurysms require close follow-up to ensure complete occlusion. It is not uncommon for basilar apex aneurysms to require delayed retreatment, especially when previously ruptured.

REFERENCES

1. Unruptured intracranial aneurysms–risk of rupture and risks of surgical intervention. International Study of Unruptured Intracranial Aneurysms Investigators. N Engl J Med 1998;339(24):1725–33.
2. Henkes H, Fischer S, Weber W, et al. Endovascular coil occlusion of 1811 intracranial aneurysms: early angiographic and clinical results. Neurosurgery 2004;54(2):268–80 [discussion: 280–5].
3. Henkes H, Fischer S, Mariushi W, et al. Angiographic and clinical results in 316 coil-treated basilar artery bifurcation aneurysms. J Neurosurg 2005;103(6):990–9.
4. Li H, Pan R, Wang H, et al. Clipping versus coiling for ruptured intracranial aneurysms: a systematic review and meta-analysis. Stroke 2013;44(1):29–37.
5. Peerless SJ, Hernesniemi JA, Gutman FB, et al. Early surgery for ruptured vertebrobasilar aneurysms. J Neurosurg 1994;80(4):643–9.
6. Lozier AP, Connolly ES Jr, Lavine SD, et al. Guglielmi detachable coil embolization of posterior circulation aneurysms: a systematic review of the literature. Stroke 2002;33(10):2509–18.
7. Liu JK, Gottfried ON, Couldwell WT. Thrombosed basilar apex aneurysm presenting as a third ventricular mass and hydrocephalus. Acta Neurochir 2005;147(4):413–6 [discussion: 417].
8. Wiebers DO, Whisnant JP, Huston J 3rd, et al. Unruptured intracranial aneurysms: natural history, clinical outcome, and risks of surgical and endovascular treatment. Lancet 2003;362(9378):103–10.
9. Schievink WI, Wijdicks EF, Piepgras DG, et al. The poor prognosis of ruptured intracranial aneurysms of the posterior circulation. J Neurosurg 1995;82(5):791–5.
10. Higashida RT, Halbach VV, Cahan LD, et al. Detachable balloon embolization therapy of posterior circulation intracranial aneurysms. J Neurosurg 1989;71(4):512–9.
11. Zeumer H, Bruckmann H, Adelt D, et al. Balloon embolization in the treatment of basilar aneurysms. Acta Neurochir 1985;78(3–4):136–41.
12. Bavinzski G, Killer M, Gruber A, et al. Treatment of basilar artery bifurcation aneurysms by using Guglielmi detachable coils: a 6-year experience. J Neurosurg 1999;90(5):843–52.
13. McDougall CG, Halbach VV, Dowd CF, et al. Endovascular treatment of basilar tip aneurysms using electrolytically detachable coils. J Neurosurg 1996;84(3):393–9.
14. Raymond J, Roy D, Bojanowski M, et al. Endovascular treatment of acutely ruptured and unruptured aneurysms of the basilar bifurcation. J Neurosurg 1997;86(2):211–9.
15. Vinuela F, Duckwiler G, Mawad M. Guglielmi detachable coil embolization of acute intracranial aneurysm: perioperative anatomical and clinical outcome in 403 patients. J Neurosurg 1997;86(3):475–82.
16. Rhoton AL Jr. Aneurysms. Neurosurgery 2002;51(Suppl 4):S121–58.

17. Moret J, Cognard C, Weill A, et al. The "remodelling technique" in the treatment of wide neck intracranial aneurysms. Angiographic results and clinical follow-up in 56 cases. Interv Neuroradiol 1997; 3(1):21–35.
18. Khatri R, Cordina SM, Hassan AE, et al. Sequential sidelong balloon remodeling technique in coil embolization of a wide-necked basilar tip aneurysm. J Vasc Interv Neurol 2013;6(1):7–9.
19. Shima H, Nomura M, Muramatsu N, et al. Embolization of a wide-necked basilar bifurcation aneurysm by double-balloon remodeling using HyperForm compliant balloon catheters. J Clin Neurosci 2009;16(4):560–2.
20. Fargen KM, Mocco J, Neal D, et al. A multicenter study of stent-assisted coiling of cerebral aneurysms with a Y configuration. Neurosurgery 2013; 73(3):466–72.
21. Mahaney KB, Chalouhi N, Viljoen S, et al. Risk of hemorrhagic complication associated with ventriculoperitoneal shunt placement in aneurysmal subarachnoid hemorrhage patients on dual antiplatelet therapy. J Neurosurg 2013;119(4):937–42.
22. Kung DK, Policeni BA, Capuano AW, et al. Risk of ventriculostomy-related hemorrhage in patients with acutely ruptured aneurysms treated using stent-assisted coiling. J Neurosurg 2011;114(4): 1021–7.
23. Kwon OK, Kim SH, Kwon BJ, et al. Endovascular treatment of wide-necked aneurysms by using two microcatheters: techniques and outcomes in 25 patients. AJNR Am J Neuroradiol 2005;26(4): 894–900.
24. Baxter BW, Rosso D, Lownie SP. Double microcatheter technique for detachable coil treatment of large, wide-necked intracranial aneurysms. AJNR Am J Neuroradiol 1998;19(6):1176–8.
25. Chalouhi N, Tjoumakaris S, Dumont AS, et al. Treatment of posterior circulation aneurysms with the pipeline embolization device. Neurosurgery 2013; 72(6):883–9.
26. Van Rooij WJ, Sluzewski M, Menovsky T, et al. Coiling of saccular basilar trunk aneurysms. Neuroradiology 2003;45(1):19–21.
27. van Oel LI, van Rooij WJ, Sluzewski M, et al. Reconstructive endovascular treatment of fusiform and dissecting basilar trunk aneurysms with flow diverters, stents, and coils. AJNR Am J Neuroradiol 2013;34(3):589–95.
28. Rinkel GJ, Djibuti M, Algra A, et al. Prevalence and risk of rupture of intracranial aneurysms: a systematic review. Stroke 1998;29(1):251–6.
29. Liu L, Jiang C, He H, et al. Delayed thrombosis of the basilar artery after stenting for a basilar trunk dissection aneurysm. A case report and review of the literature. Interv Neuroradiol 2010;16(1): 77–82.
30. Drake CG, Amacher AL. Aneurysms of the posterior cerebral artery. J Neurosurg 1969;30(4): 468–74.
31. Ciceri EF, Klucznik RP, Grossman RG, et al. Aneurysms of the posterior cerebral artery: classification and endovascular treatment. AJNR Am J Neuroradiol 2001;22(1):27–34.
32. Hallacq P, Piotin M, Moret J. Endovascular occlusion of the posterior cerebral artery for the treatment of p2 segment aneurysms: retrospective review of a 10-year series. AJNR Am J Neuroradiol 2002;23(7):1128–36.
33. Haw C, Willinsky R, Agid R, et al. The endovascular management of superior cerebellar artery aneurysms. Can J Neurol Sci 2004;31(1):53–7.
34. Uda K, Murayama Y, Gobin YP, et al. Endovascular treatment of basilar artery trunk aneurysms with Guglielmi detachable coils: clinical experience with 41 aneurysms in 39 patients. J Neurosurg 2001;95(4):624–32.
35. Bambakidis NC, Manjila S, Dashti S, et al. Management of anterior inferior cerebellar artery aneurysms: an illustrative case and review of literature. Neurosurg Focus 2009;26(5):E6.
36. Li X, Zhang D, Zhao J. Anterior inferior cerebellar artery aneurysms: six cases and a review of the literature. Neurosurg Rev 2012;35(1):111–9 [discussion: 119].
37. Yamakawa H, Hattori T, Tanigawara T, et al. Intracanalicular aneurysm at the meatal loop of the distal anterior inferior cerebellar artery: a case report and review of the literature. Surg Neurol 2004; 61(1):82–8 [discussion: 88].
38. Gonzalez LF, Alexander MJ, McDougall CG, et al. Anteroinferior cerebellar artery aneurysms: surgical approaches and outcomes–a review of 34 cases. Neurosurgery 2004;55(5):1025–35.
39. Molyneux A, Kerr R, Stratton I, et al. International Subarachnoid Aneurysm Trial (ISAT) of neurosurgical clipping versus endovascular coiling in 2143 patients with ruptured intracranial aneurysms: a randomised trial. Lancet 2002;360(9342):1267–74.
40. Molyneux AJ, Kerr RS, Yu LM, et al. International subarachnoid aneurysm trial (ISAT) of neurosurgical clipping versus endovascular coiling in 2143 patients with ruptured intracranial aneurysms: a randomised comparison of effects on survival, dependency, seizures, rebleeding, subgroups, and aneurysm occlusion. Lancet 2005;366(9488): 809–17.
41. Kawanabe Y, Sadato A, Taki W, et al. Endovascular occlusion of intracranial aneurysms with Guglielmi detachable coils: correlation between coil packing density and coil compaction. Acta Neurochir 2001; 143(5):451–5.
42. Piotin M, Mandai S, Murphy KJ, et al. Dense packing of cerebral aneurysms: an in vitro study with

detachable platinum coils. AJNR Am J Neuroradiol 2000;21(4):757–60.
43. Eskridge JM, Song JK. Endovascular embolization of 150 basilar tip aneurysms with Guglielmi detachable coils: results of the Food and Drug Administration multicenter clinical trial. J Neurosurg 1998; 89(1):81–6.
44. Guglielmi G, Vinuela F, Duckwiler G, et al. Endovascular treatment of posterior circulation aneurysms by electrothrombosis using electrically detachable coils. J Neurosurg 1992;77(4):515–24.
45. Tateshima S, Murayama Y, Gobin YP, et al. Endovascular treatment of basilar tip aneurysms using Guglielmi detachable coils: anatomic and clinical outcomes in 73 patients from a single institution. Neurosurgery 2000;47(6):1332–9 [discussion: 1339–42].
46. Johnston SC, Higashida RT, Barrow DL, et al. Recommendations for the endovascular treatment of intracranial aneurysms: a statement for healthcare professionals from the Committee on Cerebrovascular Imaging of the American Heart Association Council on Cardiovascular Radiology. Stroke 2002;33(10):2536–44.
47. Pinto Slottow TL, Bonello L, Gavini R, et al. Prevalence of aspirin and clopidogrel resistance among patients with and without drug-eluting stent thrombosis. Am J Cardiol 2009;104(4):525–30.
48. Muller-Schunk S, Linn J, Peters N, et al. Monitoring of clopidogrel-related platelet inhibition: correlation of nonresponse with clinical outcome in supra-aortic stenting. AJNR Am J Neuroradiol 2008; 29(4):786–91.
49. Fukuoka T, Furuya D, Takeda H, et al. Evaluation of clopidogrel resistance in ischemic stroke patients. Intern Med 2011;50(1):31–5.
50. Maruyama H, Takeda H, Dembo T, et al. Clopidogrel resistance and the effect of combination cilostazol in patients with ischemic stroke or carotid artery stenting using the VerifyNow P2Y12 Assay. Intern Med 2011;50(7):695–8.

Cerebral Vasospasm

Christopher D. Baggott, MD[a], Beverley Aagaard-Kienitz, MD[b,*]

KEYWORDS

- Cerebral vasospasm • Subarachnoid hemorrhage • Neurologic deficits
- Delayed ischemic neurologic injury

KEY POINTS

- Vasospasm after aneurysmal subarachnoid hemorrhage (aSAH) has long been known to cause delayed ischemic neurologic injury, and the rate of delayed ischemic neurologic injury remains unacceptably high.
- Investigating the inflammatory, genetic, and structural pathophysiology of cerebral vasospasm has translated into therapeutics that reduce delayed ischemic neurologic injury.
- Aggressive evidence-based treatment of cerebral vasospasm is essential, and this includes close neurologic monitoring, physiologic augmentation, pharmaceutical administration, and endovascular intervention.
- Understanding and treatment of cerebral vasospasm are inadequate; rigorous clinical trials and relentless basic science can make a great impact on this disease process.

INTRODUCTION

Vasospasm is defined as focal or diffuse temporarily narrowed vessel caliber due to contraction of smooth muscle in the wall of arteries as detected by angiography or imaging studies (transcranial Dopper [TCD], magnetic resonance [MR], and CT) or as seen during surgical clipping. aSAH remains the most common cause of significant cerebral vasospasm. Despite major advances over the past 3 decades in surgical and endovascular aneurysm treatment and improvements in neurologic intensive care, cerebral vasospasm remains the major cause of death and disability in patients after the initial hemorrhage. This is a significant problem because the estimated incidence of aSAH in the United States is between 21,000 and 33,000 people per year.[1] Vasospasm occurs in 67% of aSAH patients, is symptomatic in 30% to 40%, and results in ischemic infarction in 10% to 45% of patients.[2–6] The consequences of vasospasm result in disability in 25% to 50% of survivors, with only 30% to 45% of survivors returning to previous comparable jobs.[7,8] It is the cause of death in 10% to 23% of aSAH patients.[7,8]

Vasospasm and delayed neurologic deficit from aSAH remain an incompletely understood complex chain of events with as yet incompletely synthesized common pathways involving inflammation, altered vascular biomechanics, dysfunctional autoregulation, microcirculatory thromboembolism, poor collateral anatomy, and genetic influences. Currently there is no consensus on treatment modalities or treatment times, although there are published guidelines.[9]

HISTORY OF VASOSPASM

The first probable case of cerebral vasospasm was described by an English physician, Sir William Gull,[10] who in 1859 published a case report of Fanny S—, a 30-year-old female patient. Case IV, "ingravescent apoplexy from rupture of an aneurism on middle cerebral artery of left side; death on sixth day," is presented and discussed in his publication. The actual subarachnoid

Disclosures: None.
[a] Department of Neurological Surgery, University of Wisconsin Hospital and Clinics, 600 Highland Avenue, Madison, WI 53792, USA; [b] Neuroendovascular Fellowship: Endovascular Neurosurgery/Neurointerventional Surgery, Neuroendovascular Section, University of Wisconsin Hospital and Clinics, 600 Highland Avenue, Madison, WI 53792, USA
* Corresponding author.
E-mail address: BAagaard-Kienitz@uwhealth.org

Neurosurg Clin N Am 25 (2014) 497–528
http://dx.doi.org/10.1016/j.nec.2014.04.008
1042-3680/14/$ – see front matter

hemorrhage (SAH) event on November 4, 1850, was witnessed and involved initial transient loss of consciousness followed by severe headache, nausea, and vomiting. She was admitted to Guy's Hospital the next day, November 5, 1850, comatose with right hemiplegia. After admission, she improved and regained consciousness on the third hospital day, was able to eat, and attempted to speak. On the fourth hospital day, she was able to recognize a relative who visited her and was able to say, "my cousin." On the evening of the fifth hospital day (November 9, 1850), however, she exhibited a progressive neurologic decline and died, 6 days after SAH. At autopsy, a ruptured middle cerebral artery aneurysm was found, adjacent to a second unruptured aneurysm associated with a large clot in the sylvian fissure and softening in the many areas of adjacent brain. This constellation of clinical course and findings at autopsy is persuasive of cerebral infarction secondary to cerebral vasospasm, although this mechanism was not recognized at the time.[10]

Many investigators have made significant contributions over the past decades in attempting to elucidate causes for vasospasm. In 1942, Echlin[11] demonstrated that electrical and mechanical stimulation could induce vasospasm of pial arteries, reducing regional blood flow and producing temporary focal cerebral ischemia, in animals. In her 1944 article, Zucker[12] described an elaborate series of in vitro experiments in many different animal tissues, demonstrating substances in animal blood sera that stimulated smooth muscle contraction. In 1949, Robertson[13] concluded that ischemic lesions in patients with ruptured aneurysms were occasionally due to arterial spasm and suggested that this entity was a more common cause of ischemia than was realized. In 1951, Ecker and Riemenschneider[14] demonstrated vasospasm of major cerebral arteries associated with ruptured circle of Willis aneurysms in a series of angiograms. In 6 aneurysm cases, they noted that vasospasm was the most severe near the site of the ruptured aneurysm correlating to the largest amount of blood products. These investigators also noted that vasospasm was a self-limited process because, although it was seen in early angiograms, it was not seen in any angiograms performed 26 days after aSAH. Fletcher and colleagues[15] noted in their 1959 article that vasospasm not infrequently occurred after intracranial aneurysm rupture, also noting that direct observation of spastic vessels at surgery was seen more commonly as an increasing number of aneurysms were being treated with open surgical clipping. In the same year, Pool and colleagues[16] demonstrated that topical application of 3% papaverine during surgery improved vasospasm induced by surgical manipulation. In 1964, Stornelli and French[17] reported on 28 patients that the appearance of vasospasm on angiographic images was more common in patients who died than in patients who recovered after aSAH. The normal range in size of the carotid arteries and their major branches was established by Gabrielsen and Greitz in 1970.[18] This information led Weir and colleagues,[19] in 1978, to establish the time course of cerebral vasospasm in humans. Performing serial measurements on angiograms in 293 patients, they concluded that the onset of vasospasm after SAH occurred on approximately day 3, was maximal on days 6 to 8, and essentially was resolved by day 12. In 1980, Fisher and colleagues[20] noted, in an analysis of 47 ruptured aneurysm patients, "an almost exact correspondence between the site of the major subarachnoid blood clots and the location of severe vasospasm," and the Fisher CT grading system for SAH was proposed. In addition, despite the low number of cases studied, Fisher and colleagues noted that "blood localized in the subarachnoid space in sufficient amount at specific sites is the only important etiologic factor in vasospasm," thus establishing CT as an important tool to identify patients at highest risk for cerebral vasospasm.

Attempts to preserve and improve cerebral blood flow (CBF) and reduce the consequences of severe vasospasm were fully under way, both medically and endovascularly, in the 1970s and 1980s. In 1976, Hunt and Kosnik[21] published their results using hypertension postoperatively to alleviate ischemic symptoms attributed to cerebral vasospasm; additionally, they used blood volume expansion to augment vasopressor treatment. In 1979, Zervas and colleagues[22] published a randomized study to determine if administration of reserpine and kanamycin would reduce the incidence of cerebral ischemia after SAH. And in 1982, Kassell and colleagues[23] published their work using intravascular volume expansion and induced arterial hypertension to reverse neurologic deterioration in 47 of 58 patients. Balloon angioplasty to treat SAH-induced vasospasm was developed by Zubkov and colleagues[24] in 1984. Then, in 1989, Pickard and colleagues[25] published the British aneurysm nimodipine trial, a double-blind, placebo-controlled, randomized trial that is still the single-drug treatment regime for vasospasm that has class I, level A evidence as to efficacy.[26] The 1990s and 2000s saw continued intense investigations in an attempt to prevent occurrence and improve treatment of SAH-induced vasospasm but without any major breakthroughs in improved neurologic outcomes.

Numerous agents (magnesium, statins, nitroprusside, endothelin [ET] receptor antagonists, free radical scavengers, and so forth) have been tried. The lack of success in preventing/treating vasospasm and limiting neurologic injury is partly because the posthemorrhage milieu is an extremely complex series of biomechanical and inflammatory processes, influenced by an individual patient's underlying vascular anatomy and genetics. Although a single-agent approach may be appealing, such a complex problem requires a multimodality treatment approach to be successful. Additionally, it is increasingly understood that large-vessel vasospasm is only one cause of poor neurologic outcome and that a complete reevaluation of the causes of the devastating sequelae after aSAH, including microvascular spasm, microvascular thromboembolism, genetic factors, and cortical spreading depolarization (SD), to mention several, is necessary. To eliminate cerebral vasospasm and improve neurologic recovery after SAH, all of the underlying mechanisms and common pathways need to be more fully elucidated and a multimodal treatment approach developed.

The publications and studies that are presented are too numerous and detailed to be completely described in a single article; in addition, the field is so complex that not all areas or articles can be included in this review. Because the full role vasospasm plays in neurologic injury and patient outcome remains unclear, but because the effects of vasospasm are clearly involved, agents and treatments to prevent and treat it are presented. Thus, the highlights from a portion of the literature on biochemomechanical, genetic, standard, and experimental pharmacologic agents and current mechanical treatment are presented and readers are encouraged to read the original articles and delve into other ancillary articles in their particular areas of interest.

THE ROLE OF INFLAMMATION AND BIOMECHANICS OF VASOSPASM

In their 2007 article, Humphrey and colleagues[27] describe the complexity of the environment after SAH and propose a theoretic biochemomechanical framework for cerebral vasospasm. They hypothesize that "vasospasm and its potential resolution result from an acute vasoconstriction due to the initial bleed, a short-term chemo-dominated growth and remodeling (G&R) process that progresses in evolving vasoconstricted states in response to the developing extravascular clot and produces a narrowed lumen and thicker wall, which is stiffer and largely unresponsive to exogenous vasodilators, and finally a mechano-dominated G&R process that progresses in evolving vasodilated states in response to the dissolution of the clot and restores the vessel toward normal" (see Humphrey's **Figs. 1** and **2**). After hemorrhage, the organizing extracellular clot causes an increase in nitric oxide (NO) scavengers, including reactive oxygen species and oxyhemoglobin, and an increase in vasoconstrictors, including serotonin, thromboxane A2, ET-1, and thrombin, which shifts the vascular mechanics toward vasoconstriction. Clot-related mitogens, including platelet-derived

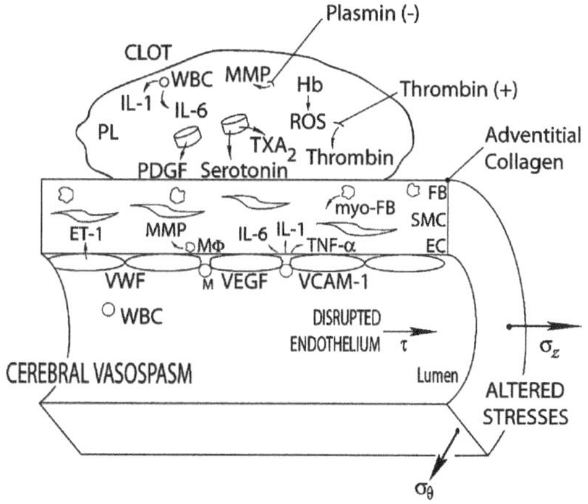

Fig. 1. This schematic from Humphrey et al illustrates some of the molecules involved in the development and dissolution of a clot outside of the blood vessels. As the clot organizes via the thrombin-fibrin cascade, platelets are activated, releasing vasoconstrictors. Meanwhile, there is a free radical chain reaction at play as nitic oxide and oxyhemoglobin interact, resulting in reactive oxygen species (ROS). This process exacerbates smooth muscle contraction and vasoconstriction. The shear stress of blood flow through the lumen of the constricted vessel can disrupt endothelium, leading to increased monocyte (M) and macrophage (M-ϕ) accumulation at the site of endothelial injury. Resultant matrix metalloproteases (MMPs) perpetuate damage to the vessel wall and stimulate production of disruptive chemokines and proteases. EC, endothelial cell; ET-1, endothelin-1; FB, fibroblast; Hb, hemoglobin; IL, interleukin; myo-FB, myofibroblast; Mϕ, macrophage; M, monocte; MMP, matrix metalloproteinase; PDGF, platelet-derived growth factor; ROS, reactive oxygen species; SMC, smooth muscle cell; TXA_2, Thromboxane A_2; TNF, Tumor necrosis factor; VCAM, vascular cell adhesion molecule; VEGF, vascular endothelial growth factor; VWF, von Willebrand factor; WBC, white blood cell; σ_z, mean axial load-induced wall stress; σ_θ, mean pressure-induced circumferential wall stress; τ, flow induced wall shear stress. (*From* Humphrey JD, Baek S, Niklason LE. Biochemomechanics of cerebral vasospasm and its resolution: I. A new hypothesis and theoretical framework. Ann Biomed Eng 2007;35(9):1486; with permission.)

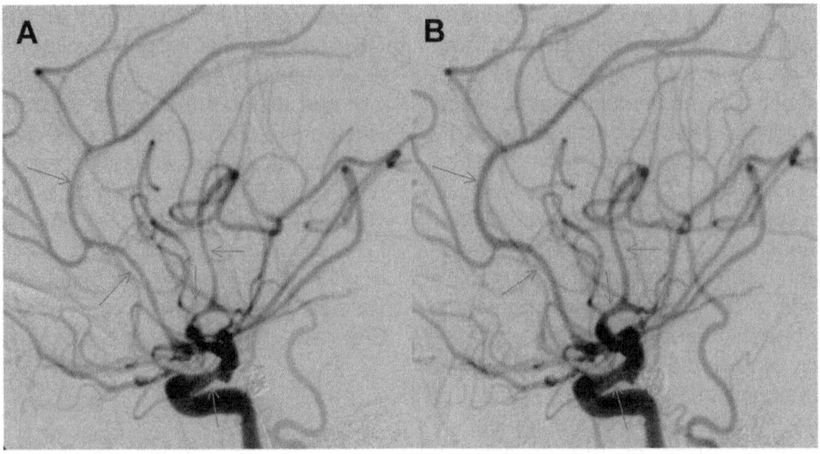

Fig. 2. Infusion of verapamil improves luminal caliber in small vessels not amenable to balloon angioplasty. (*A*) Preinfusion of IA verapamil (15 mg). (*B*) Postinfusion angiogram 20 minutes after drug infusion. Arrows demonstrate vessels in vasospasm that narrower in caliber before infusion of IA verapamil (*A*), and are larger in caliber (dilated) after infusion of IA verapamil (*B*).

growth factor, transforming growth factor B, and ET-1, promote proliferation/migration of medial smooth muscle cells and adventitial fibroblasts. These changes may result in synthesis of additional collagen, increase the mass/thickness of the vessel wall, and increase the structural stiffness. Severe vasoconstriction may disrupt endothelial cells, causing a decrease in endothelial cell production of NO and prostacyclin (PGI2) and also result in a decreased responsiveness to circulating vasodilators, further promoting constriction. Up-regulation of multiple adhesion and chemotactic factors (cell adhesion molecules—vascular cell adhesion molecule 1 and intracellular cell adhesion molecule 1, and monocyte chemoattractant protein 1) promote inflammatory responses (interleukins—IL-1, IL-6, and IL-8, and tissue necrosis factor a) and degradatory responses (macrophages and matrix metalloproteinases [MMPs]—MMP-1, MMP-2, and MMP-9) by sequestering/activating leukocytes and mononuclear phagocytes. Thus, the subarachnoid clot and endothelial disruptions sets off a cascade of factors that results in changes in smooth muscle cells and the extracellular matrix, the end result of which is a narrowed lumen and thickened vessel wall. The altered biomechanics of the vessel wall (decreased intramural stress and increased wall shear stress) may, however, in turn, stimulate production of vasodilators (NO), platelet inhibitors (PGI2), and growth factors (vascular endothelial growth factors [VEGFs]). These factors, in conjunction with clearing of the extravascular clot and endothelial recovery, promote remodeling of the vascular wall, eventually restoring the normal luminal diameter.

The complexity of this cascade as described (and even more complex than currently understood) with promoting and resolving factors demonstrates why a single agent or target is unlikely to be effective. In addition, vasospasm seems to occur in concert with microthrombosis[28] and spreading cortical depolarizations,[29] which further underscores the complexity of the process and the necessity of a multimodal treatment.

THE GENETICS OF VASOSPASM

An increasing area of research is what effect mutations and polymorphisms have on the development of cerebral vasospasm. Several genes are under evaluation as to their association with vasospasm: eNOS, Hp, PAI-1, ApoE, RyR1, and CBS (see Table 1 in ref[30]).

Nitric Oxide

NO, an endothelium-derived relaxing factor, is synthesized by NO synthase (NOS). Endothelial NOS (eNOS), found on chromosome 7q35, is present in the endothelium of cerebral arteries. Decreased bioavailability of eNOS is linked to cerebral vasospasm. Several mutations and polymorphisms of eNOS are known, which may at least partly predispose patients to vasospasm. In coronary literature, Nakayama and colleagues[31] found that the 786T>C mutation resulted in a significant reduction in eNOS gene promoter activity and the incidence of the mutations was significantly greater in patients with coronary spasm than in the control group ($P<.0001$). In the cerebral vasculature, Khurana and colleagues[32] evaluated 51 SAH patients with genomics DNA assays for 3 eNOS gene polymorphisms. Of the 28 patients presenting with Fisher 3 SAH, 21 developed vasospasm and 90% (19/21) of these patients were either cytosine allele heterozygous (18/19) or homozygous (1/19). The abnormal allele was positive in 4 of 7 patients without vasospasm, 8 of 10 patients with asymptomatic vasospasm, and 11 of 11 patients with symptomatic vasospasm ($P = .046$).

Ko and colleagues[33] also found that the 786T>C single-nucleotide polymorphism (SNP) was an increased risk for aSAH vasospasm. In their prospective cohort study of 347 SAH patients, 181 were diagnosed with vasospasm as documented by catheter angiography. Three eNOS polymorphisms were genotyped: an intron 4 variable-number tandem repeat, a promoter SNP (786T>C SNP), and a coding SNP in exon 7 (894G>T encoding E298D). Using multivariable logistic regression, they quantified the association of eNOS polymorphisms in patients with documented vasospasm. For the eNOS promoter 786T>C SNP, they found that the presence of the CC genotype, compared with any T genotype (CT or TT), was associated with increased risk of vasospasm (odds ratio [OR] 2.97; 95% CI, 1.32 – 6.67; $P = .008$). There was no association with vasospasm for the eNOS 894G>T or variable-number tandem-repeat polymorphisms. They concluded that genetic variation influencing NO regulation contributes to the risk of angiographic vasospasm and that the specific role of the promoter SNP (786T>C) may determine the effect of NO regulated by this pathway.

Starke and colleagues[34] also reported that alterations in the eNOS T-786 SNP may increase the risk of cerebral vasospasm after aSAH. In their prospective study, genetic material was obtained from 77 aSAH patients who were then observed for vasospasm. They found a significant increase in vasospasm with the TT genotype (61%) compared with the CT (35%) or CC genotype (0%) ($P = .003$). Fisher grade and genotype were the only significant predictors of vasospasm in univariate analysis, and genotype was the only independent predictor of vasospasm multivariable analysis. Patients with the T allele of the eNOS gene were also more likely to have severe vasospasm. OR for symptomatic vasospasm in patients with 1 T allele was 3.3 and 10.9 for TT. Patients with angiographic vasospasm were 3.6 times more likely to have a T allele. Patients requiring endovascular therapy for severe vasospasm were also more likely to have a T allele (OR 3.5; 95% CI, 1.3–9.5; $P = .016$; TT OR 12.0). There was no significant difference, however, in infarction based on genotype. The investigators concluded that genetic analysis could stratify a patient's risk to develop vasospasm; thus, early identification of patients with a T allele could lead to earlier treatment and potentially improve patient outcomes.

Ryanodine

Ryanodine receptors (RyRs) are a class of calcium release channels located at the endoplasmic reticulum that regulate luminal calcium concentration by mediating calcium-induced calcium release. There are 3 subtypes present in vascular smooth muscle (RyR1, RyR2, and RyR3).[35,36] RyRs are involved in regulating cerebral artery luminal diameter,[37,38] and RyRs, especially RyR1, are associated with symptomatic vasospasm after SAH. In a pilot gene association study of 46 patients, Rueffert and colleagues[39] found that SAH patients who were heterozygous carriers for the G>T genotype of RyR1 c.6178G>T polymorphism had an increased risk of developing symptomatic vasospasm (OR 6.4; 95% CI, 1.1%–37.8%; $P = .04$) compared with C>T or G>A. In the patients without vasospasm ($n = 30$), there were only 6.7% G>T carriers ($P = .04$). In the patients with symptomatic vasospasm ($n = 16$), 31.3% carried the c.6178G>T polymorphism. In the 7 patients who were heterozygous for G>T, 5 (71.4%) developed symptomatic vasospasm: 3 died due to severe complications from vasospasm, 1 survived with serious disability, and 1 survived with moderate recovery. The other 2 patients with c.6178G>T polymorphism had no symptomatic vasospasm.

Further evidence implicating RyR1 in vasospasm is found in studies using RyR1 antagonists. Dantrolene, a specific RyR1 antagonist, may prevent cerebral vasoconstriction in basilar and femoral arteries in rats[40] and has been shown to reduce vasoconstriction after dantrolene infusion in 3 human patients as measured by TCD velocities.[41]

INFLAMMATORY BIOMARKERS

The development of genomics and proteomics may lead to identifying biomarkers highlighting inflammatory changes to predict vasospasm and neurologic outcomes. One possible marker is the 25-kDa protein, high-mobility group box 1 protein ($HMGB_1$), a nonhistone DNA-binding protein that facilitates gene transcription in the nucleus.[42] $HMGB_1$ stimulates proinflammatory cytokines when it is in the extracellular space.[43] $HMGB_1$ is passively released into the cerebrospinal fluid (CSF) by necrotic neurons and thus may provide an early marker for cerebral ischemia and neurologic injury. King and colleagues[44] evaluated CSF for $HMGB_1$ and found it in all CSF samples from SAH patients ($n = 9$) and not present in CSF from any of the control patients (n = 7). Although the full functions of $HMGB_1$ are as yet incompletely elucidated they postulate, "$HMGB_1$ may represent a clinically-relevant, mechanistic link between acute injury and secondary neurovascular injury following SAH."

Another potential biomarker is MMP-9 from the class of MMPs. Metalloproteinases regulate the extracellular matrix and basal lamina; these extracellular and membrane-bound proteases are major extracellular degrading enzymes and remodel all of the components in the matrix and perform essential functions at the cell surface, including signaling and cell death.[27,45] The activity of MMPs is regulated by gene transcription, proenzyme activation, and the action of tissue inhibitors of metalloproteinases.[46] McGirt and colleagues[47] studied von Willebrand factor (vWF), MMP-9, and VEGF levels as prognostic markers in predicting cerebral vasospasm. Venous serum vWF, MM-9, and VEGF levels were prospectively measured in 38 aSAH patients as well as 7 unruptured aneurysm controls (admitted for clipping). To ascertain if these markers were specific for vasospasm versus ischemia, blood samples from a concurrent group of 42 nonhemorrhagic stroke patients within 24 hours after stroke onset were also obtained; 22 of the 38 patients (57%) developed vasospasm. They found that cerebral vasospasm was preceded by increases in serum vWF, MMP-9, and VEGF levels and were predictive of the onset of cerebral vasospasm after SAH. Moreover, these factors were not elevated by the presence of SAH alone nor were they elevated in control patients or patients with ischemic stroke. In their study, vWF levels of more than 5500 ng/mL, VEGF levels of more than 0.12 ng/mL, and MMP-9 levels of more than 700 ng/mL each independently increased the odds of subsequent vasospasm (18-, 20-, and 25-fold, respectively).

Recent animal work reported by Wang and colleagues[48] showed that the expression of MMP-9 peaked on postbleed day 3 and returned to normal on day 14 in an experimental SAH rat model. They also evaluated the effect of a selective MMP-9 inhibitor, SB-3CT, on the maximum time point of vasospasm (day 3). Using the cross-sectional area of the basilar artery and intracisternal administration of SB-3CT, they found that vasospasm was markedly reduced on postbleed day 3. Thus, there was a parallel time course between increasing MMP-9 levels and the development of cerebral vasospasm and that administration of an MMP-9 inhibitor could prevent or reduce vasospasm in this experimental rat model of SAH.

DETECTION/MONITORING OF VASOSPASM

Symptomatic cerebral vasospasm manifests most objectively as a new focal deficit not explained by hydrocephalus or rebleeding. Clinicians must also have a high index of suspicion, however, in the proper clinical circumstance when subtle change in neurologic examination, elevation of mean arterial blood pressure (MABP) from a cerebrally driven autopressor effect, or mild symptoms, like worsening headache, elevated temperature, worsening neck stiffness, or progressive hyponatremia, are encountered.[20,26,49,50]

Angiographic vasospasm has been detected as early as 48 hours after SAH in 10% of cases reported in a prospective trial.[51] Symptomatic vasospasm is rare within 3 days of SAH and peaks at approximately day 8. Symptomatic vasospasm occurs in approximately 4% of cases after day 13[50,52,53]; however, multiple episodes of aSAH may prolong this course. Fisher grading is a commonly used tool to help predict the likelihood of vasospasm.[20]

In the event of delayed neurologic deterioration after SAH, it is important to have a fairly broad differential diagnosis, particularly when the deterioration is nonfocal. In addition to vasospasm, there must be consideration of hyponatremia, hypoxia, hypercarbia, pneumonia, urinary tract infection, bacteremia, medication reaction, uremia, fever, aneurysmal rebleed, hydrocephalus, postoperative complication (stroke, hematoma, infection, and so forth), cerebral edema, seizure, and postictal state as possible causes in the differential diagnosis for delayed neurologic deficit after SAH.

Frequent careful assessment of the neurologic examination is essential but not in itself sufficient for the detection of symptomatic cerebral vasospasm, notably in high-grade patients with significant posthemorrhagic alterations in alertness. Patients requiring sedation for intracranial pressure (ICP) or respiratory management also may suffer delayed ischemia related to vasospasm that can be difficult to detect by neurologic examination alone.

Tools for evaluation of large-vessel caliber, such as TCD and perfusion imaging with CT angiography (CTA) and MR angiography, as well as tools for evaluation of the physiologic impact of vasospasm, such as electroencephalogram (EEG), near-infrared spectroscopy (NIRS), and brain tissue oxygen monitoring, are appropriate adjuncts in the detection of symptomatic cerebral vasospasm.[26,54–67] More work needs to be done to clarify the role of these neurologic examination adjuncts in the diagnosis of vasospasm. TCD, CTA, perfusion imaging, and EEG are discussed, because these modalities are used commonly in the authors' institution for evaluation of cerebral vasospasm.

Transcranial Doppler

Introduced by Aaslid and colleagues in 1982,[67] TCD has become a mainstay in the detection of cerebral vasospasm. TCD is an inexpensive portable noninvasive ultrasonic technique that measures blood flow velocity and direction in the proximal portions of the larger cerebral arteries via a transtemporal acoustic window. According to an American Academy of Neurology expert committee, there is level A, class II level evidence supporting the use of TCD given that severe spasm can be identified fairly reliably, despite variable sensitivity and specificity.[64] Normal mean velocity for the MCA is 62 ± 12 cm/s. Significant spasm on angiogram of the MCA corresponds to a mean velocity of 120 cm/s. Mean velocities of the MCA of 200 cm/s or greater indicate severe spasm and correlate with 50% or greater narrowing on angiogram.[68] The advantages of TCD are that it can be performed at a patient's bedside (thus not needing to move a critically ill patient with many lines/tubes), is highly specific to detecting vascular narrowing, has no side effects, and can be repeated as frequently as necessary or desired. Limitations of TCD include that it is operator dependent, requires a good acoustic window, has less than 60% sensitivity,[69] can be falsely positive with induced hypertension,[70] may have poor correlation with cerebral angiography in the anterior cerebral artery territory,[71] and poorly reflects smaller vessel vasospasm compared with perfusion imaging.[72] Guidelines for the management of aneurysmal subarachnoid hemorrhage: a statement for healthcare professionals from a special writing group of the Stroke Council, American Heart Association (Stroke guidelines) state that TCD has not adequately demonstrated improved outcome in treatment of SAH, and other adjuncts "have been advantageous in guiding management and may be complementary."[26]

CT, CT Angiography, and CT Perfusion

CTA and CT perfusion (CTP) imaging is increasingly used to assess patients for clinically relevant vasospasm and ischemia, in particular those with poor neurologic status. Advantages of CT include noninvasive accurate assessment, rapid imaging acquisition and reconstruction, and no anatomic limitation to imaging (like TCD). In a recently published meta-analysis, CTA pooled estimates had 79.6% sensitivity (95% CI, 74.9%–83.8%) and 93.1% specificity (95% CI, 91.7%–94.3%). CTP pooled estimates had 74.1% sensitivity (95% CI, 58.7%–86.2%) and 93.0% specificity (95% CI, 79.6%–98.7%).[73] Although metallic implants (clips, coils, and other metallic devices) can cause image degradation on CT/CTA images from beam hardening artifacts, the use of corrective algorithms are increasingly reducing these artifacts and improving imaging quality, which also is true for C-arm CT.[74] Additionally, CT, CTA, and CTP can be acquired at the same examination, combining the imaging strength of each study to provide rapid and more accurate diagnosis. Although portable CT scanners are becoming more widely used in neuro-ICUs, currently most patients are still transported to a radiology department for imaging, a disadvantage of this type of study for unstable and critically ill patients.

CT angiography

CTA was first used in the assessment of cerebral vasospasm in 1997 when Ochi and colleagues[75] published 2 cases demonstrating that noninvasive vessel imaging correctly identified vasospasm as confirmed with catheter angiography. CT imaging technology continued to develop and, with the advent of multidetector CTA, significantly improved spatial resolution at lower contrast doses was possible. Yoon and colleagues[76] studied 251 vessel segments in 17 patients suspected of having vasospasm and found that the agreement between the degree of vasospasm revealed by CTA and digital subtraction angiography (DSA) in the overall, proximal, and distal segments of the cerebral arteries was 95.2%, 96.0%, and 94.1%, respectively. Otawara and colleagues[77] studied 20 patients with multislice CTA and DSA for severity of vasospasm and found that the agreement between the severity between CTA and DSA in the overall, proximal, and distal segments of the cerebral arteries was 91.6%, 90.8%, and 92.3%, respectively. CTA technique involves intravenous (IV) injection of an iodinated contrast bolus followed by rapid scanning. Although CTA still does not match the resolution of DSA, CTA is fast, noninvasive, and inexpensive compared with catheter angiography and can be used as a surrogate for DSA for screening purposes. This is especially advantageous for critically ill or unstable patients in whom longer imaging procedures may be problematic. Correctly timing the bolus injection of contrast during acquisition is critical and has an impact on the quality of image reconstruction. The iodinated contrast requirement for this study can be a problem in patients with significant renal insufficiency; however, newer algorithms using less contrast are being developed. Additional renal protective methods, such as hydration with sodium bicarbonate,[78] hydration and oral acetylcysteine,[79] and hydration with use of isoosmolar noninonic contrast,[80] may limit renal injury.

CT perfusion

CTP studies are increasingly used to assess patients for evidence of poor perfusion secondary to vasospasm. Validation studies comparing CTP CBF measurements with positron emission tomography and with stable xenon CT have been performed and, with proper processing techniques, show good correlation.[81] CTP is a functional imaging study at the capillary level of the brain performed during the rapid infusion of IV contrast; repeated scanning is performed throughout the wash-in and washout of contrast and the resultant change in attenuation of the brain parenchyma is measured. Time-attenuation curves can be obtained for arterial, venous, and parenchymal regions of interest (ROIs). Postprocessing methods are then used to calculate the quantitative perfusion parameters of CBF in milliliters per 100 g/min, cerebral blood volume (CBV) in milliliters per 100 g, and mean transit time (MTT). The accepted normal range for CBV is 4.4 ± 0.9 mL/100 g in gray matter and 2.3 ± 0.4 mL/100 g in white matter. The normal range of values for MTT is less than 5 s.

Although no definitive diagnostic threshold values of cerebral perfusion have been established, several studies have evaluated and suggested thresholds to detect cerebral ischemia after SAH. Dankbaar and colleagues[82] found CBF was significantly lower, MTT higher, and perfusion asymmetry larger in patients with delayed cerebral ischemia (DCI) after SAH compared with clinically stable patients. Diagnostic threshold values with optimal sensitivity and specificity were an MTT of 5.9 seconds and an MTT difference of 1.1. The sensitivity and specificity were 70% and 77% for MTT. A CBF threshold of 36.3 mL/100 g/min or a CBF ratio of 0.77 between abnormal and normal contralateral hemisphere yielded sensitivity and specificity values of 74% and 76% and 63% and 63%, respectively.[82]

A study by Wintermark and colleagues[83] retrospectively evaluated 27 patients with acute SAH who had undergone CTA/CTP, TCD, and DSA within 12 hours of each other and these examinations were independently reviewed and quantified for vasospasm. Correlation with patients' charts for treatment of vasospasm was also performed; 35 examinations were performed on 27 patients. They found qualitative assessment of CTA and the CTP MTT threshold at 6.4 seconds represented the most accurate (93%) combination for the diagnosis of vasospasm and thus represented an accurate screening test for patients with suspected vasospasm. MTT considered alone was the most sensitive parameter (negative predictive value, 98.7%). A cortical regional CBF value less than or equal to 39.3 (mL $\times$ 100 g^{-1} $\times$ min^{-1}) represented the most accurate (94.8%) indicator for endovascular therapy. CTP had significantly higher positive predictive value (89.9%) than TCD (62.9%).

Electroencephalography

EEG has been used to detect reversible cerebral ischemia in carotid endarterectomy since the 1970s.[63] Specific EEG patterns show high correlation with vasospasm.[54,55,61] Real-time quantitative analysis has emerged as a way to elicit clinically useful objective data in the diagnosis of cerebral vasospasm.

Labar and colleagues[59] recorded 11 ischemic events with continuous quantitative EEG in 11 patients after SAH. The sensitivity of the trend analysis parameter of change in total power was 91%. This suggests the EEG may be an indicator of vasospasm that correlates with clinical symptoms of ischemia.

Continuous quantitative EEG monitoring focusing on the ratio of fast alpha activity and slow delta activity, the alpha-delta ratio (ADR), has been applied by Claassen and colleagues[54] with intriguing results. The group presented a series of 34 Hunt-Hess SAH Classification Grade 4 or 5 SAH patients. Of the 34 patients, 9 patients (26%) developed DCI as diagnosed by the study neurologist and confirmed retrospectively by 2 additional study physicians. The clinically useful cutoffs defined by the group were any single ADR decrease greater than 50% from baseline (sensitivity 89% and specificity 84%) as well as 6 consecutive recordings with less than 10% decrease in ADR from baseline (sensitivity 100% and specificity 76%).

Even more intriguing, Vespa and colleagues[65] present evidence that EEG change may precede clinical signs of cerebral ischemia. In all patients with angiographically documented vasospasm (n = 19 from a total of 32 patients), evaluation of relative alpha variability was decreased with vasospasm and increased with resolution of vasospasm. Relative alpha variability preceded clinical diagnosis of vasospasm by almost 3 days, although there were nondiagnostic signs of cerebral ischemia at the time of alpha variability decrease in 12 of the 19 patients. "Decreased variability was 100% sensitive but only 50% specific for vasospasm."

Continuous quantitative EEG may be useful to rule out vasospasm at the time of a delayed neurologic deficit during the vasospasm period after SAH given the suggestion of good sensitivity and a strong negative predictive value. Furthermore, earlier intervention based on EEG may be worth investigating; however, the lack of specificity with continuous quantitative EEG may be inhibitory. The ADR and alpha variability seem the most promising quantitative tools currently, but more investigation into the potential of real-time spectral analysis of EEG is appropriate.

MEDICAL THERAPY FOR VASOSPASM

Catheter-based angiography not only is the gold standard for diagnosis of cerebral vasospasm but also is a critical tool in the rapid treatment of a delayed neurologic deficit after SAH. Prior to discussion of medical therapy for vasospasm, it should be clear that early progression to endovascular therapy is reasonable in patients "who deteriorate neurologically secondary to suspected vasospasm and who do not improve rapidly after hemodynamic optimization" or where the diagnosis is uncertain and hemodynamic therapy is difficult or risky, such as in the elderly or those with cardiac disease.[50] Goals of medical management after SAH include optimizing CBF, reducing cerebral metabolic demand, and preventing secondary injury from either hydrocephalus or cerebral ischemia.

Hemodynamic Therapy

Hemodynamic therapy, popularized as triple-H therapy, is "one reasonable approach to symptomatic vasospasm."[26] Triple-H therapy includes hypervolemia, hypertension, and hemodilution.

Hypervolemia has been studied in 2 randomized trials. Lennihan and colleagues[84] conducted a blinded randomized trial of prophylactic hypervolemia versus normovolemia. There was no improvement in outcome and no reduction in delayed ischemia in the group randomized to prophylactic hypervolemia. There was no change in CBF by xenon washout but elevated cardiac filling pressures. Outcomes at 14 days and 90 days were no different. Egge and colleagues[85] conducted a randomized trial of triple-H therapy versus normovolemia without hyperdynamic therapy. Triple-H therapy included prophylactic hypervolemia (with goal central venous pressure [CVP] 8–12 cm H_2O), induced hypertension (with goal mean arterial pressure [MAP] >20 mm Hg higher than preoperative values), and hemodilution (with goal hematocrit 30%–35%). Outcomes at 12 days by single-photon emission CT and clinical examination were no different. There was no difference in 1-year clinical follow-up. Complications and costs were higher with prophylactic hypervolemic and hypertensive therapy. From the available literature, the Stroke guidelines state: "Avoiding hypovolemia is advisable, but there is no evidence that prophylactic hyperdynamic therapy is of any utility."[26]

A reasonable approach in the management of cerebral vasospasm should include monitoring volume status and treating volume contraction with isotonic fluids (class IIa, level of evidence B). Hyponatremia, likely a result of cerebral salt wasting and a cause for volume contraction, may be an independent risk factor of poor outcome. In addition to administration of large volumes of isotonic fluids to deal with volume contraction, fludrocortisone and hypertonic saline are reasonable for reducing or correcting hyponatremia due to naturesis.[26]

Permissive hypertension and induced hypertension are tools commonly used despite no literature to support practice. This practice stems from the relatively certain reversal of delayed neurologic deficit in patients with cerebral vasospasm with the induction of hypertension. Most practitioners support induced hypertension in the setting of symptomatic vasospasm.[50] There is not strong evidence that prophylactic hypertension lessens the incidence of symptomatic vasospasm.

Hemodilution remains controversial. There is evidence that CBF can be increased but oxygen delivery capacity is decreased with isovolemic hemodilution.[26] There are no convincing data to support an ideal hematocrit in the treatment of cerebral vasospasm, although many practitioners advocate a hematocrit of 28% to 32%.[50]

To conclude, in light of the available literature and guidelines, early management of the ruptured aneurysm is reasonable to facilitate permissive or induced hypertension as a first-response to a new delayed neurologic deficit diagnosed clinically as symptomatic vasospasm. Avoidance of hyponatremia and hypovolemia is appropriate. Prophylactic hypertension and hypervolemia are not well supported by available literature. Hemodilution is controversial and not well supported.

Oral Nimodipine

Regarding other established treatments for symptomatic vasospasm, oral nimodipine is clearly associated with improved neurologic outcomes after SAH, but the underlying mechanism remains uncertain.[86] Oral nimodipine (60 mg every 4 hours) has been shown to improve outcomes compared with placebo in the randomized double-blinded British aneurysm nimodipine trial. Demographic and clinical data at entry were similar in the 2 groups, 278 treated with nimodipine and 276 given placebo. In patients given nimodipine, the incidence of cerebral infarction was 22% (61/278) compared with 33% (92/276) in those given placebo, a significant reduction of 34% (95% CI, 13%–50%). Poor outcomes were also significantly reduced by 40% (95% CI, 20%–55%) with nimodipine 20% (55/278) versus 33% (91/278) in those given placebo.[25] Furthermore, a meta-analysis of 7 trials and a total of 1202 patients also demonstrated that nimodipine improved outcome on all measures examined.[86] Bederson and colleagues[26] in the Stroke guidelines recommend oral nimodipine citing level of evidence A, class I evidence.

The Stroke guidelines recommend endovascular therapy as a reasonable treatment of symptomatic vasospasm "after, together with, or in place of triple-H therapy."[26] Other methods under investigation to reduce the incidence of vasospasm include cardiac output augmentation, cisternal application of pharmaceuticals, and clot evacuation.[3,5,41,87–94]

Cardiac Augmentation

Cardiac output augmentation has been considered by investigators seeking a pharamacologic method of increasing CBF in light of the disappointing results of hypervolemic therapy, which is associated with higher complication rates and no change in CBF compared with normovolemic therapy. Joseph and colleagues[94] showed an increase in CBF with augmentation of cardiac index from 4.1 L/min/m^2 to 6.0 L/min/m^2 with dobutamine. The CBF increase was similar to the CBF increase found when MAP was increased from 102 to 132 mm Hg with phenylephrine. To clarify the relative roles for hypertension and cardiac output augmentation, Kim and colleagues[89] looked retrospectively at 174 patients, finding that hypervolemia (CVP >8 mm Hg) and hypertension (MAP goal 110–130 mm Hg) showed greater sepsis, pulmonary edema, and mortality than did normovolemic optimization of cardiac output (>4.5 L/min/m^2).

Intracisternal Agents

Cisternal application of vasoactive agents, such as papaverin, milrinone, and nicardipine, have been investigated, given promising results in in vitro and in vivo animal studies as well as in limited human trials.[88,89,93] Application of thrombolytic agents, such as urokinase and tissue plasminogen activator (tPA), likewise have been used with provocative results. Although there is no consensus regarding the role of these agents in vasospasm treatment, further investigation is ongoing.

Kim and colleagues[89] conducted a prospective study of cisternal irrigation with papaverin (n = 40), cisternal irrigation with urokinase (n = 39), and simple cisternal drainage (n = 42); notably, endovascularly treated SAH was excluded. This study did show a significant reduction in vasospasm with urokinase and papaverin compared with simple continuous drainage. There was no significant difference, however, in 6-month Glasgow Outcome Scale (GOS) scores among the 3 groups.

Nicardipine prolonged-release pellets have been placed in humans safely with promising results in a cohort study (n = 20).[88] Cisternal milrinone has been shown effective in a canine model of cerebral vasospasm by Nishiguchi and colleagues[93]; there is suggestion in their work that cisternal administration is more effective than IV administration, but this is not clearly established because the enhanced effect may also be dose dependent to some degree.

Milrinone and calcium channel antagonists are discussed in more detail later, because the experience with intra-arterial (IA) administration has been more thoroughly reported in the literature to date.

Clot clearance either mechanically or aided by thrombolytic agents may be useful given the association of clot thickness with vasospasm coupled with the numerous vasoactive substances released in the process of clot breakdown.

Urokinase administration was promoted by Yoshida and colleagues[95] in 1985. Kodama and colleagues have published a very low vasospasm rate (2.8%) in patients with Fisher grade 3 SAH and clot density greater than 60 Houndsfield units who undergo cisternal irrigation with urokinase and ascorbic acid. This rate of delayed neurologic deficit is compared with a rate of 32.5% according to a review of 30,000 cases by Dorsch and King.[96] Findlay and colleagues[87] and Seifert and colleagues[97] transitioned the work of cisternal thrombolytics to use tPA.

Cisternal administration of tPA via cisternal catheters placed at the time of craniotomy was investigated prospectively by Mizoi and colleagues.[92] After removal of as much clot as possible at the time of surgery, cisternal catheters were placed; tPA was administered into the subarachnoid space daily until all cisterns showed low density on CT, with catheters left in place for 2 weeks total, regardless of the duration of tPA administration. There was a significant reduction in delayed ischemic neurologic deficit in the tPA group, although the SAH in the control group was significantly more severe than in the tTPA group.

TIMING OF INTERVENTIONAL TREATMENT

There is as yet no consensus regarding the timing for treatment despite evidence that the timing of intervention is critical and earlier intervention before irreversible ischemia occurs results in better outcomes. Medical treatment to prevent and treat vasospasm should commence with the diagnosis of aSAH. As discussed previously, with the development of new neurologic symptoms, other entities (infection, seizure, hyponatremia, and ventricular drain malfunction) should be quickly considered and eliminated. Imaging may be necessary to exclude completed infarction or nonvasospasm causes for neurologic decline. If vasospasm is detected or if clinical suspicion remains high without another plausible explanation, catheter-based angiography should be performed and medically refractory symptomatic vasospasm aggressively treated (balloon angioplasty, IA vasodilator infusion, or both); this should occur with the same concern and urgency as acute ischemic stroke. Early aggressive treatment in less than 2 hours seems the most effective way to prevent cerebral infarction and improve neurologic function in medically refractory patients. In 1999, Rosenwasser and colleagues[98] studied 466 Hunt-Hess SAH Classification Grades 1–4 patients with aSAH treated with either open surgical clipping or endovascular coiling. Of these, 93 developed medically refractory vasospasm and underwent balloon angioplasty and, for distal vasospasm, IA papaverine infusion; 84 of the 93 were available for follow-up at 6 months. They observed that 70% of the 51 patients treated within 2 hours demonstrated sustained clinical improvement whereas only 40% of the 33 patients treated more than 2 hours (up to 18 hours) had sustained improvement. They concluded that a 2-hour window may exist for restoration of blood flow to ultimately improve a patient's outcome.

There is additional evidence, however, that delayed treatment (>2 hours) may benefit some patients and should be considered even 12 to 24 hours after symptom onset. Forty percent of Rosenwasser and colleagues[98] patients treated up to 18 hours had sustained improvement. Eskridge and colleagues[99] found that 61% of patients treated with balloon angioplasty within 18 hours of symptom onset demonstrated objective neurologic improvement. Bejjani and colleagues[100] found a clear tendency toward more significant improvement in patients with angioplasty less than 24 hours from onset of neurologic deficit ($P = .0038$).

Relative contraindications to endovascular treatment include a fixed neurologic deficit greater than or equal to 24 hours, imaging studies demonstrating completed infarction without significant penumbra, and large existing infarction at risk for reperfusion hemorrhage. Additionally, patients should not be considered for balloon angioplasty if TCD, CTA, and/or angiographic demonstrates evidence of vasospasm in a neurologically intact and asymptomatic patient. Results from 2 studies[101,102] have been published on prophylactic balloon angioplasty; however, the current literature and guidelines[9,103] do not support prophylactic invasive treatment of asymptomatic patients.

ENDOVASCULAR THERAPY FOR VASOSPASM

For those patients with medically refractory vasospasm or those with cardiac, renal, or pulmonary comorbidities precluding aggressive medical management, endovascular therapy can be performed. Current accepted standard endovascular treatment consists of mechanical dilatation with balloon-mounted microcatheters, selective or superselective pharmacologic vasorelaxation with IA drug infusion, or a combination of both. The most common IA agents currently in use include papaverine, calcium channel blockers nicardipine and verapamil, and milrinone. Of the other IA agents used, only fasudil is discussed here.

Angioplasty

Angioplasty is a controlled injury to the wall of the vasospastic vessel produced by endoluminal inflation of a balloon to the normal or just subnormal diameter to temporarily impair the functionality of vascular smooth muscle. Meygyesi and colleagues[104] studied in vivo distal cervical carotid arteries in canines with balloon angioplasty compared with controls and found durable enlargement of the carotid lumen on angiography in the canines treated with angioplasty and functional impairment of the vascular smooth muscle that persisted at least 7 days. Scanning and transmission electron microscopy demonstrated flattening of the intima and internal elastic lamina associated with patch loss of endothelial cells. A larger, longer, and more extensive canine study by the same investigators evaluated the long-term effects of balloon angioplasty up to 56 days. Scanning electron microscopy findings correlated well with angiographic studies, with dilated normal and vasospastic vessels showing enlargement of the vessel lumen to near-normal size, patchy endothelial denudation, and straightening/thinning of the internal elastic lamina. These changes in the angioplastied vessels essentially resolved after 28 days. Again, noted after angioplasty was immediate functional impairment of vascular smooth muscle with minimal or no response to vasoconstricting agents for 2 weeks.[105] Similar changes are seen in human vessels postangioplasty on autopsy studies. Honma and colleagues[106] evaluated the cerebral vessels in 2 patients, both of whom died 5 days after uncomplicated balloon angioplasty. In both patients, the extracellular matrix, including collagen, and the medial muscle components were stretched. In 1 patient, intramural hemorrhages and torn/thinned areas in the wall were found, which the investigators attributed to overinflation.

Zubkov and colleagues[107] reported compression of connective tissue, stretching of the internal elastic lamina, and compression and stretching of smooth muscle in a woman who failed to improve after angioplasty and died from aneurysm rerupture. Also noted was that the distal small arteries and arterioles that had been treated with an infusion of IA papaverine remained vasoconstricted and exhibited a thickened intimal layer.

Currently, utility of balloon angioplasty is based on positive anecdotal evidence; however, many case series have been published over the years demonstrating the safety and efficacy of balloon angioplasty to treat refractory vasospasm in the larger basal cerebral vessels. Reduction in TCD velocities, improved CBF on perfusion studies, and improved neurologic condition have been reported in many publications after balloon angioplasty for vasospasm.[100,108–111] In 1989, Newell and colleagues[112] reported 10 patients treated with angioplasty for symptomatic vasospasm not responsive to hypervolemic hypertensive therapy: 8 patients (80%) had sustained neurologic improvement after angioplasty and 2 patients underwent postangioplasty TCD evaluation, which showed decreased mean blood flow velocities after angioplasty treatment. Firlik and colleagues[113] studied14 consecutive patients, 13 of whom who underwent pre- and postangioplasty xenon-enhanced CT scanning, measuring 55 to 65 ROIs per patient. Angiographic improvement after angioplasty was seen in 13 (93%) patients. Mean CBF increased in at-risk ROIs in 12 (92%) of patients (13 mL/100 g/min preangioplasty vs 44 mL/100 g/min postangioplasty; $P = .00005$). Oskouian and colleagues[110] studied CBF, TCD velocities, and vessel diameter measurements in patients treated endovascularly for vasospasm; in the 12 patients treated with angioplasty alone, CBF increased from 27.8 $\pm$ 2.8 mL/100 g/min to 28.4 $\pm$ 3.0 mL/100 g/min ($P = .87$); the middle cerebral artery blood flow velocity was 157.6 $\pm$ 9.4 cm/s and decreased to 76.3 $\pm$ 9.3 cm/s ($P = .05$), with a mean increase in cerebral artery diameters of 24.4%. In 13 patients treated with both balloon angioplasty and IA infusion of papaverine (thus also treating the distal vasculature) the CBF significantly increased from 33.3 $\pm$ 3.2 mL/100 g/min to 41.7 $\pm$ cm/s to 111.4 $\pm$ 10.6 cm/s ($P<.05$) and decreased the TCD velocities from 148.9 $\pm$ 12.7 cm/s to 111.4 $\pm$ 10.6 cm/s ($P<.05$), with a mean increase in vessel diameters of 42.2%. Hoh and Ogilvy[114] published a review of the existent clinical series of the English language literature up to 2005 on angioplasty and clinical improvement; of 530 patients treated with angioplasty, 328 (62%) showed measureable clinical improvement. In their literature review, they also found 92 of 108 (85%) patients who underwent CBF perfusion studies before and after angioplasty had an improvement in CBF.[114]

Current standards[9] classify balloon angioplasty as class IIa, level B evidence and state, "Cerebral angioplasty and/or selective IA vasodilator therapy is reasonable in patients with symptomatic cerebral vasospasm, particularly those who are not rapidly responding to hypertensive therapy."

Recently, however, a controlled randomized trial in Germany (Vatter H, personal communication, 2014) comparing invasive endovascular rescue therapy for patients with severe vasospasm (angioplasty and IA infusion) versus conventional (unspecified but no intra-arterial therapy) has been halted. The aim of the study, as listed on the Web site, is to investigate if "rescue treatment can significantly reduce new delayed ischemic cerebral deficits after SAH." The hypothesis is that "the occurrence of delayed infarcts can be reduced by repetitive IA therapy to more than 50%." Results from the trial will be published soon.[114]

The overall advantage of balloon angioplasty is that it is more durable than selective drug infusion to treat vasospasm and has been reported to improve cerebral perfusion, which is the goal of treatment. The disadvantage of balloon angioplasty is that it is invasive and, despite advances in imaging and catheter/wire/balloon technology, continues to be associated with risks of microwire vessel perforation, thrombus formation, vessel dissection, vessel occlusion, vessel rupture, ischemic or hemorrhagic stroke, and aneurysm clip displacement, all of which may result in a patient's demise. Vessel rupture from balloon angioplasty ranges in the literature are 1.1%[114] to 4%.[115,116]

Currently, there is no consensus as to the type of balloon (compliant vs semicompliant), method of treatment (starting proximal to distal in the spastic vessel or vice versa), or type of anesthesia for angioplasty but there is wide agreement that the larger vessels 2 to 3 mm in diameter, including intradural internal carotid artery, M1 segment middle cerebral artery, A1 segment of the anterior cerebral artery, intradural vertebral artery, basilar artery, and P1 segment of the posterior cerebral artery, are the target vessels for angioplasty treatment.[103] Smaller and more distal vasopastic vessels (A2, A3, M2, P2, anterior communicating artery, and posterior communicating artery) should be treated with infused IA agents, although, rarely, angioplasty may be performed on the more distal vessels. Given the higher risks involved with distal balloon angioplasty, it is not recommended except on rare occasions and only in highly experienced hands. To reduce the risk of thromboembolism during angioplasty, effective anticoagulation is required; systemic anticoagulation with IV heparin is used most commonly because of its rapid onset of action, reversibility with protamine, and short half-life if not reversed. ACTs can be easily and quickly measured in the angiography suite and ranges from 2 to 2.5 times baseline (usually 250–300 seconds) are obtained. To minimize patient motion during the procedure, optimize safety while passing small catheters and wires intracranially, and to improve visualization of small vessels and vessel bifurcations, many investigators advocate general anesthesia with intubation and paralytics during angioplasty. Using road mapping and digital fluoroscopy while navigating and performing balloon angioplasty also improves visualization and enhance safety. Care should be taken to ensure balloon inflation is occurring in the target vessel and that a portion of the balloon is not in a smaller branch, such as a bifurcation, because failure to recognize this during balloon inflation risks vessel rupture. Particular care should be taken when angioplasty is performed around curved areas of the vessel to treat smaller lengths at a time and not to straighten the vessel to any appreciable degree when the balloon is inflated. The balloon should also not be retracted when substantially inflated, particularly in vessels with perforators (M1, for example) because this may not only increase endothelial injury but also, if perforators are present, may lead to injury or occlusion of the small perforating vessels. Angioplasty should also not be performed subjacent to an aneurysm clip, particularly if it has been recently placed, because there is a risk the clip may be displaced. Balloon inflation diameter should match or be slightly less than the expected normal diameter of the target vessel that has normal vascular architecture; balloon angioplasty in hypoplastic segments (ie, distal vertebral artery or A1 segments of the anterior cerebral artery) is not recommended. If the vasospasm is so severe that advancing the wire and balloon catheter are problematic, then a small infusion of vasorelaxant drug may allow entry of the wire/catheter after a few minutes. The authors have observed in practice that if the entire dose of drug infusion is given prior to angioplasty, then the angioplasty results may not be as durable; thus, the minimal amount of drug is given to facilitate angioplasty and subsequently the rest of the drug is infused to treat the distal vascular bed. If entry into a vessel, such as the A1 segment of the anterior cerebral artery, still cannot be accomplished or it is hypoplastic, the balloon catheter may be inflated transiently in the M1 segment of the middle cerebral artery while the pharmacologic agent is injected into the guide catheter; this allows directed preferential infusion of the agent into the target spastic segment.

Whether treating with balloon angioplasty alone, in combination with pharmacologic agents (which treats both large-vessel and distal vascular and microvascular beds) or with infused agents alone, care must be given to ensuring adequate cerebral perfusion pressure throughout the procedure. Careful attention to MABP and ICP is essential even in patients undergoing angioplasty only. The authors' current treatment protocol, and those of many other investigators, is virtually always to perform IA infusion either alone or after any necessary balloon angioplasty to treat the distal small vessels and microvasculature.

Intra-arterial Agents

Papaverine

Papaverine, a benzylisoquinoline alkaloid, is a potent nonspecific smooth muscle relaxant[117] that affects arteries and veins. Due to side effects, other agents are now used more frequently than papaverine; however, it continues to be the primary agent in some institutions. Published dosing varies from 3 to 5 mg/mL diluted in normal saline, hand injected through a microcatheter, with an approximate 1 to 2 mL/min infusion over 30 to 60 minutes for total dose of 100 to 600 mg/vessel[118] to 300 to 500 mg/vessel infused via microcatheter over 20 to 35 minutes with the rate and dose-dependent MABP and ICP recordings. Papaverine crystallization in heparin or contrast (in particular, ionic) has been reported[118] and can cause crystalline microembolization; visual changes possibly due to crystal microembolism is one reason microcatheter placement was recommended to be distal to the ophthalmic artery prior to infusion. Limitations during infusion are caused by hypotension and elevation of ICP[119] and ICP monitoring during infusion is recommended. Postinfusion of papaverine has reported to result in partial or complete resolution of spasm with increased mean arterial diameter by 26.5%,[120] 30.1%,[110] and between 40% to 100% in 76% of patients.[119] Increased CBF of 60%

with clinical improvement was reported in 43% of patients[114] and decreased cerebral mean circulation time was noted in 38% of patients[121] and 36% in 90 of 91 papaverine treatments.[122] Papaverine has a short half-life of approximately 2 hours and short-acting effect of approximately 24 hours or less with a recurrence of elevated TCDs[109] and a return to prepapaverine delayed cerebral circulation time.[120,123] The transient effect may result in multiple daily trips to the angiography suite while a patient is symptomatic. Elevation of ICP with papaverine infusion has been widely reported, occasionally resulting in poor neurologic outcome,[124] and ICP monitoring during infusion should be used whenever possible. Other serious deleterious effects have been reported, including disruption of the blood-brain barrier with neurologic decline[125]; brain stem depression with respiratory arrest[126]; neurotoxicity resulting in neurologic deterioration, with selective gray matter changes on MRI and neuronal injury on histologic analysis[127]; paradoxic exacerbation of vasospasm[128–130]; and seizure.[131]

Fasudil

Fasudil (hexahydro-1-[5-isoquinolinesulfonyl]-1H-1,4-diazepine hydrochloride) is a protein kinase inhibitor and a potent vasodilator that has shown to effectively treat cerebral vasospasm. Fasudil and its active metabolite, hydroxyl fasudil, cause vasodilation by selective inhibition of rho kinase[132] and rho-associated kinase, thus disinhibiting myosin light chain phosphatase.[133] In 1999, Tachibana and colleagues[134] were the first to report IA fasudil infusion for cerebral vasospasm. Initial IA infusion of fasudil was 1.5 mg/min for a total of 30 mg. Ten patients with 24 vascular territories (21 internal carotid and 3 vertebral) were treated; 3 patients were clinically symptomatic. Two of the 3 symptomatic patients (66.7%) had resolution of symptoms without sequelae; in the third symptomatic patient, the benefit of fasudil was temporary and this patient subsequently developed a cerebral infarction. Nine of the 10 patients demonstrated angiographic improvement in 16 arterial territories postinfusion and none showed later progression vasospasm. No adverse events occurred and no significant hypotension was noted.

In 2005 Tanaka and colleagues[135] published their results treating 23 consecutive patients with focal and/or diffuse moderate to severe symptomatic vasospasm in 34 procedures. Thirteen patients underwent the first fasudil infusion within 12 hours of the onset of clinical symptoms, 4 patients underwent treatment between 12 and 24 hours, and 6 patients were treated after 24 hours. Angiographic improvement was seen in all vessel territories postinfusion, with complete resolution of vasospasm in 3 sessions (11.8%) and partial resolution of spasm in 30 sessions. Nine patients developed recurrent vasospasm in the previously treated territories and underwent multiple fasudil infusions, ranging from 2 to 4 treatments. The dose of fasudil hydrochloride in the initial infusion treatment ranged from 15 to 45 mg (mean 22.5 mg). In the repeat treatments, the dose ranged from 15 to 45 mg (mean 23.2 mg). A significant decrease in MAP was noted from 139.0 $\pm$ 3.4 to 126.8 $\pm$ 3.6 mm Hg ($P<.0001$). ICP was monitored 8 times in 6 patients and the increase in ICP ranged from 1.1 to 5.2 mm Hg. Immediate clinical improvement was seen in 15 patients (65%). Two of the patients developed a "disturbance in consciousness" that resolved in approximately 1 hour. Fifteen patients (65%) demonstrated either a good recovery or moderate disability on GOS score at 3 months' clinical follow-up. Enomoto and colleagues[136] retrospectively analyzed patients with symptomatic cerebral vasospasm for the incidence and dose-related cause of seizure during fasudil infusion. Twenty-three patients underwent 31 procedures in 49 vessels via superselective infusion through a microcatheter at the proximal portion of the spastic artery. In 13 procedures, fasudil was manually infused (30 to 75 mg [1.2–3.7 mg/min]) over approximately 10 minutes. In 18 procedures, fasudil was administered by continuous infusion (60 mg [1.2 mg/mL]) using an infusion pump at a constant rate of 3 mg/min. General or simple partial seizures occurred in 4 patients during infusion who were being infused manually ($P<.05$). Additionally infusion rates greater than 3 mg/min ($P<.01$) were also associated with a higher incidence of seizure. Neurologic improvement after fasudil infusion was observed in 18 of 22 procedures. No changes in MAP were reported.

Milrinone

Milrinone, a selective inhibitor of cyclic adenosine monophosphate (cAMP)-specific phosphodiesterase, is a derivative of amrinone but has up to 30 times greater potency and fewer side effects than the parent drug.[137] It is used primarily to treat acute and chronic heart failure in that it has inotropic activity producing enhanced cardiac contractility, reduced afterload, and improved diastolic compliance.[138,139] Vasodilation occurs because the increase in cAMP in vascular smooth muscle facilitates calcium uptake into the sarcoplasmic reticulum, resulting in a reduction in the amount of calcium available for contraction and thus reducing vascular tone.[140] The half-life is approximately 50 minutes.

The first clinical use of milrinone IA infusion to treat cerebral vasospasm was published by Arakawa and colleagues[137] where 7 patients with symptomatic refractory vasospasm underwent either superselective or selective cervical carotid or vertebral infusion. Milrinone was diluted with physiologic saline to a 25% concentration level, and a total dose of 5 to 15 mg was infused IA at a rate of 1 mL/min (0.25 mg/min). The mean percentage change in vessel diameter infused at the cervical portion of internal carotid artery was 76.8%, and the mean change just proximal to the intracranial vasospastic artery was 78.1%; thus, there was no statistical difference in the effectiveness of IA infusion of milrinone between cervical and superselective infusion. Regional CBF value ipsilateral to the infusion increased significantly, from 32.5 ± 3.5 to 39.3 ± 3.3 mL/100 g/min. No significant changes were observed in patients' mean heart rate or blood pressure. Three of 5 patients required retreatment and in each case satisfactory redilation was achieved by the same protocol. Because of its pharmacologically short half-life and because of the approximate 2-week duration of vasospasm after aSAH, IV infusion of milrinone (0.50 or 0.75 mg/kg/min) was added to help prevent vasospasm recurrence and maintain a hyperdynamic state.

Fraticelli and colleagues[141] treated 22 consecutive patients (16 World Federation of Neurosurgical Societies [WFNS] grades 1–3 and 6 WFNS grade 4) with 34 selective IA milrinone infusion followed by continuous IV milrinone infusion until 14 days after initial SAH. In this study, early detection of cerebral vasospasm was based on serial neurologic examination, body temperature monitoring, and TCD assessment; vasospasm was suspected when patients exhibited neurologic alteration, hyperthermia, or TCD changes, either separately or in combination. Vasospasm was confirmed angiographically. IA milrinone was infused (8 mg over 30 minutes) in the main artery supplying the vasospastic territory (internal carotid, dominant vertebral artery). If there was still residual vasospasm, the infusion could be repeated once more in the same main vessel. For vasospasm in other vascular territories, milrinone infusion could also be performed with a maximum total milrinone dose of 24 mg. All patients also received continuous IV infusion of milrinone; the dose was incrementally increased in patients who tolerated it from 0.5 μg/kg/min to 1.5 μg/kg/min. IV infusion was performed to maintain the plasma concentrations of the drug after IA infusion was completed. The dose escalation was stopped when tachycardia (heart rate >100 bpm) or blood pressure reduction (>20%) occurred. There was a significant improvement in vasospasm after IA milrinone with a 53 ± 37% overall increase in vessel diameter ($P<.0001$). IA milrinone infusion resulted in moderately increased heart rate with stable arterial pressures. Within 48 hours after the procedure, 5 patients (23%) developed angiographically proved recurrence. Two recurrences were treated with IA infusion of milrinone with vasospasm resolution. The remaining 3 patients underwent mechanical angioplasty; 82% of patients had a good neurologic outcome.

Romero and colleagues[142] treated 8 patients with refractory symptomatic cerebral vasospasm with IA infusion of milrinone (rate 0.25 mg/min with total dose 10–15 mg) without an IV supplement. All patients had a significant angiographic response. Three patients developed recurrent vasospasm that improved after a second IA milrinone infusion. None of the patients developed neurologic or systemic complications related to the drug infusion. At 3-months' follow-up, the mean modified Rankin scale was 2 ± 1.

Recently, a short report from Anand and colleagues[143] describes their experience in a single patient with recurrent severe symptomatic proximal and distal left internal carotid artery territory vasospasm despite 3 sessions of IA nimodipine and milrinone, who was then treated with dual continuous IA nimodipine (2 mg/h) and milrinone (1 mg/h) via an indwelling microcatheter as well as IV milrinone at 1 μg/kg/min and 1000 U/h IV heparin. The microcatheter was kept in situ for 72 hours, then removed after giving a final dose of nimodipine (3 mg) and milrinone (3 mg). No discussion of adverse blood pressure changes or other cardiovascular parameters are described. The patient fully recovered without neurologic deficits, and CT imaging reportedly did not demonstrate any significant infarction. The investigators concluded that exceptional cases can be treated with this aggressive approach using higher doses when there is severe refractory vasospasm.

Calcium channel blockers

As a class, calcium channel blockers are agents that reduce the influx of calcium through L-type voltage-gated calcium channels in smooth muscle cells resulting in decreased smooth muscle contraction and subsequent vascular dilation. They may have direct neuroprotective properties by blocking free radical attacks on mitochondria, improving carbon dioxide reactivity and cerebral oxygen metabolism, and possibly reducing apoptosis in ischemic neurons. As a class, they provide effective but transient treatment of vasospasm with the effect time of 12 to 24 or more hours when used IA. There is an apparent high first-pass extraction of the drug when infused IA with a notable differences in cardiovascular dynamics when these agents are injected selectively than less selectively (ie, internal carotid artery, vertebral artery vs common carotid artery); for verapamil this may reflect its lipophilicity,[144] which may allow a large distribution and slow release from the brain. All calcium channel blockers potentially produce significant transient hypotension and systemic blood pressure support using may be needed during infusion. Significant elevated ICP has been reported with IA infusion nicardipine but has rarely been associated with verapamil in a majority of reports.

Nimodipine Nimodipine is a dihydropyridine calcium channel blocker originally developed for the treatment of high blood pressure but is most commonly used in aSAH patients to prevent and treat cerebral vasospasm. In addition to oral administration, nimodipine can be used IA to treat vasospasm. Biondi and colleagues[145] published a retrospective study of 30 procedures in 25 consecutive patients using doses of 1–3 mg nimodipine per vessel (5–15 mL of nimodipine infused after dilution with physiologic saline to obtain a 25% dilution). Slow continuous infusion of the solution at a rate of 2 mL/min (0.1 mg/min nimodipine) was achieved using an electric pump. Dilation of infused vessels was seen in 43% of procedures (13/30) and clinical improvement postprocedure was seen in 76% of patients (19/25). At 3- to 6-month follow-up, 72% of patients had a favorable outcome (Glasgow Coma Scale outcome score 1–2 and modified Rankin scale score 0–2). Hui and Lau[146] published a retrospective study of 9 patients with a reported 66% increased vessel diameter after IA nimodipine; 8 of 9 patients improved clinically (89%) and this was sustained in 7 of 9 patients (78%). Cho and colleagues[147] published their retrospective study of 42 patients and 101 sessions of IA nimodipine and found angiographic improvement in 82.2%, immediate clinical improvement in 68.3%, and a favorable clinical outcome in 76.2% at discharge and 84.6% at 6 months. Transient hypotension (<90 systolic blood pressure) occurred in 14% of patients. Successful treatment of vasospasm using IA nimodipine has also been reported by Kim and colleagues[148] and combination therapy using both nimodipine and milrinone by Anand and colleagues.[143] Although widely considered safe, IA nimodipine has been associated with blood-brain barrier disruption[149] and, in one report, basal ganglia vasogenic edema with deleterious consequences from blood-brain barrier disruption.[150]

Nicardipine Nicardipine is a dihydropyridine calcium channel blocker similar to nimodipine and can significantly improve TCD velocities and neurologic condition in medically refractory patients. Initial dose-escalation studies of IV nicardipine demonstrated notable improvement in angiographic and symptomatic vasospasm[151]; however, these and subsequent IV studies were hampered by significant systemic hypotension. More selective IA nicardipine infusion was then investigated. Badjatia and colleagues noted that although Kaku and colleagues[117] treated vasospastic patients with IA papaverine, all vessels were also treated with IA nicardipine (0.5 to 1.0 mg). Based on this report, Badjatia and colleagues[152] decided to treat with low-dose IA nicardipine only. Under continuous ICP monitoring, 44 vessels in 18 patients were treated with IA nicardipine (0.1 mg/mL) for a maximum of 5 mg/vessel as monotherapy. Significant improvement in TCD velocities were noted in all patients for 4 days after infusion and 42% also improved neurologically. Increased ICP was observed in 6 patients but only persistently elevated in 1 patient; no clinical deterioration occurred in any patient. Tejada and colleagues[153] reported a higher IA nicardipine dose in their retrospective review of 11 symptomatic patients and 20 cases using 0.425 to 0.81 mg/min for total doses between 10 and 40 mg. Doses were given based on the angiographic resolution of spasm. Vessel caliber improved 60% in all cases and neurologic examination improved in 10 of 11 patients (91%). No ICP elevations were reported during treatment but only 2 of 11 patients had a ventriculostomy. Blood pressure monitoring was fully documented in 8 of 20 cases with hypotension occurring in some cases. "Mean SBP was 180 (range, 150–201 mm Hg) at the beginning of the procedure and 148 (range, 75–192 mm Hg) at the end of the procedure."[154] The SBP drop was less than or equal to 25% in 4 patients, between 26% and 30% in 2 patients, and up to 35% in 1 patient. Four complications without sequelae were reported: 3 thromboembolic events and 1 acute transient spasm of a middle cerebral artery. Pandey and colleageus[154] reported a simplified high-dose method for IA infusion through a cervical catheter instead of via microcatheter. Over a 4-year period, 27 patients and 48 procedures in 72 different arterial territories were treated with IA nicardipine infusion (20 mg/h) for 30 to 60 minutes. Mean dose infused per session was 19.2 mg with a range of 5 to 50 mg. Four patients with severe spasm also underwent angioplasty. Angiographic improvement was seen in 86.1% and clinical improvement was seen in 85.1%. Overall 62.9% had a good outcome at discharge.

Eighteen of 19 patients available at follow-up were doing well. The investigators concluded that infusion could be safely and effectively performed via the cervical catheter in carotid and vertebral arteries with microcatheter infusion and angioplasty reserved for severe and less responsive cases.

Nicardipine is metabolized extensively by the liver; less than 1% of intact drug is detected in the urine. Because of this, plasma levels of the drug are influenced by changes in hepatic function. Nicardipine plasma levels are higher in patients with severe liver disease than in normal subjects. Although this medication is effective in preventing angina, in approximately 7% of patients in short-term oral nicardipine placebo-controlled angina trials have developed increased frequency, duration, or severity of angina on starting nicardipine or at the time of dosage increases compared with 4% of patients on placebo. Reportedly this may progress to myocardial infarction in patients with severe cardiac disease. The mechanism for this is not understood. This has been not reported in IA infusion of nicardipine for vasospasm publications.

Verapamil Verapamil is an L-type calcium channel blocker of the phenylalkylamine class and has actions on smooth muscle similar to other calcium channel blockers to produce vasodilation. The following is Food and Drug Administration official drug information and specifically pertains to oral verapamil; however, once absorbed and plasma levels are achieved, the following side effects could reasonably be expected from the IA dosed drug to some degree. Verapamil reduces afterload and myocardial contractility. Improved left ventricular diastolic function in patients with idiopathic hypertrophic subaortic stenosis and those with coronary heart disease has also been observed with verapamil therapy. In most patients, including those with organic cardiac disease, the negative inotropic action of verapamil is countered by reduction of afterload, and cardiac index is usually not reduced. The effect of verapamil on atrioventricular conduction and the sinoatrial node may cause asymptomatic first-degree AV block and transient bradycardia, sometimes accompanied by nodal escape rhythms. In clinical trials for oral verapamil, cardiac side effects of bradycardia, congestive heart failure, or 1°, 2°, or 3° heart block occurred only in less than or equal to 1.8% of patients.

Verapamil publications are divided into low-dose, moderate-dose, and high-dose publications. The initial human studies of IA verapamil in the cervical and intracranial cerebral vasculature were low-dose studies performed at Columbia University. It is not surprising that these initial studies started with low dosing of the medication because the only human IA cases at the time were in the cardiac literature or animal studies.[155] Based on widespread uncomplicated use of IA verapamil to treat coronary vasospasm,[156,157] Joshi and colleagues[158] used IA verapamil (first using 2 mg and then increasing the dose up to 7.5 mg) in a dose-escalation study in patients undergoing balloon test occlusion to augment CBF. During trial occlusion in 9 patients, CBF and other physiologic parameters were evaluated before and after intracarotid verapamil. Postinfusion, increased CBF was observed without significant systemic effects, suggesting that intracarotid injection of verapamil had the potential to augment CBF during acute cerebral hypotension. Increased CBF was also seen during superselected IA verapamil infusion intracranially with adverse effects in a separate study, further supporting the safety and vasodilatory effects of verapamil.[159] A retrospective analysis of 2 years (1998–2000) of IA verapamil for cerebral vasospasm was reported by Feng and colleagues.[160] Thirty-four procedures in 29 patients in patients with aSAH were performed. IA verapamil was administered in 3 settings: (1) before balloon angioplasty to prevent catheter-induced vasospasm (1–2 mg), (2) for treatment of mild vasospasm that did not require angioplasty (2 mg), and (3) treatment of moderate to severe vasospasm that could not be safely treated with balloon angioplasty (up to 8 mg/vessel). There was little systemic effect at any dose of verapamil with no significant change in MAP or bradycardia. In 10 of 34 procedures, repeat angiograms were performed 10 to 15 minutes after verapamil infusion; the average change in spastic vessel segments was 44% $\pm$ 9% and the effect was most notable in patients with severe vasospasm. As seen in the dose-escalating study, verapamil was more effect in the 6- to 8-mg/vessel range. Although ICP was not directly measured, there was no evidence of any significant ICP elevation due to verapamil: no change in output in those patients with ventriculostomies, no secondary signs of sudden increase blood pressure or bradycardia, and no evidence of altered levels of consciousness in those patients treated under conscious sedation. Post-treatment, there was no deterioration on neurologic examinations of the 17 patients treated with verapamil alone and, even at low doses, 5 patients improved neurologically and did not require additional intervention.

A contrary report of 18 infusions in 15 patients was published by Mazumdar and colleagues[161] using hand-injected doses of verapamil from 2.5 to 10 mg (mean 7.4 mg) over a period of 5 to

10 minutes through a diagnostic catheter in the cervical carotid. In 14 cases, images were obtained within approximately 5 minutes after infusion of verapamil. In 4 cases, follow-up post-treatment images were obtained after 15 and 33 minutes after infusion of verapamil. No significant change in blood pressure or ICP was seen in 14 of 15 patients; in 1 patient significant systemic hypotension occurred but this resolved after infusion was stopped. Six of 15 patients showed some degree of clinical improvement within 24 hours after intra-arterial verapamil administration. Instead of focusing on the most spastic vessels preinfusion and measuring the response of these areas postinfusion, predetermined sites were chosen to represent the proximal, intermediate, and distal arteries. Using this system, they found no significant change in the diameters of proximal, intermediate, or distal vessels after verapamil infusion. The main concerns with this study are the markedly short interval between drug infusion and follow-up angiography, the slow delivery of verapamil infusion, and the methodology in vessel measurement because, as Feng and colleagues[160] noted, the most significant change occurs in the more severely spastic vessels. The investigators recognized these limitations in their article, noting that animal studies showed the effect of calcium channel blockers was dose dependent and that large-vessel dilation peaks at 15 to 30 minutes where the effect on small vessels may be more rapid; thus, they recognized that delayed angiography (at least 15 minutes after verapamil infusion) might demonstrate the responses more accurately.

The true effective dose of IA verapamil is not known for vasospasm. Some postulate that higher doses of Verpamil would be more effective in treating severe refractory vasospasm if associated systemic hypotension could be resolved. Keuskamp and colleagues[162] retrospectively reported the results of 10 patients who underwent 12 procedures using 20 mg or more of IA verapamil infused over 1.5 to 2.0 hours. Although the highest total dose is not explicitly stated, the mean verapamil dose per procedure was calculated at 41 $\pm$ 29 mg, and the mean verapamil dose over time was 0.24 $\pm$ 0.09 mg per minute. Improvement in the degree of vasospasm was seen in 10 of 12 procedures and was statistically significant. Eight of 12 procedures resulted in improvement in neurologic condition and no patient suffered a neurologic decline. Additionally, no statistically significant changes in MAP, heart rate, or ICP were observed. Albanese and colleagues[163] retrospectively reported extremely high doses of IA verapamil in 12 patients and 27 treatments in 36 vessels of 25 to 360 mg per vessel (for a range of total treatment dose of 70–720 mg) delivered over an average of 7.8 hours (1–20.5 hours) via a microcatheter and continuous infusion. This continuous infusion was effective in 32 of the 36 vessels and partially effective in 4 vessels. One of the infusions was stopped after the ICP reached 20 cm H_2O and subsequently normalized, no other elevations in ICP were described. Two patients had transient hypotension of MAP below 80 mm Hg. No other adverse effects of the IA verapamil infusion were noted. No new ischemic events were noted on CT in 9 of 12 patients treated. At clinical follow-up 6 to 12 months after discharge, 8 of 11 patients had a modified Rankin scale score less than or equal to 2.

Stuart and colleagues[164] studied the longer-term effect of IA verapamil infusion in 22 poor-grade aSAH in which hourly intracerebral microdialysis measurements and continuously recorded MAP, ICP, cerebral perfusion pressure, and brain tissue oxygen tension were analyzed for 6 hours before and 12 hours after treatment. Infused verapamil doses ranged from 15 to 55 mg (median 23 mg). Compared with baseline measurements, maximal reductions in cerebral perfusion pressure and MAP occurred 3 hours postinfusion (from 105 $\pm$ 13 mm Hg to 95 $\pm$ 15 mm Hg and from 116 $\pm$ 12 mm Hg to 106 $\pm$ 16 mm Hg; $P<.01$) and persisted for up to 6 hours ($P<.04$). Increased vasopressor therapy was required in 8 procedures (53%). Unlike other studies, they found that ICP increased by 30% to a peak of 14 $\pm$ 9 mm Hg after infusion and remained elevated until 3 hours post-angiography ($P<.03$). Brain glucose increased 33% by 9 hours postangiography ($P<.01$) but there were no significant changes in brain tissue oxygen tension or lactate/pyruvate ratios. They concluded that patients undergoing high-dose IA verapamil infusion required close hemodynamic and ICP monitoring for at least 12 hours after treatment.

At the authors' institution, verapamil has been the first drug of choice for IA infusion to treat refractory cerebral vasospasm since 2000. The authors' patients with vasospasm refractory to medical therapy are treated with endovascular therapy as early as possible targeting less than 2 hours after neurological change. Balloon angioplasty is performed in larger vessels for greater than 50% luminal narrowing. IA verapamil is infused for smaller or hypoplastic vessels and to empirically treat the microcirculation. Pre- and post-treatment angiograms are also reconstructed with syngo iFlow (Siemens). The dose of IA verapamil infused depends on the degree of vasospasm but generally ranges between 5 and 20 mg/vessel territory. This is usually bolused in 5-mg aliquots through the diagnostic or guide catheter but superselective and balloon-directed infusions are also performed as needed. Follow-up post-treatment angiogram is greater than 15 minutes (≥20 minutes even better) after drug infusion to assess response. Careful attention to systemic blood pressure and cerebral perfusion pressure is maintained throughout the procedure. In general, the authors attempt to keep the use of vasopressors as low as possible (ie, phenylephrine 0.1–0.2 mg/min and below 0.4 mg/min) and use other agents, such as IV infusion of 250 mL of 5% albumin plus IV calcium, and transfuse if hematocrit is less than 30 (preferably during the procedure). In addition, the authors closely monitor ICP during treatment and keep the ventriculostomy open for drainage as much as possible.

In 2004, the authors reviewed their experience performing 75 procedures in 21 patients for refractory symptomatic aSAH. In this group, 1 patient was treated with angioplasty only, 2 had no evidence of vasospasm and were not treated, IA verapamil as monotherapy was performed in 61 procedures, and combined angioplasty and IA verapamil infusion was performed in 11 procedures. Vessel caliber improved significantly (up to 66%) after verapamil infusion after measuring the areas of most severe vasospasm. Although blood pressure support was needed with the higher verapamil doses in some patients, elevations in ICP during and after the procedures were not seen. No adverse cardiac reactions to verapamil occurred. In 2006, to assess the efficacy and safety in the multitreatment (frequent flyer) patients, the authors retrospectively evaluated 12 (9 female and 3 male) patients who underwent 86 procedures for severe refractory vasospasm; 0 patients had either 2 or 3 procedures and12 patients had between 4 and 9 procedures. Infused doses ranged from 5 mg to 35 mg per vascular territory (average 15 mg). Maximum total dose administered in a single procedure was 60 mg. Increase in vessel caliber was 25% to 66%. No change in ICP was noted during or after the procedure. No adverse cardiovascular events occurred; however, blood pressure support was required for the larger verapamil doses. All patients were either neurologically stable or improved postinfusion. From this, the authors concluded that in a select subset of patients, repetitive IA verapamil infusion was a safe and effective adjunct for the treatment of recurrent severe vasospasm.

Rarely, IA verpamail infusion has been associated with seizure. In 2007, Westhout and Nwagwu[165] reported a single case of a 24-year-old woman who experienced seizures on 2 occasions after IA verapamil infusion. The first event occurred on SAH day 7 during infusion of IA verapamil (15 mg) when the patient developed a right-sided focal motor seizure. The second event occurred 7 days later (SAH day 14) when a generalized seizure occurred 90 minutes after IA verapamil (25 mg) was infused. In both instances, the patient was therapeutic on Phenytoin. Significant improvement in vessel caliber was noted after each verapamil infusion. The patient made an uneventful recovery and no further seizures were noted at a 3-month follow-up. At the authors' institution, 1 patient experienced a seizure that seemed related to verapamil infusion. In this case, the patient had a generalized seizure within 5 minutes of IA verapamil infusion in the angiography suite; the patient recovered without incident and had no further seizures after discharge.

IFLOW AND C-ARM CT PERFUSION (CTP) FOR MONITORING/ASSESSING TREATMENT

Recently, the authors have been using color-coded blood flow imaging (syngo iFlow) in the angiography suite to assist in treatment of patients with vasospasm. Background and initial evaluation as to the usefulness of color-encoded DSA have been previously reported from the authors' institution.[166] The technique and rapidity of reconstruction have dramatically improved since the initial work in 2007; this technology is commercially available and the authors currently use it as a surrogate for MTT. In the future, the authors will also incorporate C-arm CT measurement of CBV and CBF[167] during some of these clinical cases to replace conventional CTP pre- and post-treatment. Using iFlow adds to the information seen with standard DSA images; however, the color images often improve the conspicuity of the perfusion changes after treatment (**Figs. 3** and **4**). Partial resolution of vasospasm and improvement in perfusion can also be seen better with iFlow than conventional DSA (**Fig. 5**). iFlow is a dynamic tool and reflects either improved flow or decreased flow after treatment; this may reflect overall systemic factors, such as decreased systemic blood pressure secondary to the infused agent.

INTRAVENOUS AGENTS

Magnesium

Magnesium sulfate is a neuroprotective agent via its inhibition of the release of excitatory amino acids and blockade of the *N*-methyl-D-aspartate glutamate receptor (NMDAR). Magnesium is also a noncompetitive antagonist of voltage-dependent calcium channels, has cerebrovascular dilatory activity, and is an important cofactor of

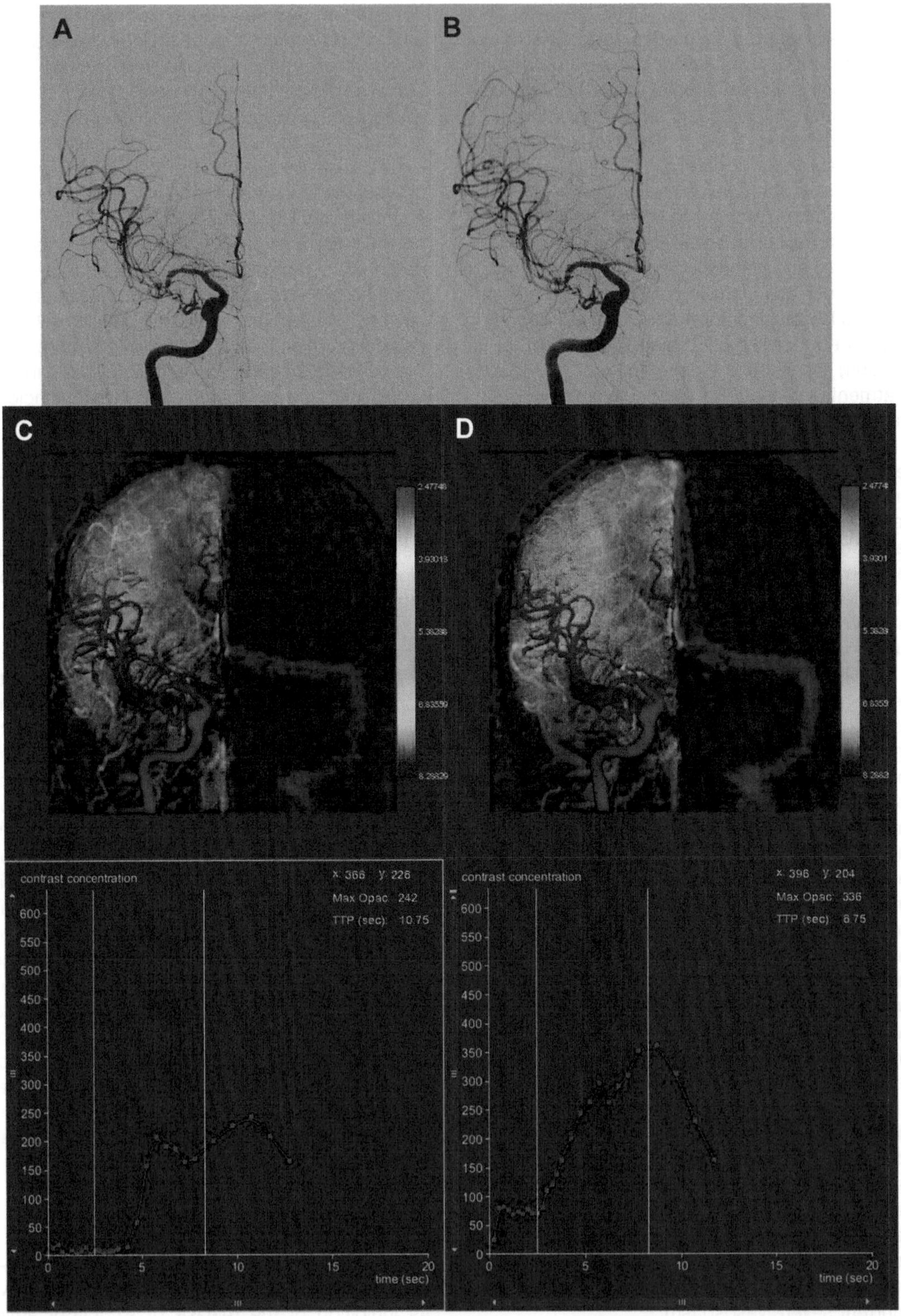

Fig. 3. Changes in flow after IA verapamil are seen better with iFlow than with conventional DSA. (*A*) Preverapamil infusion. (*B*) Postverapamil infusion. (*C*) Preverapamil infusion time to peak at 10.75 seconds. (*D*) Postverapamil infusion time to peak at 8.75 seconds demonstrating the improved transit time after treatment.

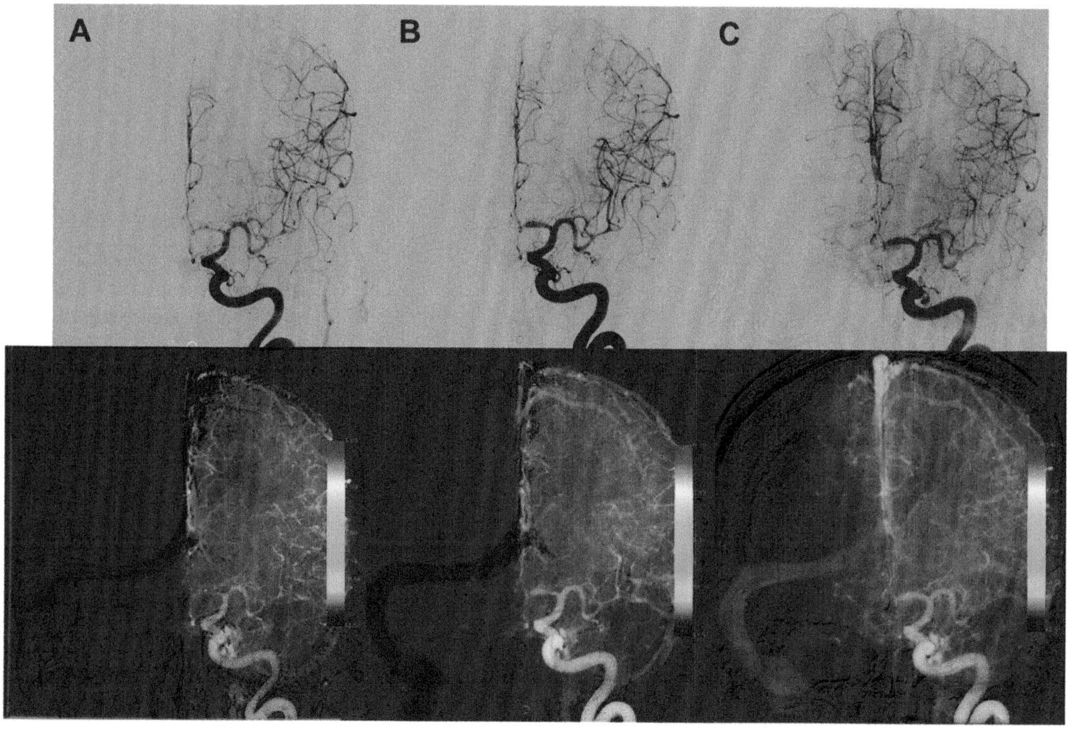

Fig. 4. Angioplasty followed by infusion of IA verapamil in a patient with symptomatic refractory vasospasm. (*A*) Pretreatment angiogram with corresponding iFlow directly below. (*B*) Postangioplasty angiogram and corresponding iFlow directly below. (*C*) Postangioplasty and post-IA verapamil infusion angiogram and corresponding iFlow directly below demonstrating further improvement in perfusion in the right anterior cerebral territory after verapamil infusion. Note the more rapid transit time in the draining veins as well.

cellular ATPases, including the Na/K-ATPase.[168] Although clinical studies have shown that IV magnesium is safe, the efficacy of this agent has not been proved. Recent trials to assess efficacy have all been completed: Magnesium in Aneurysmal Subarachnoid Hemorrhage (MASH), Intravenous Magnesium Sulphate for Aneurysmal Subarachnoid Hemorrhage, and MASH-2. MASH was a randomized, double-blind, placebo-controlled multicenter trial of 283 patients who were randomized, on SAH day 4, to magnesium versus placebo and acetylsalicylic acid versus placebo. The primary outcome was DCI, which was defined as the occurrence of a new hypodense lesion on CT scan with clinical features of DCI. The study results showed that magnesium reduced DCI by 34% and poor outcome risk reduction was 23% but the differences with placebo were not definitive.[169] MASH-2, a phase III, randomized, placebo-controlled multicenter trial, studying 1204 patients, has recently been completed. In addition, the authors performed an updated meta-analysis of 7 randomized trials. Dorhout Mees and colleagues[170] reported that 158 patients (26.2%) had poor outcome in the magnesium group compared with 151 (25.3%) in the placebo group. Their meta-analysis of 7 randomized trials with 2047 patients demonstrated that magnesium was not superior to placebo for reduction of poor outcome after aSAH (relative risk [RR] 0.96; 95% CI, 0.86–1.08). The conclusion of these trials is that IV magnesium sulfate does not improve outcomes in SAH patients.

Statins

Tseng[171] and the participants in the International Multidisciplinary Consensus Conference on the Critical Care Management of Subarachnoid Hemorrhage have written a review summarizing the evidence of statin effectiveness in statin-naïve patients with SAH. Statins, inhibitors of 3-hydroxy-3-methylglutaryl coenzyme A reductase, have been discovered to have neuroprotection independent of cholesterol reduction and exclusively associated with up-regulation of eNOS.[172] A literature search of all studies published through October 2010 where statin-naïve patients were treated with statins after aSAH was performed. Six randomized controlled clinical trials and 4

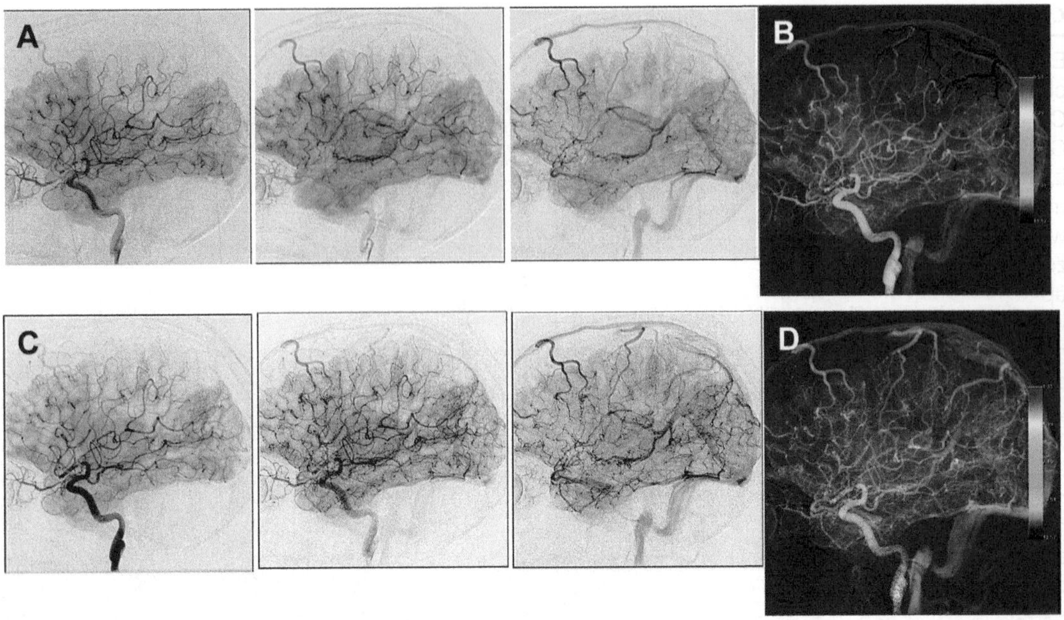

Fig. 5. Preverapamil out of phase, where there is lack of uniformity in one portion of the vascular territory on DSA (*A*) and the corresponding iFlow (*B*), and the more in-phase appearance postverapamil infusion, where the capillary blush is more uniform on DSA (*C*) and the corresponding iFlow (*D*). Note how much better iFlow shows perfusion in this slow flow area after treatment with improved transit times in the corresponding venous system (dark blue, 13.57 seconds, to green, 7.45 seconds).

observational studies were included in the analysis. Although there were inconsistent results between the studies, a meta-analysis of randomized controlled data demonstrated a significant reduction in delayed ischemic deficits with statin therapy. Different definitions used among studies, small sample sizes, historical controls, and treatment variability hampered data interpretation. The authors were able to conclude, however, that immediate statin therapy in statin-naïve patients seems safe and that there is some supporting evidence that statins may be beneficial to in reducing delayed ischemic deficits and possibly beneficial for cerebral vasospasm. Thus, this therapy may reduce early mortality in patients with aSAH.[171]

Endothelin Receptor Antagonists

ETs are a family of 3 peptides (ET-1, ET-2, and ET-3) that act primarily on ETA and ETB receptors. Experimental data show that ETs are involved in the development of arterial and arteriolar vasospasm after SAH.[173] A variety of ET receptor antagonists have been developed. TAK-044 is a nonselective antagonist of ETA and ETB receptors.[174] Clazosentan is an ET receptor antagonist with high ETA receptor selectivity for prevention of angiographic vasospasm.[175] Promising early work suggested that ET receptor antagonists reversed experimental SAH-induced vasospasm in animals.[176,177]

TAK-044

The ET antagonist, TAK-044, acts on both ETA and ETB receptors and has lost favor to more ETA-selective agents. A multicenter, randomized, double-blind, placebo-controlled, parallel-group phase II trial of TAK-044 was published in 2000 where 420 patients were studied.[178] The primary endpoint was whether a delayed ischemic event occurred within 3 months after the first dose of the study drug. Secondary endpoints included determining whether a delayed ischemic event occurred by 10 days after the first dose of the study drug, whether a new cerebral infarct was demonstrated on a CT scan or at postmortem examination by 3 months after administration after the initial dose, and the patients' GOS scores at 3 months after the initial dose. The investigators found a lower incidence of delayed ischemic events at 3 months in the TAK-044–treated group: 29.5% compared with 36.6% in a group of patients receiving placebo (estimated RR was 0.8 with a 95% CI, 0.61–1.06). There were no significant differences in the secondary endpoints, including clinical outcomes in the placebo-treated and TAK-044–treated groups.

Clazosentan

Early human data initially appeared promising with clazosentan after a phase IIa trial[5] and the CONSCIOUS-1 trial.[179] In 2011, the results from CONSCIOUS-2 were published.[180] In this randomized, double-blinded, placebo-controlled phase III multicenter study, ruptured aneurysm patients were randomly assigned after clipping to either clazosentan (5 mg/h; n = 768) or placebo (n = 389) for up to 14 days. The primary endpoint (week 6) included all-cause mortality, vasospasm-related new cerebral infarcts, delayed ischemic neurologic deficit due to vasospasm, and rescue therapy for vasospasm. The primary endpoint was met in in 161 (21%) of 764 clazosentan-treated patients and 97 (25%) of 383 placebo-treated patients (RR reduction 17%; 95% CI, −4 − 33; *P* = .10). The main secondary endpoint was the dichotomized extended GOS at week 12. The results showed poor functional outcome (GOS Extended [GOSE] ≤4) occurred in 224 (29%) clazosentan-treated patients and 95 (25%) placebo-treated patients (−18%, −45 to 4; *P* = .10). In subgroup analysis, patients receiving clazosentan had a greater risk reduction if they had a poor WFNS grade or diffuse thick SAH at baseline; however, this did not translate into better outcome at week 12, as measured by the GOSE. As seen in previous trials with clazosentan, lung complications, anemia, and hypotension were again more common in patients who received clazosentan than placebo.

The endovascular coiling counterpart to the clipping group, CONSCIOUS-3, was published in 2012.[181] This was a double-blind, placebo-controlled, phase III trial that randomized ruptured aneurysm patients treated with endovascular coiling to less than or equal to 14 days IV clazosentan (5 or 15 mg/h) or placebo. The primary and secondary endpoints were the same as in CONSCIOUS-2. CONSCIOUS-3 was halted prematurely after the results of CONSCIOUS-2 were analyzed; 38% (577) of the planned 1500 patients were enrolled at the time the trial was stopped. Of the 571 patients who were treated, 189 patients received placebo, 194 patients received clazosentan (5 mg/h), and 188 patients received clazosentan (15 mg/h). The primary endpoint occurred in 27% of placebo-treated patients (50/189) compared with 24% of patients (47/194) treated with clazosentan, 5 mg/h (OR 0.786; 95% CI, 0.479–1.289; *P* = .340), and 15% of patients (28/188) treated with clazosentan, 15 mg/h (OR 0.474; 95% CI, 0.275–0.818; *P* = .007). Poor outcome (GOSE score ≤4) occurred in 24% of patients with placebo; 25% of patients with clazosentan, 5 mg/h (OR 0.918; 95% CI, 0.546–1.544; *P* = .748); and 28% of patients with clazosentan, 15 mg/h (OR 1.337; 95% CI, 0.802–2.227; *P* = .266). At week 12, mortality was 6% with placebo, 4% with clazosentan (5 mg/h), and 6% with clazosentan (15 mg/h). As seen in previous trials with clazosentan, pulmonary complications and hypotension were again more common in patients who received clazosentan. Thus, analysis of patients enrolled prior to cessation of the trial demonstrated that although clazosentan (15 mg/h) significantly reduced post–SAH vasospasm-related morbidity and mortality, neither dose improved outcome (based on GOSE) compared with placebo. The investigators noted, however, that oral nimodipine was given to 94% of placebo patients and 95% of both clazosentan (5 mg/h) and clazosentan (15 mg/h) patients; they suggested that restricting nimodipine could help determine the influence of each drug in future studies. Additionally they noted that higher-dose clazosentan (15 mg/h) did prevent delayed ischemic neurologic deficits and reduced rescue therapy compared with the placebo group, with an OR of 0.474 (*P* = .007), which could be evaluated in future studies.

INVESTIGATIONAL APPROACHES

Spreading Depolarization and NMDAR Antagonists

An increasingly important area of research is determining the role that SD and subsequent spreading depression plays in the development of DCI. These phenomena are casting doubt on the traditional large-vessel vasospasm model as the etiologic agent for DCI and turning the focus on the microenvironment to elucidate mechanisms and find ways to block or reduce the vascular and neuronal response. This is the case particularly because of the observed temporal discordance between vasospasm and the development of DCI[182] and reports that delayed infarcts can occur without evidence of vasospasm (albeit using large-vessel vasospasm as the definition of vasospasm and not the microcirculation).[183] SDs have been recorded in patients with brain injury and correlate with outcome. SD has been described as "a wave in the gray matter of the central nervous system characterized by swelling of neurons, distortion of dendritic spines, a large change of the slow electrical potential and silencing of brain electrical activity (spreading depression)." Cortical spreading depressions after aSAH are associated with vasoconstriction and tissue hypoxia, which can result in neuronal death. The vascular response to SDs depends on whether the wave is occurring in healthy tissue or compromised tissue; a hemodynamic response with transient hyperperfusion occurs in normal brain tissue; however, severe hypoperfusion (the inverse of the normal hemodynamics) occurs in at-risk brain tissue, resulting in spreading ischemia. This represents dysfunction in the microvasculature.[184,185] The NMDAR is a specific glutamate receptor implicated in synaptic plasticity and memory function. *N*-methyl-D-aspartate (NMDA), an amino acid derivative, binds to and regulates the NMDAR and does not bind to other glutamate receptors. NMDA is an excitotoxin causing nerve cell death by overexcitation allowing influx of calcium ions (Ca^{2+}) to enter the cell. NMDA antagonists reduce the SDs, and also reduce the hypoperfusion associated with the paradoxic hemodynamic response.[186]

An intriguing possible reason that cerebral infarction and improved outcomes are better with nimodipine, as documented in the British nimodipine trial, may be due to its ability to reverse hypoperfusion seen with depolarization back to the hyperemic response. Dreier and colleagues[187] were able to induce cortical spreading depression in an in vivo rat model by adding hemoglobin (NO scavenger) and K^+ in artificial CSF, leading to decreased CBF and ischemia. Nimodipine (2 μg/kg body weight/min) administered IV transformed the ischemia back to hyperemia ($n = 4$). The investigators suggest that release of hemoglobin and K^+ from erythrocytes, as occurs after aSAH, simulates the same microenvironment because they were able to experimentally induce in the rats. Thus, the combination of decreased NO levels and increased subarachnoid K^+ levels induces spreading depression and results in an acute ischemic CBF response.

To better understand the correlation between SD and DCI, a nontherapeutic multicenter diagnostic phase III single-arm study is being performed: Depolarisations in ISCHaemia after aneurysmal subARachnoid haemorrhaGE: a multicentre diagnostic phase III single-arm study (DISCHARGE-1). The hypothesis is that recording of cortical SDs at the bedside allows real-time detection of delayed ischemia in patients with aSAH. More information can be found on this trial on controlled-trials.com Web site (ISRCTN05667702). Although the trial is listed as completed on the Web site, this is actually not the case; Dr Jens Dreier stated that the trial is ongoing because the recruitment was slower than expected (Dreier JP, personal communication, 2014).

Near-Infrared Spectroscopy

Continuous measurement of blood flow has not typically been performed with imaging. In the past, jugular venous sampling via a catheter was placed into the jugular vein, and sampling of blood was performed. The results were prone to error because the blood sampling reflected the brain as a whole rather than just the vascular distribution exhibiting vasospasm. The consequence was that the normally perfused areas would dilute the poorly perfused area limiting the sensitivity and specificity of the study. Consequently, devices to measure tissue oxygen, CBF, and brain chemistry via microdialysis were developed, which have shown some promise. They are continuous monitors but are invasive and are only capable of measuring an area of approximately 1 cm^3. This is problematic given the different vascular distributions that are not measured because they are more than 1 cm away from the sensor.[56,57,188–193]

NIRS is a noninvasive, continuous monitoring modality performed at the bedside that uses the illumination properties and flow kinetics of hemoglobin chromophores to provide noninvasive, continuous, real-time assessments of cerebral cortical perfusion. This existing technology is frequently used in the pediatric ICU for detection of global cerebral hypoperfusion in neonates with cardiac malformations. NIRS measures a tissue oxygenation index within the brain, which serves as an indicator of cerebral cortical blood flow and cerebral cortex oxygen extraction. Cerebral oxygen extraction increases in cases of increased oxygen demand or reduced oxygen supply. NIRS measurement in a vascular distribution occurs using an oximetry strip that contains both a laser light source and 2 sensors that receive wavelength specific signals. The triangulation of these signals allows the sensor to detect changes in tissue oxygenation at an average of 3 cm deep. This strategy allows the sensor to bypass reading potential background data from the blood flow within the bone, scalp, and CSF. With each detector strip, 3 near-infrared wavelengths at 775, 810, and 850 nm are generated per laser light source. The wavelengths penetrate through the scalp and bone and are absorbed by chromophores, primarily oxygenated and deoxygenated hemoglobin within the vascular system of the cerebral cortex. This depth measurement permits cortical blood flow assessment as the signals are directed back toward the sensor. A mathematical model is used to determine tissue oxygenation based on the light diffusion equation. Corresponding values are transferred from the monitor to a computer for displaying and recording real-time data.[56,57,60,66,188,194]

At the authors' institution, Drs Azam Ahmed, Joshua Medow, and Yiping Li from the Department of Neurosurgery are investigating NIRS in adults with aSAH to ascertain if it is a highly correlative measure for cerebral perfusion as well as an early sensitive screening tool for cerebral vasospasm compared with DSA and CTA. If proved, NIRS could be used for earlier detection and treatment of cerebral vasospasm after aSAH, which could improve patient outcomes.

SUMMARY

In summary, delayed neurologic deterioration after aSAH is a highly complex, poorly understood cascade of events that has an impact neurologic outcome. Vasospasm, autoregulatory dysfunction, inflammation, genetic predispositions, microcirculatory failure, and spreading cortical depolarization are aspects of the pathophysiology that can be exploited with multimodal treatment to achieve improved neurologic outcomes. Moving forward, the mechanism, diagnosis, and treatment of delayed ischemic neurologic injury need to be explored with rigorous and thoughtful science that can be efficiently translated to real and substantive interventions.

REFERENCES

1. Suarez JI, Tarr RW, Selman WR. Aneurysmal subarachnoid hemorrhage. N Engl J Med 2006;354:387–96.
2. Kassell NF, Sasaki T, Colohan AR, et al. Cerebral vasospasm following aneurysmal subarachnoid hemorrhage. Stroke 1985;16:562–72.
3. Lanzino G, Kassell NF. Double-blind, randomized, vehicle-controlled study of high-dose tirilazad mesylate in women with aneurysmal subarachnoid hemorrhage. Part II. A cooperative study in North America. J Neurosurg 1999;90:1018–24.
4. Song MK, Kim MK, Kim TS, et al. Endothelial nitric oxide gene T-786C polymorphism and subarachnoid hemorrhage in Korean population. J Korean Med Sci 2006;21:922–6.
5. Vajkoczy P, Meyer B, Weidauer S, et al. Clazosentan (AXV-034343), a selective endothelin a receptor antagonist, in the prevention of cerebral vasospasm following severe aneurysmal subarachnoid hemorrhage: results of a randomized, double-blind, placebo-controlled, multicenter phase IIa study. J Neurosurg 2005;103:9–17.
6. Wurm G, Tomancok B, Nussbaumer K, et al. Reduction of ischemic sequelae following spontaneous subarachnoid hemorrhage: a double-blind, randomized comparison of enoxaparin versus placebo. Clin Neurol Neurosurg 2004;106:97–103.
7. Ropper AH, Zervas NT. Outcome 1 year after SAH from cerebral aneurysm. Management morbidity, mortality, and functional status in 112 consecutive good-risk patients. J Neurosurg 1984;60:909–15.
8. Solenski NJ, Haley EC Jr, Kassell NF, et al. Medical complications of aneurysmal subarachnoid hemorrhage: a report of the multicenter, cooperative aneurysm study. Participants of the multicenter cooperative aneurysm study. Crit Care Med 1995;23:1007–17.
9. Connolly ES Jr, Rabinstein AA, Carhuapoma JR, et al. Guidelines for the management of aneurysmal subarachnoid hemorrhage: a guideline for healthcare professionals from the American Heart Association/American Stroke Association. Stroke 2012;43:1711–37.
10. Gull SW. Cases of aneurism of the cerebral vessels. Guys Hospital Reports 1859;5:281–304.
11. Echlin F. Vasospasm and focal cerebral ischemia: an experimental study. Arch Neurol Psychiatry 1942;47(1):77–96.
12. Zucker MD. A study of the substances in blood serum and platelets which stimulate smooth muscle. Am J Physiol 1944;142:12–26.
13. Robertson EG. Cerebral lesions due to intracranial aneurysms. Brain 1949;72:150–85.
14. Ecker A, Riemenschneider PA. Arteriographic demonstration of spasm of the intracranial arteries, with special reference to saccular arterial aneurysms. J Neurosurg 1951;8:660–7.
15. Fletcher TM, Taveras JM, Pool JL. Cerebral vasospasm in angiography for intracranial aneurysms. Incidence and significance in one hundred consecutive angiograms. Arch Neurol 1959;1:38–47.
16. Pool JL, Ransohoff J, Yahr MD, et al. Early surgical treatment of aneurysms of the circle of Willis. Neurology 1959;9:478–86.
17. Stornelli SA, French JD. Subarachnoid hemorrhage–factors in prognosis and management. J Neurosurg 1964;21:769–80.
18. Gabrielsen TO, Greitz T. Normal size of the internal carotid, middle cerebral and anterior cerebral arteries. Acta Radiol Diagn (Stockh) 1970;10:1–10.
19. Weir B, Grace M, Hansen J, et al. Time course of vasospasm in man. J Neurosurg 1978;48:173–8.
20. Fisher CM, Kistler JP, Davis JM. Relation of cerebral vasospasm to subarachnoid hemorrhage visualized by computerized tomographic scanning. Neurosurgery 1980;6:1–9.
21. Kosnik EJ, Hunt WE. Postoperative hypertension in the management of patients with intracranial arterial aneurysms. J Neurosurg 1976;45:148–54.
22. Zervas NT, Candia M, Candia G, et al. Reduced incidence of cerebral ischemia following rupture of intracranial aneurysms. Surg Neurol 1979;11:339–44.
23. Kassell NF, Peerless SJ, Durward QJ, et al. Treatment of ischemic deficits from vasospasm with intravascular volume expansion and induced arterial hypertension. Neurosurgery 1982;11:337–43.

24. Zubkov YN, Nikiforov BM, Shustin VA. Balloon catheter technique for dilatation of constricted cerebral arteries after aneurysmal SAH. Acta Neurochir (Wien) 1984;70:65–79.
25. Pickard JD, Murray GD, Illingworth R, et al. Effect of oral nimodipine on cerebral infarction and outcome after subarachnoid haemorrhage: British aneurysm nimodipine trial. BMJ 1989;298:636–42.
26. Bederson JB, Connolly ES Jr, Batjer HH, et al. Guidelines for the management of aneurysmal subarachnoid hemorrhage: a statement for healthcare professionals from a special writing group of the Stroke Council, American Heart Association. Stroke 2009;40:994–1025.
27. Humphrey JD, Baek S, Niklason LE. Biochemomechanics of cerebral vasospasm and its resolution: I. A new hypothesis and theoretical framework. Ann Biomed Eng 2007;35:1485–97.
28. Vergouwen MD, Vermeulen M, Coert BA, et al. Microthrombosis after aneurysmal subarachnoid hemorrhage: an additional explanation for delayed cerebral ischemia. J Cereb Blood Flow Metab 2008;28:1761–70.
29. Dreier JP, Major S, Manning A, et al. Cortical spreading ischaemia is a novel process involved in ischaemic damage in patients with aneurysmal subarachnoid haemorrhage. Brain 2009;132:1866–81.
30. Ladner TR, Zuckerman SL, Mocco J. Genetics of cerebral vasospasm. Neurol Res Int 2013;2013:291895.
31. Nakayama M, Yasue H, Yoshimura M, et al. T-786->C mutation in the 5'-flanking region of the endothelial nitric oxide synthase gene is associated with coronary spasm. Circulation 1999;99:2864–70.
32. Khurana VG, Fox DJ, Meissner I, et al. Update on evidence for a genetic predisposition to cerebral vasospasm. Neurosurg Focus 2006;21:E3.
33. Ko NU, Rajendran P, Kim H, et al. Endothelial nitric oxide synthase polymorphism (-786T->C) and increased risk of angiographic vasospasm after aneurysmal subarachnoid hemorrhage. Stroke 2008;39:1103–8.
34. Starke RM, Kim GH, Komotar RJ, et al. Endothelial nitric oxide synthase gene single-nucleotide polymorphism predicts cerebral vasospasm after aneurysmal subarachnoid hemorrhage. J Cereb Blood Flow Metab 2008;28:1204–11.
35. Ledbetter MW, Preiner JK, Louis CF, et al. Tissue distribution of ryanodine receptor isoforms and alleles determined by reverse transcription polymerase chain reaction. J Biol Chem 1994;269:31544–51.
36. Neylon CB, Richards SM, Larsen MA, et al. Multiple types of ryanodine receptor/Ca2+ release channels are expressed in vascular smooth muscle. Biochem Biophys Res Commun 1995;215:814–21.
37. Wellman GC, Nathan DJ, Saundry CM, et al. Ca2+ sparks and their function in human cerebral arteries. Stroke 2002;33:802–8.
38. Knot HJ, Standen NB, Nelson MT. Ryanodine receptors regulate arterial diameter and wall [Ca2+] in cerebral arteries of rat via Ca2+-dependent K+ channels. J Physiol 1998;508(Pt 1):211–21.
39. Rueffert H, Gumplinger A, Renner C, et al. Search for genetic variants in the ryanodine receptor 1 gene in patients with symptomatic cerebral vasospasm after aneurysmal subarachnoid hemorrhage. Neurocrit Care 2011;15:410–5.
40. Salomone S, Soydan G, Moskowitz MA, et al. Inhibition of cerebral vasoconstriction by dantrolene and nimodipine. Neurocrit Care 2009;10:93–102.
41. Muehlschlegel S, Rordorf G, Bodock M, et al. Dantrolene mediates vasorelaxation in cerebral vasoconstriction: a case series. Neurocrit Care 2009;10:116–21.
42. Bustin M. Regulation of DNA-dependent activities by the functional motifs of the high-mobility-group chromosomal proteins. Mol Cell Biol 1999;19:5237–46.
43. Andersson U, Wang H, Palmblad K, et al. High mobility group 1 protein (HMG-1) stimulates proinflammatory cytokine synthesis in human monocytes. J Exp Med 2000;192:565–70.
44. King MD, Laird MD, Ramesh SS, et al. Elucidating novel mechanisms of brain injury following subarachnoid hemorrhage: an emerging role for neuroproteomics. Neurosurg Focus 2010;28:E10.
45. Candelario-Jalil E, Yang Y, Rosenberg GA. Diverse roles of matrix metalloproteinases and tissue inhibitors of metalloproteinases in neuroinflammation and cerebral ischemia. Neuroscience 2009;158:983–94.
46. Yong VW, Krekoski CA, Forsyth PA, et al. Matrix metalloproteinases and diseases of the CNS. Trends Neurosci 1998;21:75–80.
47. McGirt MJ, Lynch JR, Blessing R, et al. Serum von Willebrand factor, matrix metalloproteinase-9, and vascular endothelial growth factor levels predict the onset of cerebral vasospasm after aneurysmal subarachnoid hemorrhage. Neurosurgery 2002;51:1128–34 [discussion: 1134–5].
48. Wang Z, Fang Q, Dang BQ, et al. Potential contribution of matrix metalloproteinase-9 (mmp-9) to cerebral vasospasm after experimental subarachnoid hemorrhage in rats. Ann Clin Lab Sci 2012;42:14–20.
49. Fisher CM, Roberson GH, Ojemann RG. Cerebral vasospasm with ruptured saccular aneurysm–the clinical manifestations. Neurosurgery 1977;1:245–8.
50. Weyer GW, Nolan CP, Macdonald RL. Evidence-based cerebral vasospasm management. Neurosurg Focus 2006;21:E8.

51. Baldwin ME, Macdonald RL, Huo D, et al. Early vasospasm on admission angiography in patients with aneurysmal subarachnoid hemorrhage is a predictor for in-hospital complications and poor outcome. Stroke 2004;35:2506–11.
52. Dorsch N. A clinical review of cerebral vasospasm and delayed ischaemia following aneurysm rupture. Acta Neurochir Suppl 2011;110:5–6.
53. Dorsch NW. Therapeutic approaches to vasospasm in subarachnoid hemorrhage. Curr Opin Crit Care 2002;8:128–33.
54. Claassen J, Hirsch LJ, Kreiter KT, et al. Quantitative continuous EEG for detecting delayed cerebral ischemia in patients with poor-grade subarachnoid hemorrhage. Clin Neurophysiol 2004;115:2699–710.
55. Claassen J, Vu A, Kreiter KT, et al. Effect of acute physiologic derangements on outcome after subarachnoid hemorrhage. Crit Care Med 2004;32: 832–8.
56. Gomez H, Torres A, Polanco P, et al. Use of non-invasive NIRS during a vascular occlusion test to assess dynamic tissue O(2) saturation response. Intensive Care Med 2008;34:1600–7.
57. Keller E, Nadler A, Imhof HG, et al. New methods for monitoring cerebral oxygenation and hemodynamics in patients with subarachnoid hemorrhage. Acta Neurochir Suppl 2002;82:87–92.
58. Klingelhofer J, Dander D, Holzgraefe M, et al. Cerebral vasospasm evaluated by transcranial Doppler ultrasonography at different intracranial pressures. J Neurosurg 1991;75:752–8.
59. Labar DR, Fisch BJ, Pedley TA, et al. Quantitative EEG monitoring for patients with subarachnoid hemorrhage. Electroencephalogr Clin Neurophysiol 1991;78:325–32.
60. Poon WS, Wong GK, Ng SC. The quantitative time-resolved near infrared spectroscopy (TR-NIRs) for bedside cerebrohemodynamic monitoring after aneurysmal subarachnoid hemorrhage: can we predict delayed neurological deficits? World Neurosurg 2010;73:465–6.
61. Rivierez M, Landau-Ferey J, Grob R, et al. Value of electroencephalogram in prediction and diagnosis of vasospasm after intracranial aneurysm rupture. Acta Neurochir (Wien) 1991;110:17–23.
62. Schuknecht B, Fandino J, Yuksel C, et al. Endovascular treatment of cerebral vasospasm: assessment of treatment effect by cerebral angiography and transcranial colour Doppler sonography. Neuroradiology 1999;41:453–62.
63. Sharbrough FW, Messick JM Jr, Sundt TM Jr. Correlation of continuous electroencephalograms with cerebral blood flow measurements during carotid endarterectomy. Stroke 1973;4:674–83.
64. Sloan MA, Alexandrov AV, Tegeler CH, et al. Assessment: transcranial doppler ultrasonography: report of the therapeutics and technology assessment subcommittee of the American Academy of Neurology. Neurology 2004;62:1468–81.
65. Vespa PM, Nuwer MR, Juhasz C, et al. Early detection of vasospasm after acute subarachnoid hemorrhage using continuous EEG ICU monitoring. Electroencephalogr Clin Neurophysiol 1997;103: 607–15.
66. Yokose N, Sakatani K, Murata Y, et al. Bedside monitoring of cerebral blood oxygenation and hemodynamics after aneurysmal subarachnoid hemorrhage by quantitative time-resolved near-infrared spectroscopy. World Neurosurg 2010;73: 508–13.
67. Aaslid R, Markwalder TM, Nornes H. Noninvasive transcranial doppler ultrasound recording of flow velocity in basal cerebral arteries. J Neurosurg 1982;57:769–74.
68. Newell DW, Winn HR. Transcranial doppler in cerebral vasospasm. Neurosurg Clin N Am 1990;1: 319–28.
69. Sloan MA, Haley EC Jr, Kassell NF, et al. Sensitivity and specificity of transcranial doppler ultrasonography in the diagnosis of vasospasm following subarachnoid hemorrhage. Neurology 1989;39: 1514–8.
70. Manno EM, Gress DR, Schwamm LH, et al. Effects of induced hypertension on transcranial doppler ultrasound velocities in patients after subarachnoid hemorrhage. Stroke 1998;29:422–8.
71. Fontanella M, Valfre W, Benech F, et al. Vasospasm after SAH due to aneurysm rupture of the anterior circle of Willis: value of TCD monitoring. Neurol Res 2008;30:256–61.
72. Minhas PS, Menon DK, Smielewski P, et al. Positron emission tomographic cerebral perfusion disturbances and transcranial Doppler findings among patients with neurological deterioration after subarachnoid hemorrhage. Neurosurgery 2003;52: 1017–22 [discussion: 1022–4].
73. Greenberg ED, Gold R, Reichman M, et al. Diagnostic accuracy of CT angiography and CT perfusion for cerebral vasospasm: a meta-analysis. AJNR Am J Neuroradiol 2010;31:1853–60.
74. Prell D, Kyriakou Y, Struffert T, et al. Metal artifact reduction for clipping and coiling in interventional C-arm CT. AJNR Am J Neuroradiol 2010;31:634–9.
75. Ochi RP, Vieco PT, Gross CE. CT angiography of cerebral vasospasm with conventional angiographic comparison. AJNR Am J Neuroradiol 1997;18:265–9.
76. Yoon DY, Choi CS, Kim KH, et al. Multidetector-row CT angiography of cerebral vasospasm after aneurysmal subarachnoid hemorrhage: comparison of volume-rendered images and digital subtraction angiography. AJNR Am J Neuroradiol 2006;27: 370–7.

77. Otawara Y, Ogasawara K, Ogawa A, et al. Evaluation of vasospasm after subarachnoid hemorrhage by use of multislice computed tomographic angiography. Neurosurgery 2002;51:939–42 [discussion: 942–3].
78. Merten GJ, Burgess WP, Gray LV, et al. Prevention of contrast-induced nephropathy with sodium bicarbonate: a randomized controlled trial. JAMA 2004;291:2328–34.
79. Shyu KG, Cheng JJ, Kuan P. Acetylcysteine protects against acute renal damage in patients with abnormal renal function undergoing a coronary procedure. J Am Coll Cardiol 2002;40:1383–8.
80. Adolph E, Holdt-Lehmann B, Chatterjee T, et al. Renal insufficiency following radiocontrast exposure trial (REINFORCE): a randomized comparison of sodium bicarbonate versus sodium chloride hydration for the prevention of contrast-induced nephropathy. Coron Artery Dis 2008;19:413–9.
81. Wintermark M, Thiran JP, Maeder P, et al. Simultaneous measurement of regional cerebral blood flow by perfusion CT and stable xenon CT: a validation study. AJNR Am J Neuroradiol 2001;22:905–14.
82. Dankbaar JW, de Rooij NK, Rijsdijk M, et al. Diagnostic threshold values of cerebral perfusion measured with computed tomography for delayed cerebral ischemia after aneurysmal subarachnoid hemorrhage. Stroke 2010;41:1927–32.
83. Wintermark M, Ko NU, Smith WS, et al. Vasospasm after subarachnoid hemorrhage: utility of perfusion CT and CT angiography on diagnosis and management. AJNR Am J Neuroradiol 2006;27:26–34.
84. Lennihan L, Mayer SA, Fink ME, et al. Effect of hypervolemic therapy on cerebral blood flow after subarachnoid hemorrhage: a randomized controlled trial. Stroke 2000;31:383–91.
85. Prophylactic hyperdynamic postoperative fluid therapy after aneurysmal subarachnoid hemorrhage: a clinical, prospective, randomized, controlled study 2001;49(3):593.
86. Barker FG 2nd, Ogilvy CS. Efficacy of prophylactic nimodipine for delayed ischemic deficit after subarachnoid hemorrhage: a meta analysis. J Neurosurg 1996; 84:405–14.
87. Findlay JM, Weir BK, Kassell NF, et al. Intracisternal recombinant tissue plasminogen activator after aneurysmal subarachnoid hemorrhage. J Neurosurg 1991;75:181–8.
88. Kasuya H, Onda H, Takeshita M, et al. Efficacy and safety of nicardipine prolonged-release implants for preventing vasospasm in humans. Stroke 2002;33:1011–5.
89. Kim JH, Yi HJ, Ko Y, et al. Effectiveness of papaverine cisternal irrigation for cerebral vasospasm after aneurysmal subarachnoid hemorrhage and measurement of biomarkers. Neurol Sci 2014;35: 712–22.
90. Kodama N. Cisternal irrigation with UK to prevent vasospasm. Surg Neurol 2000;54:95.
91. Kodama N, Sasaki T, Kawakami M, et al. Cisternal irrigation therapy with urokinase and ascorbic acid for prevention of vasospasm after aneurysmal subarachnoid hemorrhage. Outcome in 217 patients. Surg Neurol 2000;53:110–7 [discussion: 117–8].
92. Mizoi K, Yoshimoto T, Takahashi A, et al. Prospective study on the prevention of cerebral vasospasm by intrathecal fibrinolytic therapy with tissue-type plasminogen activator. J Neurosurg 1993;78: 430–7.
93. Nishiguchi M, Ono S, Iseda K, et al. Effect of vasodilation by milrinone, a phosphodiesterase III inhibitor, on vasospastic arteries after a subarachnoid hemorrhage in vitro and in vivo: effectiveness of cisternal injection of milrinone. Neurosurgery 2010;66:158–64 [discussion: 164].
94. Joseph M, Ziadi S, Nates J, et al. Increases in cardiac output can reverse flow deficits from vasospasm independent of blood pressure: a study using xenon computed tomographic measurement of cerebral blood flow. Neurosurgery 2003;53: 1044–51 [discussion: 1051–2].
95. Yoshida Y, Ueki S, Takahashi A, et al. Intrathecal irrigation with urokinase in ruptured cerebral aneurysm cases. Basic study and clinical application. Neurol Med Chir (Tokyo) 1985;25:989–97 [in Japanese].
96. Dorsch NW, King MT. A review of cerebral vasospasm in aneurysmal subarachnoid haemorrhage Part I: incidence and effects. J Clin Neurosci 1994;1:19–26.
97. Seifert V, Eisert WG, Stolke D, et al. Efficacy of single intracisternal bolus injection of recombinant tissue plasminogen activator to prevent delayed cerebral vasospasm after experimental subarachnoid hemorrhage. Neurosurgery 1989;25:590–8.
98. Rosenwasser RH, Armonda RA, Thomas JE, et al. Therapeutic modalities for the management of cerebral vasospasm: timing of endovascular options. Neurosurgery 1999;44:975–9 [discussion: 979–80].
99. Eskridge JM, McAuliffe W, Song JK, et al. Balloon angioplasty for the treatment of vasospasm: results of first 50 cases. Neurosurgery 1998;42:510–6 [discussion: 516–7].
100. Bejjani GK, Bank WO, Olan WJ, et al. The efficacy and safety of angioplasty for cerebral vasospasm after subarachnoid hemorrhage. Neurosurgery 1998;42:979–86 [discussion: 986–7].
101. Muizelaar JP, Zwienenberg M, Rudisill NA, et al. The prophylactic use of transluminal balloon angioplasty in patients with Fisher grade 3 subarachnoid hemorrhage: a pilot study. J Neurosurg 1999;91: 51–8.
102. Zwienenberg-Lee M, Hartman J, Rudisill N, et al. Effect of prophylactic transluminal balloon

angioplasty on cerebral vasospasm and outcome in patients with Fisher grade III subarachnoid hemorrhage: results of a phase II multicenter, randomized, clinical trial. Stroke 2008;39:1759–65.
103. Abruzzo T, Moran C, Blackham KA, et al. Invasive interventional management of post-hemorrhagic cerebral vasospasm in patients with aneurysmal subarachnoid hemorrhage. J Neurointerv Surg 2012;4:169–77.
104. Megyesi JF, Findlay JM, Vollrath B, et al. In vivo angioplasty prevents the development of vasospasm in canine carotid arteries. Pharmacological and morphological analyses. Stroke 1997;28:1216–24.
105. Megyesi JF, Vollrath B, Cook DA, et al. Long-term effects of in vivo angioplasty in normal and vasospastic canine carotid arteries: pharmacological and morphological analyses. J Neurosurg 1999; 91:100–8.
106. Honma Y, Fujiwara T, Irie K, et al. Morphological changes in human cerebral arteries after percutaneous transluminal angioplasty for vasospasm caused by subarachnoid hemorrhage. Neurosurgery 1995;36:1073–80 [discussion: 1080–1].
107. Zubkov AY, Lewis AI, Scalzo D, et al. Morphological changes after percutaneous transluminal angioplasty. Surg Neurol 1999;51:399–403.
108. Newell DW, Eskridge J, Mayberg M, et al. Endovascular treatment of intracranial aneurysms and cerebral vasospasm. Clin Neurosurg 1992;39:348–60.
109. Elliott JP, Newell DW, Lam DJ, et al. Comparison of balloon angioplasty and papaverine infusion for the treatment of vasospasm following aneurysmal subarachnoid hemorrhage. J Neurosurg 1998;88: 277–84.
110. Oskouian RJ Jr, Martin NA, Lee JH, et al. Multimodal quantitation of the effects of endovascular therapy for vasospasm on cerebral blood flow, transcranial doppler ultrasonographic velocities, and cerebral artery diameters. Neurosurgery 2002;51:30–41 [discussion: 41–3].
111. Polin RS, Coenen VA, Hansen CA, et al. Efficacy of transluminal angioplasty for the management of symptomatic cerebral vasospasm following aneurysmal subarachnoid hemorrhage. J Neurosurg 2000;92:284–90.
112. Newell DW, Eskridge JM, Mayberg MR, et al. Angioplasty for the treatment of symptomatic vasospasm following subarachnoid hemorrhage. J Neurosurg 1989;71:654–60.
113. Firlik AD, Kaufmann AM, Jungreis CA, et al. Effect of transluminal angioplasty on cerebral blood flow in the management of symptomatic vasospasm following aneurysmal subarachnoid hemorrhage. J Neurosurg 1997;86:830–9.
114. Hoh BL, Ogilvy CS. Endovascular treatment of cerebral vasospasm: transluminal balloon angioplasty, intra-arterial papaverine, and intra-arterial nicardipine. Neurosurg Clin N Am 2005;16: 501–16. vi.
115. Eskridge JM, Song JK. A practical approach to the treatment of vasospasm. AJNR Am J Neuroradiol 1997;18:1653–60.
116. Eskridge JM, Song JK, Elliott JP, et al. Balloon angioplasty of the A1 segment of the anterior cerebral artery narrowed by vasospasm. Technical note. J Neurosurg 1999;91:153–6.
117. Kaku Y, Yonekawa Y, Tsukahara T, et al. Superselective intra-arterial infusion of papaverine for the treatment of cerebral vasospasm after subarachnoid hemorrhage. J Neurosurg 1992;77:842–7.
118. Clouston JE, Numaguchi Y, Zoarski GH, et al. Intraarterial papaverine infusion for cerebral vasospasm after subarachnoid hemorrhage. AJNR Am J Neuroradiol 1995;16:27–38.
119. McAuliffe W, Townsend M, Eskridge JM, et al. Intracranial pressure changes induced during papaverine infusion for treatment of vasospasm. J Neurosurg 1995;83:430–4.
120. Milburn JM, Moran CJ, Cross DT 3rd, et al. Increase in diameters of vasospastic intracranial arteries by intraarterial papaverine administration. J Neurosurg 1998;88:38–42.
121. Milburn JM, Moran CJ, Cross DT 3rd, et al. Effect of intraarterial papaverine on cerebral circulation time. AJNR Am J Neuroradiol 1997;18:1081–5.
122. Liu JK, Tenner MS, Gottfried ON, et al. Efficacy of multiple intraarterial papaverine infusions for improvement in cerebral circulation time in patients with recurrent cerebral vasospasm. J Neurosurg 2004;100:414–21.
123. Vajkoczy P, Horn P, Bauhuf C, et al. Effect of intra-arterial papaverine on regional cerebral blood flow in hemodynamically relevant cerebral vasospasm. Stroke 2001;32:498–505.
124. Andaluz N, Tomsick TA, Tew JM Jr, et al. Indications for endovascular therapy for refractory vasospasm after aneurysmal subarachnoid hemorrhage: experience at the University of Cincinnati. Surg Neurol 2002;58:131–8 [discussion: 138].
125. Platz J, Barath K, Keller E, et al. Disruption of the blood-brain barrier by intra-arterial administration of papaverine: a technical note. Neuroradiology 2008;50:1035–9.
126. Barr JD, Mathis JM, Horton JA. Transient severe brain stem depression during intraarterial papaverine infusion for cerebral vasospasm. AJNR Am J Neuroradiol 1994;15:719–23.
127. Smith WS, Dowd CF, Johnston SC, et al. Neurotoxicity of intra-arterial papaverine preserved with chlorobutanol used for the treatment of cerebral vasospasm after aneurysmal subarachnoid hemorrhage. Stroke 2004;35:2518–22.
128. Clyde BL, Firlik AD, Kaufmann AM, et al. Paradoxical aggravation of vasospasm with papaverine

infusion following aneurysmal subarachnoid hemorrhage. Case report. J Neurosurg 1996;84:690–5.

129. Tsurushima H, Kamezaki T, Nagatomo Y, et al. Complications associated with intraarterial administration of papaverine for vasospasm following subarachnoid hemorrhage–two case reports. Neurol Med Chir (Tokyo) 2000;40:112–5.
130. Tsurushima H, Hyodo A, Yoshii Y. Papaverine and vasospasm. J Neurosurg 2000;92:509–11.
131. Carhuapoma JR, Qureshi AI, Tamargo RJ, et al. Intra-arterial papaverine-induced seizures: case report and review of the literature. Surg Neurol 2001;56:159–63.
132. Nagumo H, Sasaki Y, Ono Y, et al. Rho kinase inhibitor HA-1077 prevents Rho-mediated myosin phosphatase inhibition in smooth muscle cells. Am J Physiol Cell Physiol 2000;278:C57–65.
133. Nakamura K, Nishimura J, Hirano K, et al. Hydroxyfasudil, an active metabolite of fasudil hydrochloride, relaxes the rabbit basilar artery by disinhibition of myosin light chain phosphatase. J Cereb Blood Flow Metab 2001;21:876–85.
134. Tachibana E, Harada T, Shibuya M, et al. Intra-arterial infusion of fasudil hydrochloride for treating vasospasm following subarachnoid haemorrhage. Acta Neurochir (Wien) 1999;141:13–9.
135. Tanaka K, Minami H, Kota M, et al. Treatment of cerebral vasospasm with intra-arterial fasudil hydrochloride. Neurosurgery 2005;56:214–23 [discussion: 214–23].
136. Enomoto Y, Yoshimura S, Yamada K, et al. Convulsion during intra-arterial infusion of fasudil hydrochloride for the treatment of cerebral vasospasm following subarachnoid hemorrhage. Neurol Med Chir (Tokyo) 2010;50:7–11 [discussion: 11–2].
137. Arakawa Y, Kikuta K, Hojo M, et al. Milrinone for the treatment of cerebral vasospasm after subarachnoid hemorrhage: report of seven cases. Neurosurgery 2001;48:723–8 [discussion: 728–30].
138. Monrad ES, Baim DS, Smith HS, et al. Milrinone, dobutamine, and nitroprusside: comparative effects on hemodynamics and myocardial energetics in patients with severe congestive heart failure. Circulation 1986;73:III168–74.
139. Monrad ES, McKay RG, Baim DS, et al. Improvement in indexes of diastolic performance in patients with congestive heart failure treated with milrinone. Circulation 1984;70:1030–7.
140. Honerjager P. Pharmacology of bipyridine phosphodiesterase III inhibitors. Am Heart J 1991;121:1939–44.
141. Fraticelli AT, Cholley BP, Losser MR, et al. Milrinone for the treatment of cerebral vasospasm after aneurysmal subarachnoid hemorrhage. Stroke 2008;39:893–8.
142. Romero CM, Morales D, Reccius A, et al. Milrinone as a rescue therapy for symptomatic refractory cerebral vasospasm in aneurysmal subarachnoid hemorrhage. Neurocrit Care 2009;11:165–71.
143. Anand S, Goel G, Gupta V. Continuous intra-arterial dilatation with nimodipine and milrinone for refractory cerebral vasospasm. J Neurosurg Anesthesiol 2014;26:92–3.
144. Cheymol G. Clinical pharmacokinetics of drugs in obesity. An update. Clin Pharmacokinet 1993;25:103–14.
145. Biondi A, Ricciardi GK, Puybasset L, et al. Intra-arterial nimodipine for the treatment of symptomatic cerebral vasospasm after aneurysmal subarachnoid hemorrhage: preliminary results. AJNR Am J Neuroradiol 2004;25:1067–76.
146. Hui C, Lau KP. Efficacy of intra-arterial nimodipine in the treatment of cerebral vasospasm complicating subarachnoid haemorrhage. Clin Radiol 2005;60:1030–6.
147. Cho WS, Kang HS, Kim JE, et al. Intra-arterial nimodipine infusion for cerebral vasospasm in patients with aneurysmal subarachnoid hemorrhage. Interv Neuroradiol 2011;17:169–78.
148. Kim SS, Park DH, Lim DJ, et al. Angiographic features and clinical outcomes of intra-arterial nimodipine injection in patients with subarachnoid hemorrhage-induced vasospasm. J Korean Neurosurg Soc 2012;52:172–8.
149. Janardhan V, Biondi A, Riina HA, et al. Vasospasm in aneurysmal subarachnoid hemorrhage: diagnosis, prevention, and management. Neuroimaging Clin N Am 2006;16:483–96,. viii–ix.
150. Ryu CW, Koh JS, Yu SY, et al. Vasogenic edema of the Basal Ganglia after intra-arterial administration of nimodipine for treatment of vasospasm. J Korean Neurosurg Soc 2011;49:112–5.
151. Flamm ES, Adams HP Jr, Beck DW, et al. Dose-escalation study of intravenous nicardipine in patients with aneurysmal subarachnoid hemorrhage. J Neurosurg 1988;68:393–400.
152. Badjatia N, Topcuoglu MA, Pryor JC, et al. Preliminary experience with intra-arterial nicardipine as a treatment for cerebral vasospasm. AJNR Am J Neuroradiol 2004;25:819–26.
153. Tejada JG, Taylor RA, Ugurel MS, et al. Safety and feasibility of intra-arterial nicardipine for the treatment of subarachnoid hemorrhage-associated vasospasm: initial clinical experience with high-dose infusions. AJNR Am J Neuroradiol 2007;28:844–8.
154. Pandey P, Steinberg GK, Dodd R, et al. A simplified method for administration of intra-arterial nicardipine for vasospasm with cervical catheter infusion. Neurosurgery 2012;71:77–85.
155. Takayasu M, Bassett JE, Dacey RG Jr. Effects of calcium antagonists on intracerebral penetrating arterioles in rats. J Neurosurg 1988;69:104–9.

156. Pomerantz RM, Kuntz RE, Diver DJ, et al. Intracoronary verapamil for the treatment of distal microvascular coronary artery spasm following PTCA. Cathet Cardiovasc Diagn 1991;24:283–5.
157. Taniyama Y, Ito H, Iwakura K, et al. Beneficial effect of intracoronary verapamil on microvascular and myocardial salvage in patients with acute myocardial infarction. J Am Coll Cardiol 1997;30: 1193–9.
158. Joshi S, Young WL, Pile-Spellman J, et al. Manipulation of cerebrovascular resistance during internal carotid artery occlusion by intraarterial verapamil. Anesth Analg 1997;85:753–9.
159. Joshi S, Young WL, Pile-Spellman J, et al. Intraarterial nitrovasodilators do not increase cerebral blood flow in angiographically normal territories of arteriovenous malformation patients. Stroke 1997; 28:1115–22.
160. Feng L, Fitzsimmons BF, Young WL, et al. Intraarterially administered verapamil as adjunct therapy for cerebral vasospasm: safety and 2-year experience. AJNR Am J Neuroradiol 2002;23:1284–90.
161. Mazumdar A, Rivet DJ, Derdeyn CP, et al. Effect of intraarterial verapamil on the diameter of vasospastic intracranial arteries in patients with cerebral vasospasm. Neurosurg Focus 2006;21:E15.
162. Keuskamp J, Murali R, Chao KH. High-dose intraarterial verapamil in the treatment of cerebral vasospasm after aneurysmal subarachnoid hemorrhage. J Neurosurg 2008;108:458–63.
163. Albanese E, Russo A, Quiroga M, et al. Ultrahigh-dose intraarterial infusion of verapamil through an indwelling microcatheter for medically refractory severe vasospasm: initial experience. J Neurorsurg 2010;113:913–22.
164. Stuart RM, Helbok R, Kurtz P, et al. High-dose intraarterial verapamil for the treatment of cerebral vasospasm after subarachnoid hemorrhage: prolonged effects on hemodynamic parameters and brain metabolism. Neurosurgery 2011;68:337–45 [discussion: 345].
165. Westhout FD, Nwagwu CI. Intra-arterial verapamil-induced seizures: case report and review of the literature. Surg Neurol 2007;67:483–6 [discussion: 486].
166. Strother CM, Bender F, Deuerling-Zheng Y, et al. Parametric color coding of digital subtraction angiography. AJNR Am J Neuroradiol 2010;31: 919–24.
167. Royalty K, Manhart M, Pulfer K, et al. C-arm CT measurement of cerebral blood volume and cerebral blood flow using a novel high-speed acquisition and a single intravenous contrast injection. AJNR Am J Neuroradiol 2013;34:2131–8.
168. van den Bergh WM, Dijkhuizen RM, Rinkel GJ. Potentials of magnesium treatment in subarachnoid haemorrhage. Magnes Res 2004;17:301–13.
169. van den Bergh WM, Algra A, van Kooten F, et al. Magnesium sulfate in aneurysmal subarachnoid hemorrhage: a randomized controlled trial. Stroke 2005;36:1011–5.
170. Dorhout Mees SM, Algra A, Vandertop WP, et al. Magnesium for aneurysmal subarachnoid haemorrhage (MASH-2): a randomised placebo-controlled trial. Lancet 2012;380:44–9.
171. Tseng MY. Summary of evidence on immediate statins therapy following aneurysmal subarachnoid hemorrhage. Neurocrit Care 2011;15:298–301.
172. Sabri M, Macdonald RL. Statins: a potential therapeutic addition to treatment for aneurysmal subarachnoid hemorrhage? World Neurosurg 2010; 73:646–53.
173. Zimmermann M. Endothelin in cerebral vasospasm. Clinical and experimental results. J Neurosurg Sci 1997;41:139–51.
174. Ikeda S, Awane Y, Kusumoto K, et al. A new endothelin receptor antagonist, TAK-044, shows long-lasting inhibition of both ETA- and ETB-mediated blood pressure responses in rats. J Pharmacol Exp Ther 1994;270:728–33.
175. Roux S, Breu V, Giller T, et al. Ro 61-1790, a new hydrosoluble endothelin antagonist: general pharmacology and effects on experimental cerebral vasospasm. J Pharmacol Exp Ther 1997;283: 1110–8.
176. Zuccarello M, Boccaletti R, Romano A, et al. Endothelin B receptor antagonists attenuate subarachnoid hemorrhage-induced cerebral vasospasm. Stroke 1998;29:1924–9.
177. Zuccarello M, Lewis AI, Rapoport RM. Endothelin ETA and ETB receptors in subarachnoid hemorrhage-induced cerebral vasospasm. Eur J Pharmacol 1994;259:R1–2.
178. Shaw MD, Vermeulen M, Murray GD, et al. Efficacy and safety of the endothelin, receptor antagonist TAK-044 in treating subarachnoid hemorrhage: a report by the Steering Committee on behalf of the UK/Netherlands/Eire TAK-044 Subarachnoid Haemorrhage Study Group. J Neurosurg 2000;93: 992–7.
179. Macdonald RL, Kassell NF, Mayer S, et al. Clazosentan to overcome neurological ischemia and infarction occurring after subarachnoid hemorrhage (CONSCIOUS-1): randomized, double-blind, placebo-controlled phase 2 dose-finding trial. Stroke 2008;39:3015–21.
180. Macdonald RL, Higashida RT, Keller E, et al. Clazosentan, an endothelin receptor antagonist, in patients with aneurysmal subarachnoid haemorrhage undergoing surgical clipping: a randomised, double-blind, placebo-controlled phase 3 trial (CONSCIOUS-2). Lancet Neurol 2011;10:618–25.
181. Macdonald RL, Higashida RT, Keller E, et al. Randomized trial of clazosentan in patients with

aneurysmal subarachnoid hemorrhage undergoing endovascular coiling. Stroke 2012;43:1463–9.
182. Stein SC, Levine JM, Nagpal S, et al. Vasospasm as the sole cause of cerebral ischemia: how strong is the evidence? Neurosurg Focus 2006;21:E2.
183. Naidech AM, Drescher J, Tamul P, et al. Acute physiological derangement is associated with early radiographic cerebral infarction after subarachnoid haemorrhage. J Neurol Neurosurg Psychiatry 2006;77:1340–4.
184. Dreier JP. The role of spreading depression, spreading depolarization and spreading ischemia in neurological disease. Nat Med 2011;17:439–47.
185. Leng LZ, Fink ME, Iadecola C. Spreading depolarization: a possible new culprit in the delayed cerebral ischemia of subarachnoid hemorrhage. Arch Neurol 2011;68:31–6.
186. Shin HK, Dunn AK, Jones PB, et al. Vasoconstrictive neurovascular coupling during focal ischemic depolarizations. J Cereb Blood Flow Metab 2006; 26:1018–30.
187. Dreier JP, Korner K, Ebert N, et al. Nitric oxide scavenging by hemoglobin or nitric oxide synthase inhibition by N-nitro-L-arginine induces cortical spreading ischemia when K+ is increased in the subarachnoid space. J Cereb Blood Flow Metab 1998;18:978–90.
188. Soller BR, Yang Y, Soyemi OO, et al. Noninvasively determined muscle oxygen saturation is an early indicator of central hypovolemia in humans. J Appl Physiol (1985) 2008;104:475–81.
189. Sarrafzadeh AS, Sakowitz OW, Callsen TA, et al. Detection of secondary insults by brain tissue pO2 and bedside microdialysis in severe head injury. Acta Neurochir Suppl 2002;81:319–21.
190. Sarrafzadeh A, Haux D, Sakowitz O, et al. Acute focal neurological deficits in aneurysmal subarachnoid hemorrhage: relation of clinical course, CT findings, and metabolite abnormalities monitored with bedside microdialysis. Stroke 2003;34:1382–8.
191. Hillered L, Vespa PM, Hovda DA. Translational neurochemical research in acute human brain injury: the current status and potential future for cerebral microdialysis. J Neurotrauma 2005;22:3–41.
192. Heran NS, Hentschel SJ, Toyota BD. Jugular bulb oximetry for prediction of vasospasm following subarachnoid hemorrhage. Can J Neurol Sci 2004;31:80–6.
193. Citerio G, Cormio M, Portella G, et al. Jugular saturation (SjvO2) monitoring in subarachnoid hemorrhage (SAH). Acta Neurochir Suppl 1998;71:316–9.
194. Calderon-Arnulphi M, Alaraj A, Slavin KV. Near infrared technology in neuroscience: past, present and future. Neurol Res 2009;31:605–14.

Endovascular Approaches to Pial Arteriovenous Malformations

Matthew R. Sanborn, MD, Min S. Park, MD,
Cameron G. McDougall, MD, Felipe C. Albuquerque, MD*

KEYWORDS

• Arteriovenous malformation • AVM • Embolization • Onyx • EVOH • Endovascular • Intracranial • n-BCA

KEY POINTS

- Endovascular treatment of arteriovenous malformations requires a multidisciplinary team approach.
- Physicians must select patients carefully and consider each patient's Spetzler-Martin grade, individual lesion angioarchitecture, and high-risk features before attempting treatment.
- The goals of therapy should be established before treatment and may include preoperative, targeted, palliative, or curative embolization.
- Technical advances in endovascular techniques and embolic materials have resulted in safer, more complete embolization.

INTRODUCTION

Cerebral arteriovenous malformations (AVMs) are high-flow lesions consisting of an abnormal tangle of vessels that connect the arterial and venous systems. Although they seem to be primarily congenital in origin, these clearly dynamic lesions are capable of spontaneous growth and regression, and have often been reported arising de novo.[1] Although hemorrhage is the most common presentation, AVMs can also cause seizures, focal neurologic deficits, and headaches.[2] The goals of therapy are to eliminate or reduce the risk of bleeding and to ameliorate symptoms. Cerebral AVMs lie at a therapeutic nexus and may require treatment with open surgery, radiosurgery, or endovascular embolization, or with a multimodality approach using a combination of these techniques.

NATURAL HISTORY

The first step in any treatment algorithm for an AVM is deciding whether treatment is necessary, which requires weighing the risks of the natural history of the disease against the risks of treatment. The ubiquitously quoted annual rupture risk for cerebral AVMs of 2% to 4% is from a Finnish study in which unruptured AVMs were significantly underrepresented, making up only 29% of the sample.[3] More recent data suggest that the annual hemorrhage rate of unruptured AVMs without deep venous drainage or deep location may be as low as 0.9%.[4] However, the optimal approach to unruptured AVMs remains an area of controversy.

One recent study, A Randomized Trial of Unruptured Brain AVMs (ARUBA), compared the risks of

Disclosure: The authors have no conflicts of interest to disclose.
Division of Neurological Surgery, Barrow Neurological Institute, St Joseph's Hospital and Medical Center, 350 West Thomas Road, Phoenix, AZ 85013, USA
* Corresponding author. c/o Neuroscience Publications, Barrow Neurological Institute, St Joseph's Hospital and Medical Center, 350 West Thomas Road, Phoenix, AZ 85013.
E-mail address: neuropub@dignityhealth.org

Neurosurg Clin N Am 25 (2014) 529–537
http://dx.doi.org/10.1016/j.nec.2014.04.009
1042-3680/14/$ – see front matter

treating unruptured AVMs with the risks of observation. Enrollment was terminated early, after it was observed that the end point of death or stroke occurred in 10% of those randomized to medical management and in 29% of those randomized to intervention. Short follow-up and sample heterogeneity preclude any definitive recommendations from this study, although enrolled patients will continue to be followed.

In the absence of further data on the best treatment method for unruptured AVMs, the decision to offer intervention must be based on an analysis of the high-risk features of the lesion and patient symptoms. Deep location and exclusively deep venous drainage are associated with an increased risk of hemorrhage, as are anatomic features such as intranidal aneurysms, venous stenosis, and venous ectasia.[4,5] In addition, an attempt should be made to verify whether the AVM is the source the patient's symptoms.

There is more certainty regarding the role of intervention in ruptured AVMs. Once an AVM has ruptured, the risk of rerupture increases to 7% to 17% in the first year.[6,7] In this setting, prompt treatment is indicated.

RISKS OF ENDOVASCULAR TREATMENT

Endovascular therapy has associated risks. Aside from the normal complications of diagnostic angiography, which include groin or retroperitoneal hematoma, contrast-induced allergy, contrast-induced nephrotoxicity, and vessel injury, embolization is associated with a risk of intracerebral hemorrhage and infarction. Estimates of the likelihood of these complications vary widely, with reports of permanent neurologic deficits ranging from 2% to 20% and mortality ranging from 1% to 3%.[8–13] One large prospective study of 201 patients undergoing 339 embolizations showed a risk of 9% for permanent neurologic deficit per patient, with 2% mortality.[14]

GOALS OF TREATMENT

The role of endovascular treatment in patients with AVMs is evolving. Decisions regarding the optimal treatment strategy for any AVM are best made by incorporating input from a team of specialists with expertise in open, endovascular, and radiosurgical approaches.[15,16] Particularly for endovascular treatment, the ultimate goal of the intervention defines the approach taken and techniques used. These goals include preoperative embolization to facilitate a planned surgery; attempted curative embolization; prestereotactic radiosurgery to reduce target size; targeted embolization of high-risk features; and palliative embolization in cases of symptomatic, large, complex AVMs that are otherwise not amenable to treatment.

Preoperative Embolization

Preoperative embolization should be targeted toward achieving a stepwise reduction in blood flow. Of highest priority for occlusion are deep-feeding arterial pedicles and other arteries that would be problematic or difficult to access at the time of surgery or those that supply deep portions of the AVM.

The appropriate timing of surgery after AVM embolization is controversial. Although some clinicians advocate waiting for up to 3 weeks after embolization to allow for progressive thrombosis and stabilization of local and regional hemodynamic changes,[17] others perform surgery within a few days because of the perceived increased risk of hemorrhage associated with embolization.[18]

Surgical treatment of patients with Spetzler-Martin grade I and II lesions is associated with low morbidity and mortality. For these lesions, preoperative embolization may increase the risk for adverse events without significantly decreasing the risk of surgery, and therefore may be indicated only in select cases. In contrast, patients with Spetzler-Martin grade III lesions may often benefit from embolization before definitive treatment with resection or radiosurgery. Those with Spetzler-Martin grade IV and V lesions who need treatment often require multimodality therapy with embolization as one part of a larger treatment strategy.

Curative Embolization

Patients with certain types of AVMs may be amenable to curative endovascular treatment with embolization. Before the introduction of ethyl vinyl alcohol copolymer (EVOH), a small series showed that embolization using n-butyl cyanoacrylate (n-BCA) achieved complete angiographic occlusion in approximately 20% of patients.[19] More recent series using EVOH (Onyx, ev3, Irvine, CA) have achieved angiographic obliteration rates as high as 51% in patients undergoing embolization and as high as 96% in carefully selected patient cohorts with the stated goal of AVM cure.[20,21] AVM characteristics that are favorable for curative embolization are small or medium size, superficial location, a simple nidus with a single or few arterial pedicles from a single vascular territory, and an easily identifiable draining vein. The feeding pedicles must be amenable to catheterization with a microcatheter and, ideally, allow for reflux of Onyx for 2 to 3 cm before encountering a branch point supplying normal brain. However, some lesions that were thought to be angiographically cured after embolization showed residual filling at the time of surgery.[18] There is little long-term follow-up evidence regarding the durability of Onyx or its long-term effects in vivo; thus serious consideration should be given to surgical resection of the AVM nidus when feasible.

Embolization Before Radiosurgery

The role of embolization to facilitate radiosurgery is becoming limited to select cases. Embolization has been used to shrink the AVM nidus to facilitate radiosurgery, allowing a decreased integral dose to be delivered, with a corresponding reduced risk to surrounding normal brain tissue. However, many studies have now shown a reduced rate of AVM obliteration after embolization with no differences in rates of hemorrhage during the latency period.[22–24] Embolization before radiosurgery may adversely affect obliteration rates by fragmenting the nidus into discrete compartments, which makes treatment planning more difficult. There is also the potential for recanalization of previously embolized areas of nidus and difficulty during the targeting stage of radiosurgery because embolic material may introduce image distortion.[22,25] Studies have found, however, that Onyx does not significantly reduce the radiation dose delivered by linear accelerator stereotactic radiosurgery.[26]

For large, high-grade AVMs in eloquent areas, therapeutic options may be limited. Staged endovascular embolization to reduce the volume and allow stereotactic radiosurgery in large AVMs compares favorably with other treatment options in these difficult-to-treat lesions.[27] For these large and otherwise untreatable AVMs, embolization before radiosurgery also allows the treatment of high-risk features, such as intranidal aneurysms or direct fistulous connections.

Targeted Embolization

Certain angioarchitectural features are associated with an increased risk of hemorrhagic presentation. These features may include associated aneurysms, venous abnormalities such as ectasia and stenosis, and the presence of a single draining vein.[28–30] There is no evidence that partially treating an AVM, without specifically targeting high-risk features, reduces the risk of hemorrhage, whereas some evidence suggests that it may adversely affect the natural history.[31] In carefully selected patients, it may be reasonable to target high-risk features, such as aneurysms and venous ectasias, for embolization (**Fig. 1**), particularly in patients who are not surgical candidates already hemorrhaged. Partial targeted embolization of intranidal aneurysms and venous ectasias may provide some protection against hemorrhage.[11,32]

Palliative Embolization

Some investigators have attributed progressive neurologic deficits and intellectual decline in patients with AVMs to vascular steal.[33] There are limited case reports, but no large series or randomized studies, suggesting that partial embolization to reduce arteriovenous shunting may improve both perfusion and symptoms in brain adjacent to the AVM.[31,34,35] It is important to consider this option in the context of the multiple studies showing an increased risk of hemorrhage from partially treated AVMs and, if attempted, to avoid compromising venous outflow (**Fig. 2**).[36]

TECHNICAL CONSIDERATIONS

Successful endovascular treatment of AVMs begins with appropriate, careful patient selection along with clearly defined goals of embolization. Before beginning any embolization, careful evaluation of the arterial supply, nidal component, and venous drainage of the AVM is mandatory.

A small number of large feeding vessels creates a favorable environment for embolization. Multiple, small, and diffuse feeding vessels may make embolization impossible or prohibitively risky. Feeding arteries may directly supply the AVM or may supply predominantly normal cortex with small branching en-passage vessels feeding the AVM. The former are safer for embolization. When embolizing en-passage vessels there is often little leeway for tolerating reflux of embolization material; any reflux along the catheter could result in stroke. The nidus should be evaluated to delineate any distinct hemodynamic compartments.[37]

The nature of the connection between the arterial and venous compartments must also be appreciated. These connections can be nidal or fistulous. Fistulous connections require close attention to ensure that rapid progression of embolisate through the fistula to the venous side does not occlude a major draining vein.

In addition, the nature of venous drainage must be considered. Embolic material that progresses into a draining vein may result in sudden pressure changes within the AVM and precipitate rupture. This result is more likely in AVMs with a single draining vein, stenosis, or obstruction of a draining vein compared with an AVM that has multiple draining veins.

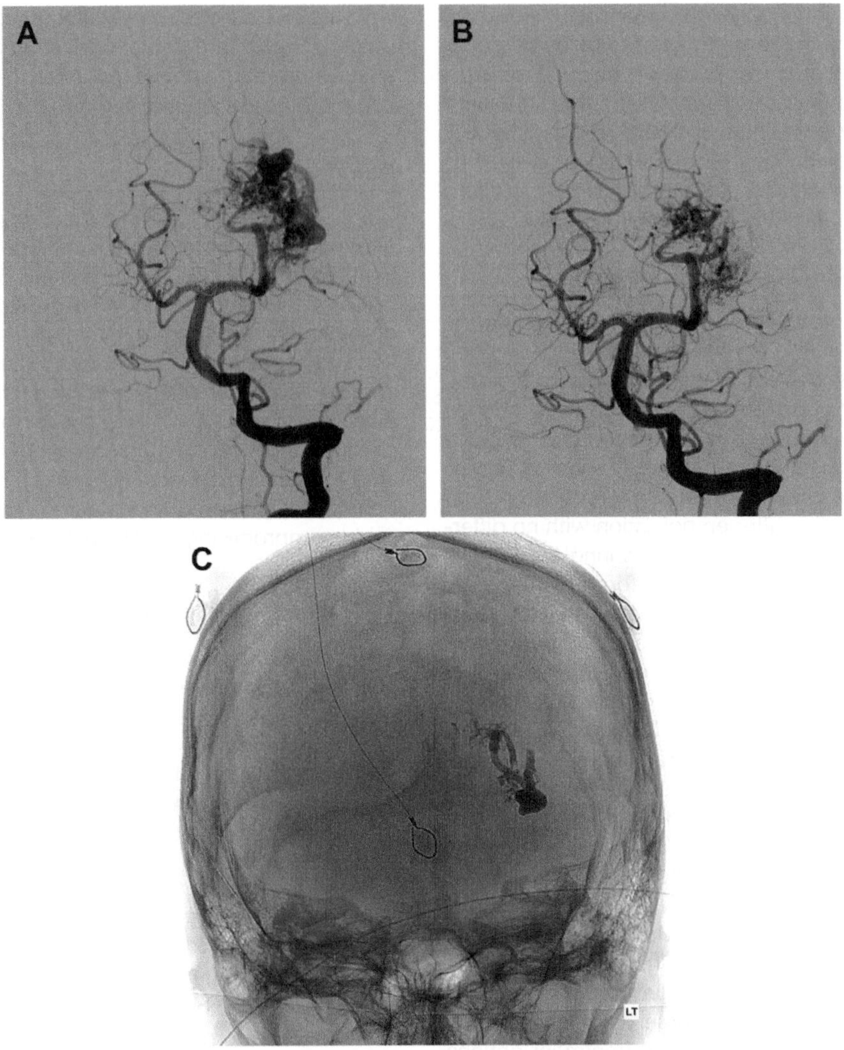

Fig. 1. Posteroanterior angiogram with a left vertebral artery injection showing an AVM measuring 3.4 × 2.4 cm abutting the thalamus with 2 intranidal aneurysms arising from the left posterior cerebral artery (*A*) in a 15-year-old girl with intraventricular hemorrhage. After targeted embolization with Onyx, the high-risk intranidal aneurysms are no longer filling (*B*). An unsubtracted posteroanterior view (*C*) shows the Onyx cast. (*Courtesy of* Barrow Neurological Institute, Phoenix AZ; with permission.)

Strong consideration should be given to routine neuromonitoring of somatosensory evoked potentials and electroencephalography for AVM embolization. In select cases the use of pharmacologic provocation with amobarbital (Amytal, Marathon Pharmaceuticals, Northbrook, IL, USA) can be a useful adjunct.[38,39]

Embolic Agents

Although a host of agents have been used to block blood flow to AVMs, including calibrated particles,[12] silk,[40] and absolute alcohol,[41] current strategies rely primarily on liquid embolic agents. The chosen embolic agent must penetrate into the nidus of the AVM; blocking arterial vessels proximal to the nidus allows vessel recruitment and persistence of the AVM. For this reason, detachable coils are minimally effective, although, in rare instances, they are a useful adjunct to liquid embolic agents to treat high-flow lesions.[42]

EVOH

EVOH, sold under the trade name Onyx, is a liquid embolic agent approved by the US Food and Drug Administration (FDA) in 2005 as a humanitarian use device for AVM embolization. The EVOH is mixed with tantalum powder to make it radiopaque and dissolved in dimethyl sulfoxide (DMSO). It requires catheters that are compatible with DMSO. When

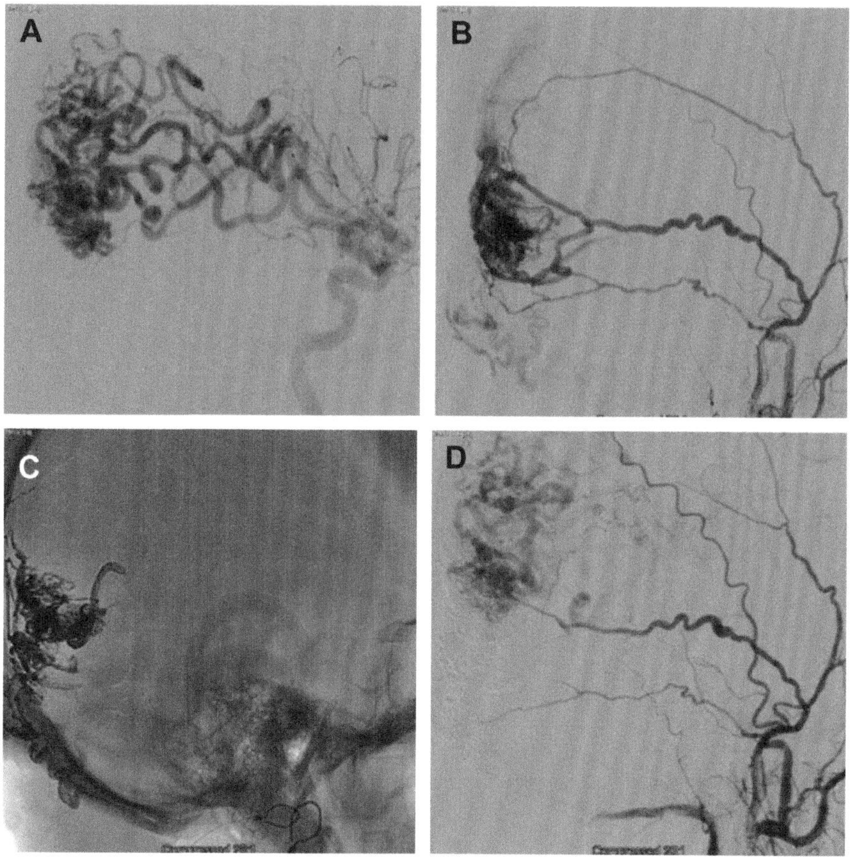

Fig. 2. Lateral angiogram with right external (*A*) and internal (*B*) carotid artery injections showing a right occipital Spetzler-Martin grade V AVM. The patient presented with worsening, intractable headaches and elected to undergo palliative embolization. After embolization of pedicles arising from the middle meningeal and occipital arteries, an angiogram shows the Onyx cast (*C*) and reduced flow into the nidus of the AVM (*D*). The patient's headaches improved. (*Courtesy of* Barrow Neurological Institute, Phoenix AZ; with permission.)

injected into an aqueous solution (eg, blood) the DMSO diffuses into the bloodstream, allowing the Onyx to precipitate. After filling the dead space of the microcatheter with DMSO, Onyx is injected slowly (typically over as long as 90 seconds). Rapid injection of DMSO is associated with angionecrosis.[43] EVOH is less adhesive than n-BCA, allowing slower injections over a longer period of time. Although long-term follow-up data are lacking, there is some evidence that recanalization can occur after embolization with EVOH.[44] Given the prolonged working time of EVOH it may be prudent to have a strategy for dealing with nidal or vessel rupture and hemorrhage, such as ready access to n-BCA.

The handling characteristics of EVOH may be altered by varying its concentration. It is currently available in 2 viscosities for AVM embolization: Onyx 18 (6% EVOH) and Onyx 34 (8% EVOH). Onyx 18 is less viscous and is used to achieve distal nidal penetration. Onyx 34 is more viscous and may be used in high-flow lesions with a fistulous component or to create a plug around the catheter. A common technique for AVM embolization with Onyx is a continuous injection to form a plug around the catheter tip with frequent pauses when reflux is observed. Once this plug is formed, Onyx 18 can be used to achieve distal nidal penetration.[20,45]

There is an increasing number of reports of using a dual lumen–compliant balloon catheter for AVM embolization. This technique may prevent unwanted proximal reflux and decrease procedure time and fluoroscopy exposure, but it is associated with the risk of vessel perforation from balloon inflation.[46,47] More proximal occlusion using a separate balloon catheter can also be used to decrease flow and minimize the risk of uncontrolled embolization into draining veins (**Fig. 3**). An alternative technique to improve efficiency, and possibly occlusion rates, in AVM embolization is positioning 2 microcatheters within separate

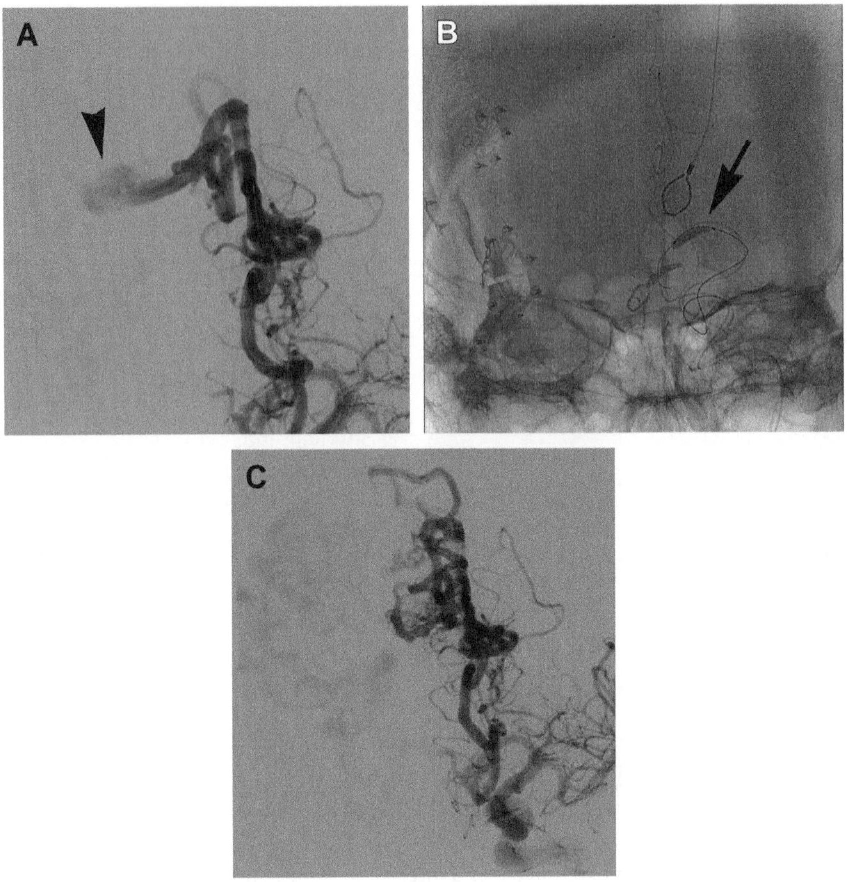

Fig. 3. Magnified posteroanterior (PA) angiogram (*A*) showing an ectatic venous pouch (*arrowhead*) arising from a fistulous connection in a patient with a Spetzler-Martin grade V AVM. Angiography was prompted by worsening seizures and headaches. An unsubtracted PA angiogram (*B*) shows microcatheters within the fistulous connection as well as an inflated hyperglide balloon, size 3 × 10 mm (*arrow*). The balloon was used to decrease flow and facilitate embolization of the fistula site while minimizing the risk of embolizing venous structures. A postembolization PA angiogram (*C*) shows obliteration of the high-risk fistula. (*Courtesy of* Barrow Neurological Institute, Phoenix AZ; with permission.)

feeding arteries and concurrently injecting Onyx.[48,49]

n-BCA

There is a long history of using cyanoacrylates to embolize AVMs. Trufill n-BCA (Codman, Raynham, MA) was approved by the FDA for use in AVM embolization in 2000. It is a monomer that polymerizes into a liquid adhesive on contact with any ionic substance. Because n-BCA polymerizes readily on contact with anything ionic, it is imperative to pay careful attention to detail throughout its use. The components are typically mixed immediately before use at a table isolated from any ionic compounds such as blood, saline, tissue, or contrast. New gloves should be used when handling the n-BCA and all material used for the glue should be new and kept separate from other angiographic supplies.[50] A 5% dextrose solution should be used for rinsing the equipment and flushing the microcatheter in preparation for injection.

Although n-BCA is radiolucent, it is frequently mixed with either tantalum powder or ethiodized oil (Ethiodol, Savage Laboratories, Melville, NY) to make the solution radiopaque. The addition of Ethiodol increases both the polymerization time and the viscosity of the n-BCA solution. Glacial acetic acid can also be used to delay polymerization.[51] The proportion of Ethiodol typically varies from 1:1 to 1:4 (glue/oil). Although higher concentrations of oil theoretically delay polymerization and may allow more distal nidal penetration, this is at least partially offset by an increase in viscosity.

The goal of any AVM embolization with n-BCA is penetration of the nidus. Proximal embolization of feeding arteries is not sufficient: recanalization occurs when the nidus is not embolized.[52] There are several important technical nuances to safely achieve this. Glue may be injected using either a continuous-column technique or a push technique. In the continuous-column technique the n-BCA is injected slowly and continuously through the microcatheter until reflux is observed around the catheter tip or the goals of embolization are met. The catheter is quickly removed to minimize the risk of catheter retention. In the push technique a 5% dextrose solution is used to push the glue, either through the microcatheter[50] or through the guide catheter.[53] When performed through a microcatheter, the amount of glue that can be used is limited to less than the dead space of the catheter. However, there is the potential to use the microcatheter for more than a single injection, provided there is no reflux of the glue around the tip of the catheter. When using a guide catheter, a 60-mL syringe is used to infuse a 5% dextrose-in-water solution at the same time as the n-BCA injection is started through the microcatheter. This method delays contact of the n-BCA with ionic substances and allows more distal penetration. Although advancing the microcatheter within the nidus is optimal, if the catheter can be wedged into position proximal to the nidus then the dextrose solution in the catheter similarly replaces the column of blood and may promote deposition within the nidus.[54]

SUMMARY

Endovascular treatment of AVMs is challenging. It requires complex decision making, thorough understanding of often complicated vascular anatomy, and technical precision. Meticulous attention to detail, from preoperative planning to diagnostic angiography to treatment and follow-up, are paramount for good clinical outcomes. AVMs should be treated in a multidisciplinary setting with open lines of communication between specialists capable of providing endovascular, open surgical, and radiosurgical treatment. Advances in techniques and technology are making endovascular treatment feasible and useful for an increasing number of patients.

REFERENCES

1. Stevens J, Leach JL, Abruzzo T, et al. De novo cerebral arteriovenous malformation: case report and literature review. AJNR Am J Neuroradiol 2009;30:111–2.
2. Hofmeister C, Stapf C, Hartmann A, et al. Demographic, morphological, and clinical characteristics of 1289 patients with brain arteriovenous malformation. Stroke 2000;31:1307–10.
3. Ondra SL, Troupp H, George ED, et al. The natural history of symptomatic arteriovenous malformations of the brain: a 24-year follow-up assessment. J Neurosurg 1990;73:387–91.
4. Stapf C, Mast H, Sciacca RR, et al. Predictors of hemorrhage in patients with untreated brain arteriovenous malformation. Neurology 2006;66:1350–5.
5. Hernesniemi JA, Dashti R, Juvela S, et al. Natural history of brain arteriovenous malformations: a long-term follow-up study of risk of hemorrhage in 238 patients. Neurosurgery 2008;63:823–9.
6. Itoyama Y, Uemura S, Ushio Y, et al. Natural course of unoperated intracranial arteriovenous malformations: study of 50 cases. J Neurosurg 1989;71:805–9.
7. Mast H, Young WL, Koennecke HC, et al. Risk of spontaneous haemorrhage after diagnosis of cerebral arteriovenous malformation. Lancet 1997;350:1065–8.
8. Jahan R, Murayama Y, Gobin YP, et al. Embolization of arteriovenous malformations with Onyx: clinicopathological experience in 23 patients. Neurosurgery 2001;48:984–95.
9. Klurfan P, Gunnarsson T, Haw C, et al. Endovascular treatment of brain arteriovenous malformations: the Toronto experience. Interv Neuroradiol 2005;11:51–6.
10. Liu HM, Huang YC, Wang YH. Embolization of cerebral arteriovenous malformations with n-butyl-2-cyanoacrylate. J Formos Med Assoc 2000;99:906–13.
11. Meisel HJ, Mansmann U, Alvarez H, et al. Effect of partial targeted N-butyl-cyano-acrylate embolization in brain AVM. Acta Neurochir (Wien) 2002;144:879–87.
12. Sorimachi T, Koike T, Takeuchi S, et al. Embolization of cerebral arteriovenous malformations achieved with polyvinyl alcohol particles: angiographic reappearance and complications. AJNR Am J Neuroradiol 1999;20:1323–8.
13. Vinuela F, Duckwiler G, Jahan R, et al. Therapeutic management of cerebral arteriovenous malformations. Present role of interventional neuroradiology. Interv Neuroradiol 2005;11:13–29.
14. Taylor CL, Dutton K, Rappard G, et al. Complications of preoperative embolization of cerebral arteriovenous malformations. J Neurosurg 2004;100:810–2.
15. Ogilvy CS, Stieg PE, Awad I, et al. AHA scientific statement: recommendations for the management of intracranial arteriovenous malformations: a statement for healthcare professionals from a special writing group of the Stroke Council, American Stroke Association. Stroke 2001;32:1458–71.
16. Richling B, Killer M, Al-Schameri AR, et al. Therapy of brain arteriovenous malformations: multimodality

treatment from a balanced standpoint. Neurosurgery 2006;59:S148–57.
17. Starke RM, Meyers PM, Connolly ES Jr. Adjuvant endovascular management of brain arteriovenous malformations. In: Winn R, editor. Youmans neurological surgery. Philadelphia: Elsevier; 2011. p. 4058.
18. Natarajan SK, Ghodke B, Britz GW, et al. Multimodality treatment of brain arteriovenous malformations with microsurgery after embolization with onyx: single-center experience and technical nuances. Neurosurgery 2008;62:1213–25.
19. Yu SC, Chan MS, Lam JM, et al. Complete obliteration of intracranial arteriovenous malformation with endovascular cyanoacrylate embolization: initial success and rate of permanent cure. AJNR Am J Neuroradiol 2004;25:1139–43.
20. Saatci I, Geyik S, Yavuz K, et al. Endovascular treatment of brain arteriovenous malformations with prolonged intranidal Onyx injection technique: long-term results in 350 consecutive patients with completed endovascular treatment course. J Neurosurg 2011; 115:78–88.
21. van Rooij WJ, Jacobs S, Sluzewski M, et al. Curative embolization of brain arteriovenous malformations with onyx: patient selection, embolization technique, and results. AJNR Am J Neuroradiol 2012;33:1299–304.
22. Andrade-Souza YM, Ramani M, Beachey DJ, et al. Liquid embolisation material reduces the delivered radiation dose: a physical experiment. Acta Neurochir (Wien) 2008;150:161–4.
23. Kano H, Kondziolka D, Flickinger JC, et al. Stereotactic radiosurgery for arteriovenous malformations after embolization: a case-control study. J Neurosurg 2012;117:265–75.
24. Schwyzer L, Yen CP, Evans A, et al. Long-term results of gamma knife surgery for partially embolized arteriovenous malformations. Neurosurgery 2012;71:1139–47.
25. Shtraus N, Schifter D, Corn BW, et al. Radiosurgical treatment planning of AVM following embolization with Onyx: possible dosage error in treatment planning can be averted. J Neurooncol 2010;98:271–6.
26. Bing F, Doucet R, Lacroix F, et al. Liquid embolization material reduces the delivered radiation dose: clinical myth or reality? AJNR Am J Neuroradiol 2012;33:320–2.
27. Blackburn SL, Ashley WW Jr, Rich KM, et al. Combined endovascular embolization and stereotactic radiosurgery in the treatment of large arteriovenous malformations. J Neurosurg 2011;114:1758–67.
28. Brown RD Jr, Wiebers DO, Forbes GS. Unruptured intracranial aneurysms and arteriovenous malformations: frequency of intracranial hemorrhage and relationship of lesions. J Neurosurg 1990;73: 859–63.
29. da Costa L, Wallace MC, Ter Brugge KG, et al. The natural history and predictive features of hemorrhage from brain arteriovenous malformations. Stroke 2009;40:100–5.
30. Kader A, Young WL, Pile-Spellman J, et al. The influence of hemodynamic and anatomic factors on hemorrhage from cerebral arteriovenous malformations. Neurosurgery 1994;34:801–7.
31. Han PP, Ponce FA, Spetzler RF. Intention-to-treat analysis of Spetzler-Martin grades IV and V arteriovenous malformations: natural history and treatment paradigm. J Neurosurg 2003;98:3–7.
32. Krings T, Hans FJ, Geibprasert S, et al. Partial "targeted" embolisation of brain arteriovenous malformations. Eur Radiol 2010;20:2723–31.
33. Batjer HH, Devous MD Sr, Seibert GB, et al. Intracranial arteriovenous malformation: relationships between clinical and radiographic factors and ipsilateral steal severity. Neurosurgery 1988;23:322–8.
34. Kusske JA, Kelly WA. Embolization and reduction of the "steal" syndrome in cerebral arteriovenous malformations. J Neurosurg 1974;40:313–21.
35. Luessenhop AJ, Mujica PH. Embolization of segments of the circle of Willis and adjacent branches for management of certain inoperable cerebral arteriovenous malformations. J Neurosurg 1981; 54:573–82.
36. Kalani MY, Albuquerque FC, Fiorella D, et al. Endovascular treatment of cerebral arteriovenous malformations. Neuroimaging Clin N Am 2013;23: 605–24.
37. Yamada S, Brauer FS, Colohan AR, et al. Concept of arteriovenous malformation compartments and surgical management. Neurol Res 2004;26: 288–300.
38. Niimi Y, Sala F, Deletis V, et al. Neurophysiologic monitoring and pharmacologic provocative testing for embolization of spinal cord arteriovenous malformations. AJNR Am J Neuroradiol 2004;25: 1131–8.
39. Sala F, Beltramello A, Gerosa M. Neuroprotective role of neurophysiological monitoring during endovascular procedures in the brain and spinal cord. Neurophysiol Clin 2007;37:415–21.
40. Schmutz F, McAuliffe W, Anderson DM, et al. Embolization of cerebral arteriovenous malformations with silk: histopathologic changes and hemorrhagic complications. AJNR Am J Neuroradiol 1997;18:1233–7.
41. Yakes WF, Krauth L, Ecklund J, et al. Ethanol endovascular management of brain arteriovenous malformations: initial results. Neurosurgery 1997;40: 1145–52.
42. Nakstad PH, Bakke SJ, Hald JK. Embolization of intracranial arteriovenous malformations and fistulas with polyvinyl alcohol particles and platinum fibre coils. Neuroradiology 1992;34:348–51.

43. Murayama Y, Vinuela F, Ulhoa A, et al. Nonadhesive liquid embolic agent for cerebral arteriovenous malformations: preliminary histopathological studies in swine rete mirabile. Neurosurgery 1998;43:1164–75.
44. Natarajan SK, Born D, Ghodke B, et al. Histopathological changes in brain arteriovenous malformations after embolization using Onyx or N-butyl cyanoacrylate. Laboratory investigation. J Neurosurg 2009;111:105–13.
45. De Keukeleire K, Vanlangenhove P, Kalala Okito JP, et al. Transarterial embolization with ONYX for treatment of intracranial non-cavernous dural arteriovenous fistula with or without cortical venous reflux. J Neurointerv Surg 2011;3:224–8.
46. Jagadeesan BD, Grigoryan M, Hassan AE, et al. Endovascular balloon-assisted embolization of intracranial and cervical arteriovenous malformations using dual-lumen coaxial balloon microcatheters and onyx: initial experience. Neurosurgery 2013;73(Suppl Operative 2):ons238–43.
47. Spiotta AM, Miranpuri AS, Vargas J, et al. Balloon augmented Onyx embolization utilizing a dual lumen balloon catheter: utility in the treatment of a variety of head and neck lesions. J Neurointerv Surg 2013. [Epub ahead of print].
48. Abud DG, Riva R, Nakiri GS, et al. Treatment of brain arteriovenous malformations by double arterial catheterization with simultaneous injection of Onyx: retrospective series of 17 patients. AJNR Am J Neuroradiol 2011;32:152–8.
49. Renieri L, Consoli A, Scarpini G, et al. Double arterial catheterization technique for embolization of brain arteriovenous malformations with onyx. Neurosurgery 2013;72:92–8.
50. Rosen RJ, Contractor S. The use of cyanoacrylate adhesives in the management of congenital vascular malformations. Semin Intervent Radiol 2004;21:59–66.
51. Spiegel SM, Vinuela F, Goldwasser JM, et al. Adjusting the polymerization time of isobutyl-2 cyanoacrylate. AJNR Am J Neuroradiol 1986;7:109–12.
52. Vinuela F, Fox AJ, Pelz D, et al. Angiographic follow-up of large cerebral AVMs incompletely embolized with isobutyl-2-cyanoacrylate. AJNR Am J Neuroradiol 1986;7:919–25.
53. Moore C, Murphy K, Gailloud P. Improved distal distribution of n-butyl cyanoacrylate glue by simultaneous injection of dextrose 5% through the guiding catheter: technical note. Neuroradiology 2006;48:327–32.
54. Nelson PK, Russell SM, Woo HH, et al. Use of a wedged microcatheter for curative transarterial embolization of complex intracranial dural arteriovenous fistulas: indications, endovascular technique, and outcome in 21 patients. J Neurosurg 2003;98:498–506.

Endovascular Management of Intracranial Dural Arteriovenous Fistulae

Stylianos Rammos, MD[a], Carlo Bortolotti, MD[b],
Giuseppe Lanzino, MD[c,*]

KEYWORDS

- Intracranial dural arteriovenous fistulae (DAVF) • Transarterial embolization
- Transvenous embolization • Indirect carotido-cavernous fistulae • Transverse-sigmoid sinus DAVF

KEY POINTS

- Endovascular embolization is the preferred treatment modality of dural arteriovenous fistulae (DAVF) with retrograde leptomeningeal drainage.
- Transarterial ethylene vinyl alcohol and *n*-butyl-2-cyanoacrylate embolization of DAVF are associated with high cure rates and low complication rates.
- Transvenous embolization of cavernous DAVF is associated with high occlusion rates and symptomatic improvement of ocular hypertension.
- Direct percutaneous access via either the orbit or the calvarial foramina may be performed in cases of difficult arterial or venous access routes.
- Transarterial particle embolization with or without adjuvant radiosurgery may improve symptoms in patients with DAVF and no retrograde leptomeningeal drainage.

INTRODUCTION

With better understanding of the pathophysiology of intracranial dural arteriovenous fistulae (DAVF) and improvement in catheter and embolic material technology, endovascular treatment has become the treatment of choice for most intracranial DAVF. The goal of endovascular treatment of intracranial DAVF depends on clinical presentation, location, and angioarchitecture of the fistula.[1]

DAVF with retrograde leptomeningeal drainage (RLVD) are associated with a high incidence of hemorrhage and symptomatic venous hypertension. Patients who originally present with hemorrhage have a risk of rebleeding as high as 33% in the first 2 weeks.[2] The treatment goal for DAVF presenting with hemorrhage or with progressive symptoms of intracranial or ocular hypertension is complete obliteration. Complete obliteration should be considered even in asymptomatic patients with RLVD, even though lack of symptoms in patients with RLVD is associated with a more benign natural history than in symptomatic patients.[3] There is no evidence to support the notion that partial or palliative treatment reduces the risk of hemorrhage, venous infarction, or visual loss in symptomatic patients with RLVD, although partial treatment may be a reasonable

Disclosure: G. Lanzino is a consultant for Covidien, Codman/Johnson and Johnson.
[a] Arkansas Neuroscience Institute, 5 Saint Vincent Circle, Suite 503, Little Rock, AR 72205, USA; [b] Division of Neurosurgery, Istituto delle Scienze Neurologiche di Bologna, IRCCS Bellaria Hospital, Via Castiglione 29, BO 40124, Italy; [c] Department of Neurologic Surgery, College of Medicine, Mayo Clinic, 200 First Street, Rochester, MN 55905, USA
* Corresponding author.
E-mail address: lanzino.giuseppe@mayo.edu

Neurosurg Clin N Am 25 (2014) 539–549
http://dx.doi.org/10.1016/j.nec.2014.04.010
1042-3680/14/$ – see front matter

compromise in selected cases. A more individualized approach may be applied to patients with DAVF without RLVD, where symptom amelioration or resolution may be achieved without necessarily obtaining an angiographic cure. This latter principle applies especially to patients with high-flow DAVF without RLVD and severe pulsatile tinnitus interfering with their quality of life.

Careful analysis and understanding of the DAVF angioarchitecture are a critical prerequisite to treatment planning. Pretreatment angiography should address the exact location of arteriovenous shunting, arterial supply (dural and pial), flow characteristics, and venous drainage of the DAVF. Particular attention should be paid to the venous drainage of normal brain during the late venous phase of angiography. The venous outflow should be scrutinized for the presence of a parallel venous pouch or compartmentalization of the involved dural sinus, which is often present in DAVF associated with a major intracranial venous sinus. It is of paramount importance to identify whether the involved sinus is functionally isolated or still serves as a conduit for normal venous drainage.

Complete and persistent obliteration of the DAVF is achieved by occlusion of its proximal venous drainage. Based on the route of access, endovascular approaches to DAVF can be schematically divided into transarterial, transvenous, combined, and percutaneous/direct. The choice of access used depends on clinical presentation, location, ease of access, operator experience, and most importantly, careful analysis of the angiographic architecture of each lesion.

TRANSARTERIAL EMBOLIZATION OF DAVF WITH ONYX

A transarterial approach has become the most frequently used initial treatment modality for DAVF with RLVD, primarily after the introduction of ethylene vinyl alcohol (Onyx; Covidien, Dublin, Ireland), a permanent, nonadhesive, liquid polymer embolic agent. DAVF with *direct* RLVD represent the ideal candidates for transarterial treatment with Onyx. DAVF with sinus *and* RLVD outflow can also be successfully treated with Onyx embolization, especially if a parallel venous pouch or compartmentalization of the involved sinus is present.

A standard transfemoral arterial route is used. An Onyx-compatible microcatheter is navigated and positioned as close as possible to the fistulous connection. The dead space of the microcatheter is filled initially with the solvent dimethyl sulfoxide. A proximal plug of Onyx is then created around the distal tip of the microcatheter to produce sufficient proximal flow arrest and allow distal penetration of Onyx into the fistula. Two separate preparations of Onyx are available: Onyx 18, the agent most commonly used, has low viscosity and allows optimal distal penetration in DAVF with low flow. On the other hand, Onyx 34 has higher viscosity, resulting in greater and more rapid cohesion of the injected material and less fragmentation in the flow stream.[4] The authors use Onyx 34 to build an optimal proximal plug and avoid premature distal migration.[5,6] A relatively long injection of Onyx will allow optimal DAVF penetration. If a "wedged" distal position of the microcatheter is achieved, Onyx may progress in an antegrade fashion with minimal or no reflux (**Fig. 1**). If excessive reflux along the microcatheter or inadvertent distal migration of Onyx is noted under fluoroscopy, the injection can be halted, the roadmap renewed, and the injection restarted after 1 to 2 minutes. The goal of treatment is to fill the DAVF proximal venous outlet while allowing retrograde occlusion of contributing arterial feeders, until no shunting is verified on control angiography (see **Fig. 1**).

Most noncavernous DAVF are supplied by transosseous branches of the occipital and meningeal arteries, most commonly the middle meningeal artery (MMA). Transosseous pedicles of scalp arteries may be quite tortuous, particularly in their distal course, in proximity to the fistula, and therefore their navigation may be difficult or even impossible. Whenever the posterior branch of the MMA provides a supply to the DAVF, microcatheter navigation and positioning are often possible in close proximity to the fistulous tract (see **Fig. 1**). This branch often provides a natural direct access to the fistula's venous collector system.[7] Furthermore, the MMA and its branches run a relatively straight course beyond the foramen spinosum, where the artery enters the cranium, and are anchored on the dura, making failed microcatheter retrieval rare despite substantial proximal Onyx reflux.[8–10] Although proximal Onyx reflux may occur with a high margin of safety[9] in the MMA, reflux should not be allowed in proximity to the level of the foramen spinosum to avoid inadvertent compromise of the arterial supply to the trigeminal and facial nerves.[6] It is therefore important to maintain a lateral view on at least one projection to have an accurate estimation of the level of the skull base.

The most common cause of inadequate fistula obliteration after transarterial Onyx embolization is failure to reach the venous side and/or failure to overfill the proximal venous side. It is important to recognize that Onyx will initially coat the endothelial surface circumferentially before obliterating the lumen of the embolized vessel. The difference

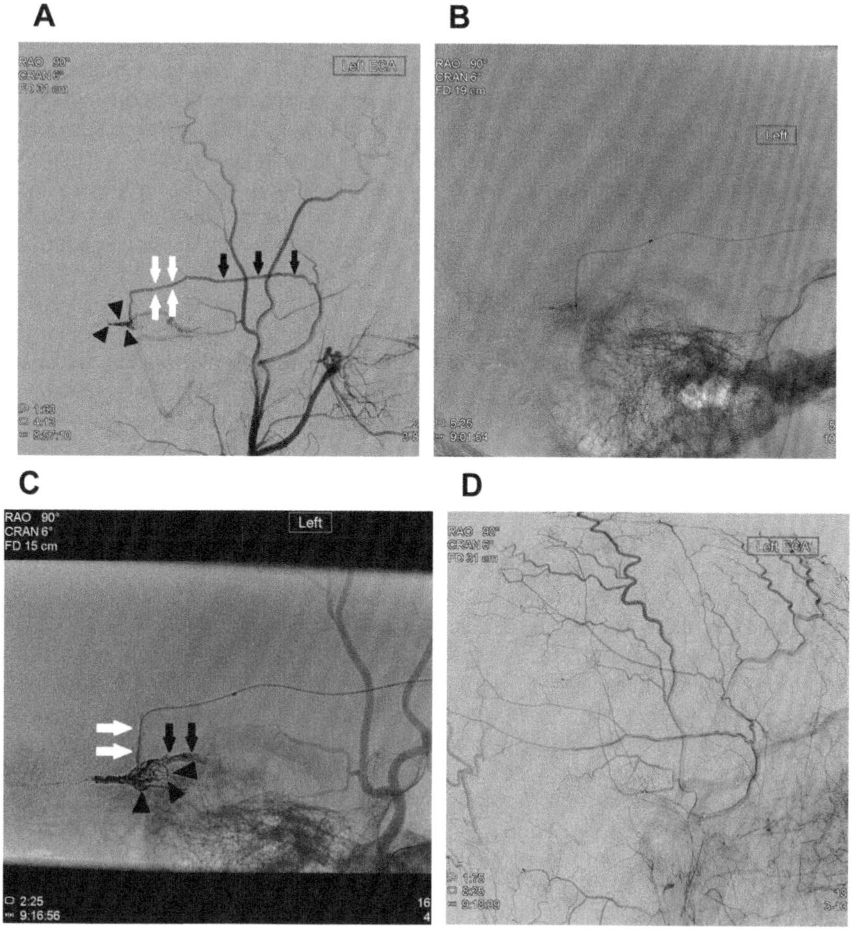

Fig. 1. Incidental tentorial DAVF discovered in an 18-year-old during investigation for a symptomatic vertebral artery dissection. (*A*) Selective right external carotid artery injection demonstrates the fistula (*arrowheads*) fed primarily by the posterior branch of the MMA (*arrows*). The posterior branch of the MMA is an "ideal" branch for catheterization because of its relatively straight course (*black arrows*). (*B*) The straight course of the posterior branch of the MMA allows for a very distal catheterization often in a "wedge" position very close to the point of fistualization (*arrows*). (*C*) Onyx cast showing filling of the "nidus" (*arrowheads*) and the proximal portion of the venous drainage (*arrows*). There is a small amount of reflux around the distal portion of the microcatheter (*white arrows*). (*D*) Selective right external carotid artery injection, late arterial phase, confirms complete angiographic obliteration of the DAVF.

may be subtle to differentiate with current angiographic resolution and it is critical to follow the immediate posttreatment angiogram well late into the venous phase to rule out persistent filling. Patients need to have follow-up catheter angiography 3 to 6 months after initial treatment to confirm persistent and complete obliteration because recurrence may develop without associated clinical symptoms.[11] However, long-term occlusion rates seem to be high after transarterial Onyx embolization: in a study of DAVF with initial complete or near complete obliteration, stability of angiographic findings at 6, 12, 24, and 46 months was 100%, 95.4%, 93.8%, and 92.3%, respectively.[12] A lower success rate after Onyx embolization may also be more prevalent after a previously failed embolization.[9]

Several recent studies have confirmed transarterial Onyx embolization to be an effective treatment of DAVF with RLVD. In a single-center prospective series of 30 patients with DAVF and RLVD, 80% experienced angiographic cure, 83% of which after a single procedure. Persistent occlusion was verified in 23 of 24 patients on follow-up angiography at 3 months. Re-hemorrhage, however, occurred in one completely cured patient because of draining vein thrombosis, and one patient developed a transient cranial nerve palsy.[9] Similarly, van Rooij and Sluzewski[10] successfully treated 8 patients with DAVF and RLVD without complications and with complete obliteration present at 6- to 12-weeks follow-up angiography. Puffer and coworkers[6] reported successful complete or near complete obliteration of tentorial DAVF with transarterial Onyx embolization in 8 of 9 patients with no periprocedural morbidity and mortality. Finally, Maimon and colleagues[13] were able to obliterate 94% of DAVF completely with RLVD in 17 patients, with a 6% morbidity.

A distinct disadvantage associated with the use of Onyx for DAVF treatment is the prolonged fluoroscopy frequently used and associated increased radiation exposure. Alopecia and cutaneous burns may therefore develop, while the delayed health risks are currently unknown. In addition, the cost of the procedure may be fairly high. Postprocedural pain is experienced by most patients, probably related to dural ischemia,[10] but is rarely unresponsive to mild oral analgesics. Procedural complications may include inadvertent microcatheter retention, pulmonary embolism, bradyarrhythmia (due to an exaggerated trigeminocardiac reflex), and palsies of the trigeminal, facial, and lower cranial nerves.[14] Arterial ischemic events are rare because dural arteries are the primary conduits used for embolization; however, particular attention should be paid to anastomoses between the external carotid and vertebral arteries that may become more pronounced during the course of embolization. Finally, venous ischemia and/or hemorrhage may result from occlusion of normal cerebral venous drainage.

TRANSARTERIAL EMBOLIZATION OF DAVF WITH ACRYLIC GLUE

Transarterial DAVF embolization can be successfully performed with acrylic embolic agents, such as *n*-butyl-2-cyanoacrylate (nBCA; Trufill, Codman, Raynham, MA, USA), although its use for this indication has decreased in the "Onyx" era, especially in the United States. Patients harboring DAVF with *direct* RLVD, and less commonly, DAVF with sinus *and* RLVD, are candidates for this treatment modality. A standard transfemoral arterial route is used. An nBCA-compatible microcatheter is navigated and positioned in close proximity to the fistulous connection in a wedged position with the tip of the microcatheter establishing flow arrest in the vessel. The microcatheter is flushed with a 5% dextrose solution before injection, to avoid glue precipitation within the microcatheter. The injection dynamic should be predicated on the catheter's distance from the fistula, flow rate, and the size of the feeding artery engaged.[15] Unlike Onyx, nBCA is adhesive and thrombogenic, and recanalization is unlikely to occur if the glue cast traverses the fistulous connection and occludes the immediate proximal venous outflow. Low-concentration nBCA is used to achieve distal penetration in the nidus, and concurrent injection of dextrose solution via the guide catheter during embolization can prevent proximal polymerization and premature proximal occlusion.[16] The angiographic cure rate for DAVF with isolated direct RLVD was shown to improve from 10% to 55% as the mean concentration of glue decreased from 37% to 23%.[16] NBCA embolization offers the advantage of shorter procedure lengths, decreased radiation exposure, and lower cost compared with Onyx-based embolization. Interestingly, delayed thrombosis of incompletely treated DVAF with transarterial acrylics has been reported, presumably because of the thrombogenic properties of nBCA.[16,17]

Transarterial nBCA embolization may be quite effective even if multiple sessions of transarterial embolization may be necessary for complete DAVF occlusion. Nelson and colleagues[15] reported 30% of cases requiring more than one attempt to occlude the DAVF completely. Although unsuccessful depositions because of inadequate venous penetration may not in and by themselves be curative, they reduce collateral inflow, making subsequent transarterial attempts more likely to be successful in achieving angiographic cure. Complete occlusion was achieved in all patients and no recurrence was encountered during a mean follow-up period of 18.7 months. Angiographic cure was accomplished in 90% (34/38 patients) with DAVF and RLVD with no permanent morbidity, whereas 2.37 arterial pedicles were embolized per patient on an average of 1.37 sessions per patient.[17] In the largest reported retrospective series of 170 patients, treated within a 16-year period, 85% of patients were treated with a single procedure (mean, 1.2 sessions) with a 66% complete occlusion rate (69% complete occlusion in DAVF with RLVD), and 2.3% had a permanent neurologic deficit.[18] Procedural complications during transarterial nBCA embolization are similar to Onyx-based treatment and more commonly include cranial nerve palsies, arterial ischemia, and venous ischemia and/or hemorrhage.

TRANSVENOUS EMBOLIZATION OF DAVF

A transvenous approach remains the predominant approach in treatment of DAVF of the cavernous sinus.[19] Furthermore, certain DAVF associated with a functionally isolated segment of the superior sagittal sinus and transverse/sigmoid junction harboring the fistulous connection may be accessible via a transvenous route. A transvenous approach may also be more suitable if multiple small arterial feeders shunt into a widely dispersed segment of the dural sinus wall.[20] A standard transfemoral or transjugular venous approach is frequently used. The major routes available for access to the cavernous sinus include anteriorly the superior ophthalmic and facial veins; superiorly the superficial middle cerebral vein and sphenoparietal sinus; posteriorly the petrosal sinuses; and inferiorly the pterygoid plexus (**Fig. 2**). If venous access to the fistulous site is difficult, direct surgical exposure of the superior ophthalmic vein may be entertained. Access to DVAF of the transverse/sigmoid junction may be established via the ipsilateral, or a patent contralateral, transverse sinus through the torcula. In rare instances, craniotomy may ultimately be necessary to provide access for endovascular occlusion of DAVF of the transverse/sigmoid sinus junction.[21] Transvenous embolization has traditionally been performed with detachable and fibered coils that promote thrombosis, and less frequently, with liquid embolic agents.[22]

Nonselective sacrifice of a dural sinus that harbors a DAVF and concurrently serves as a functional outlet for normal venous drainage may lead to venous ischemia and/or hemorrhage and could trigger the de novo development of DAVF.[23] Moreover, excessive sinus packing, frequently necessary in the treatment of cavernous DAVF, may also be responsible for the development or exacerbation of cranial neuropathies and ophthalmoplegia.[24] In most cases, however, meticulous DAVF angioarchitectural analysis will frequently uncover a parallel venous pouch that acts as the recipient of arterial inflow, and which is angiographically discrete from the involved sinus.[25] Arterial inflow will converge to a venous pouch that may have the angiographic appearance of either a compartment within the involved sinus (septation) or one outside the sinus (accessory sinus), and its superselective occlusion will lead to DAVF obliteration without compromise of the functioning portion of the sinus.[23] With selective mapping, including three-dimensional angiography, the fistulous connection in cavernous DAVF may in fact reside outside the confines of the cavernous sinus (**Fig. 3**).[26]

Using superimposed superselective arterial and venous angiography, Satow and colleagues[26] were able to confirm their venous microcatheter location in the exact shunt segment, followed by transvenous coil placement restricted in a small compartment of the cavernous sinus. Twenty-five percent of patients with selective shunt occlusion within the cavernous sinus developed a transient sixth nerve palsy that eventually resolved and

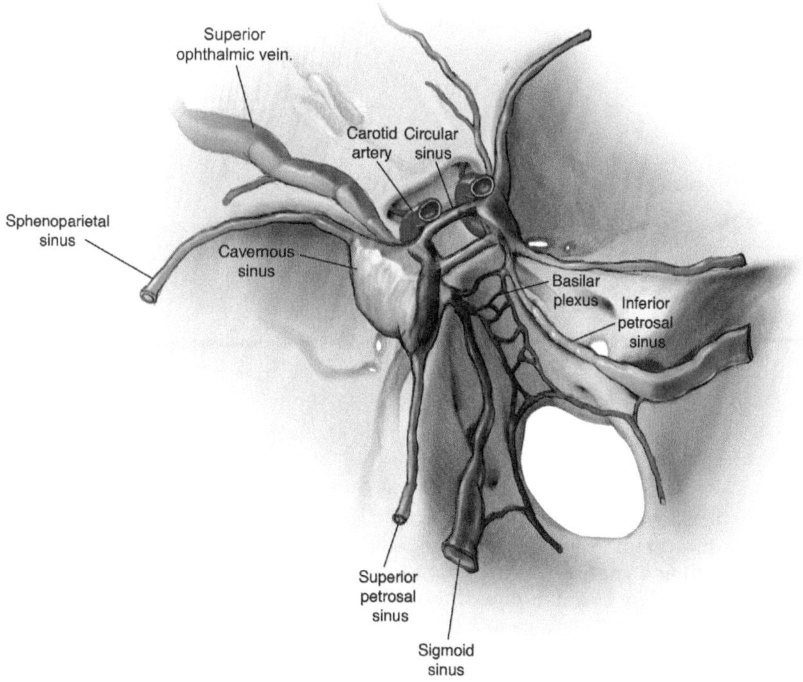

Fig. 2. Artist's depiction of a carotido-cavernous fistula and the main routes of drainage of the cavernous sinus. Various access routes can be used to access the cavernous sinus region through a transvenous approach. (*Courtesy of* Mayo Foundation for Medical Education and Research, Rochester, MN, USA © All rights reserved.)

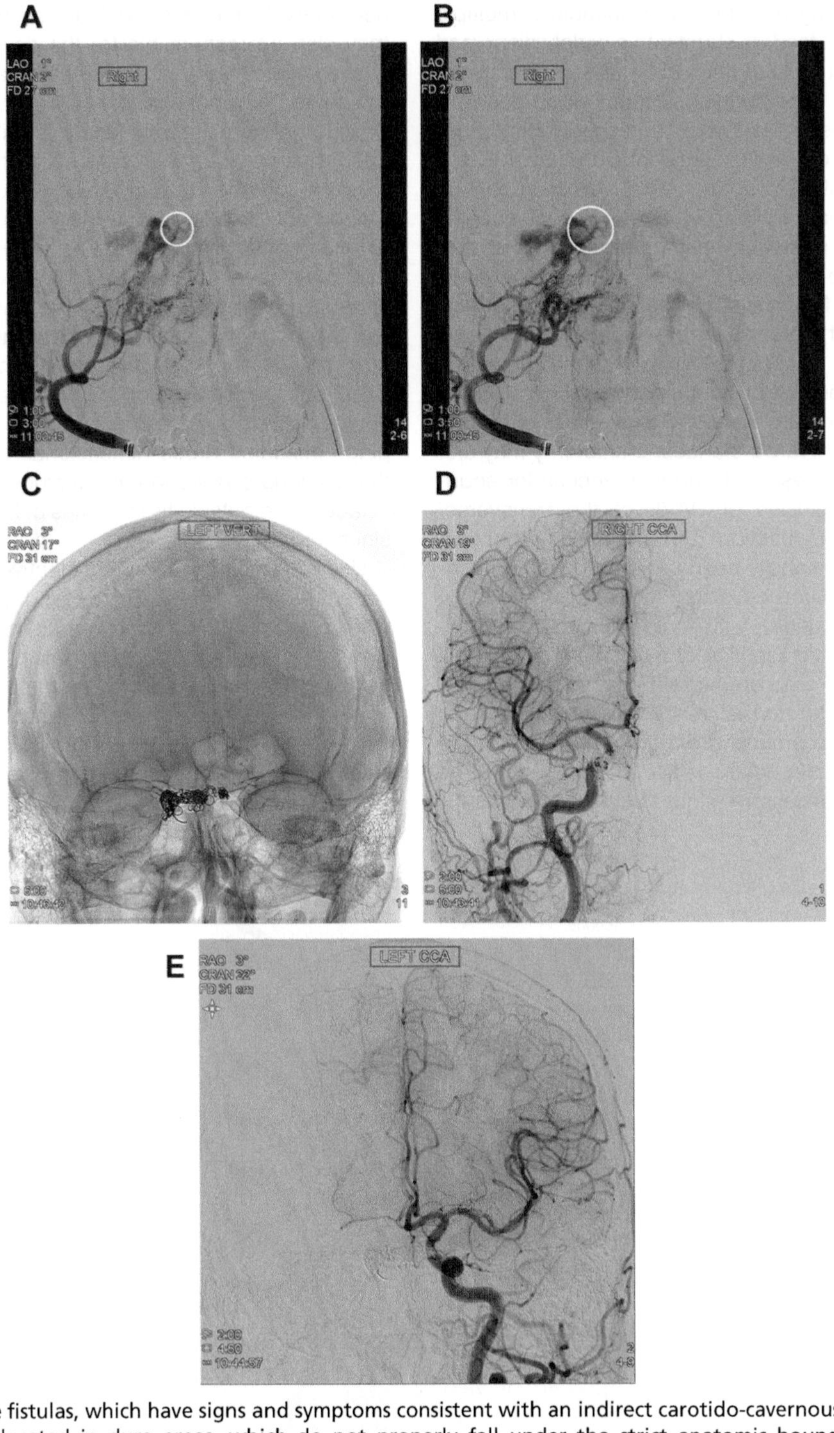

Fig. 3. Some fistulas, which have signs and symptoms consistent with an indirect carotido-cavernous fistula, may actually be located in dura areas, which do not properly fall under the strict anatomic boundaries of the "cavernous sinus." Early (*A*) and later (*B*) selective right internal maxillary artery injection demonstrate a fistula based on the right portion (*white circle*) of one of the 2 arms of the intercavernous sinus, forming the circular sinus with bilateral (right greater than left) venous drainage. The fistula was occluded with detachable and pushable coils through a transvenous approach. (*C*) The coil cast outlines the boundaries of the involved intercavernous sinus. Postoperative right (*D*) and left (*E*) common carotid artery injection 3 months later confirms persistent complete obliteration of the DAVF.

had no evidence of angiographic recurrence at a mean follow-up of 4 years, compared with 25% of patients who developed permanent ophthalmoplegia after nonselective cavernous sinus packing.

DAVF associated with an isolated sinus are characterized by a network of small arterial feeders opening into the wall of a completely thrombosed sinus that prohibits antegrade or retrograde venous access. Transvenous access may therefore be difficult to achieve. However, navigation into an isolated sinus was successful in 51 of 61 patients, as reported by Lekkhong and colleagues.[20] A 0.035-inch or 0.038-inch hydrophilic guidewire was gently advanced with continuous rotation under roadmap navigation from the arterial injection (venogram) toward the occluded sinus and hence create a visualized track for the subsequent advancement of the microcatheter. The authors were able to achieve angiographic cure in 49 of 51 patients with no permanent procedure-related morbidity.

Transvenous embolization of cavernous DAVF is associated with a high occlusion rate and symptom improvement.[19] Theaudin and colleagues[27] reported a rate of 87% complete occlusion (14/17) with 71% (10/14) of angiographically cured patients being asymptomatic at follow-up. In a series of 141 patients, complete DAVF interruption was achieved in 81% of patients, whereas cranial nerve palsies and diplopia improved slowly (65%) or did not change (11%). In a subset of 39 patients with visual impairment, vision recovered in almost all cases within the first 2 weeks after intervention.[28] It is not uncommon, however, for clinical symptoms to worsen transiently before their resolution, which may take up to 2 years.[29] Furthermore, ophthalmoplegia may persist despite successful endovascular treatment. Despite complete regression of chemosis, exophthalmos, and pulsating tinnitus in every patient with no DAVF recurrence at a mean follow-up of 4.4 years, Bink and coworkers[30] reported that 44% of patients were still troubled by persistent cranial nerve deficits. A significant correlation was found between coil volume and persistent diplopia.

A potential complication of transvenous cavernous DAVF embolization, especially when attempting access through a thrombosed venous tributary, such as the inferior petrosal sinus, is vessel injury. In a series of 56 patients, 5.4% patients had venous perforation and subarachnoid hemorrhage. The complication was managed with prompt coil occlusion of the rupture site without neurologic sequelae.[31]

The reported rate of recanalization of cavernous DAVF after complete obliteration on immediate angiography is low. Using a transvenous approach, primarily via the inferior petrosal sinus, Yoshida and colleagues[32] were able to occlude 82% of cavernous sinus DAVF. During a follow-up period between 6 to 40 months, recanalization was encountered in 9% of patients.

USE OF ADJUVANT FLOW CONTROL TECHNIQUES IN TRANSARTERIAL AND TRANSVENOUS DAVF EMBOLIZATION

Adjuvant flow control techniques have recently been introduced and are becoming increasingly popular in the endovascular treatment of DAVF. In most instances, a balloon microcatheter is used in conjunction with a liquid embolic agent during transarterial or transvenous embolization. Superselective distal arterial access may be hindered due to the presence of multiple acute bends, especially in the occipital artery and its transosseous branches. A separate balloon microcatheter may assist in "jailing" of the working microcatheter when the latter's distal advancement into a transosseous pedicle is not possible because of vessel tortuosity (**Fig. 4**). Furthermore, a dual lumen balloon microcatheter can be used in a stand-alone fashion when difficulty is expected in reaching the fistulous site or where multiple feeding arteries arise from a common trunk. Temporary balloon inflation allows the unopposed forward penetration of Onyx, without the time-consuming efforts of plug formation, while concurrently decreasing the risk of premature proximal reflux. Rapid transarterial occlusion of DAVF can therefore be achieved with a short period of fluoroscopy and potentially with a lower risk of microcatheter retention.[33,34]

In addition, a balloon microcatheter may be navigated transvenously and positioned in the recipient sinus adjacent to the fistula and be used to prevent untoward distal migration into a functional sinus and adjacent cortical veins, while at the same time directing flow of Onyx into the fistulous connection and arterial feeders.[4,35]

In the largest series to date where flow control adjuncts were used, complete obliteration was achieved in 71% (41 of 58) of patients. Complication rates were similar in procedures using adjunctive flow control techniques (19.4%) compared with stand-alone Onyx embolization (17.6%).[4] However, complications unique to the use of such adjuncts have been reported, including arterial and venous rupture during balloon inflation.[33,34]

DIRECT PERCUTANEOUS ACCESS FOR DAVF EMBOLIZATION

A direct puncture technique may be used when standard arterial or venous routes do not allow

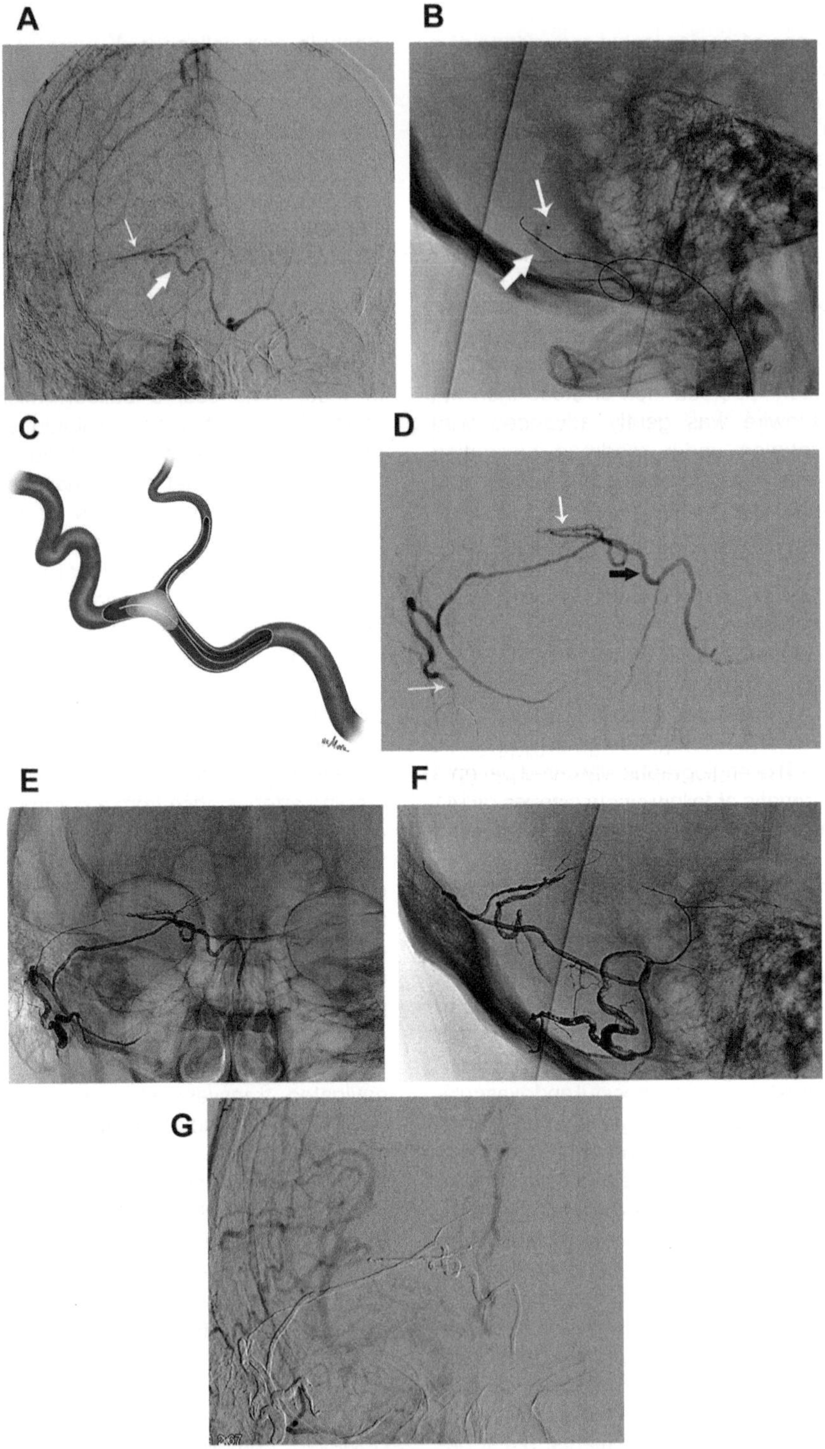

Fig. 4. Symptomatic tentorial DAVF in a 78-year-old woman with gait ataxia. (*A*) Right external carotid angiogram reveals tentorial DAVF (*small arrow*) with arterial supply by a transmastoid branch of the right occipital artery and a single retrograde leptomeningeal vein crossing the midline (*large arrow*). (*B*) A 4 × 7-mm compliant balloon microcatheter is positioned and inflated in the occipital artery (*large arrow*) with the working microcatheter "jailed" in the transmastoid branch (*small arrow*). (*C*) Artist's depiction of microcatheter position before embolization. (*D*) Superselective transmastoid artery angiogram with the balloon inflated; (*yellow arrow*) working microcatheter tip; (*white arrow*) tentorial DAVF; (*black arrow*) retrograde leptomeningeal vein. (*E, F*) Onyx 18 cast after forward, nonstop, 90-second injection that has filled the transmastoid branch, fistula, and proximal leptomeningeal vein. (*G*) Postcompletion right external carotid angiogram reveals complete obliteration of fistula.

successful navigation to the fistulous connection. A direct percutaneous transorbital approach without the need for surgical exposure was used by White and colleagues[36] to treat 8 patients with cavernous DAVF. This approach is particularly useful in the setting of pronounced anterior drainage of DVAF in the ophthalmic veins, allowing an anatomically direct avenue to the cavernous sinus for subsequent embolization without significant risk. All patients experienced alleviation of symptoms without procedural complications.

Furthermore, a direct transcranial needle puncture via parietal and mastoid foramina of the calvarium that harbor transosseous arterial DAVF feeders can be performed. Liquid embolics can then be used for embolization either directly or via an introduced microcatheter. Chapot and colleagues[37] were able to achieve cure in 4 patients with DVAF supplied by the occipital artery. Under biplane fluoroscopy, the axial view was used to identify the location of needle puncture and the lateral view to delineate the limit of progression of the needle into the cranial foramen. After selective puncture of the transosseous branch, a microcatheter was advanced and DAVF were injected with acrylic glue. Similarly, Saura and colleagues[38] treated 5 patients achieving complete occlusion at 6-month angiographic follow-up by using direct needle puncture of transosseous arterial feeders and subsequent Onyx embolization.

TRANSARTERIAL PARTICLE EMBOLIZATION OF SYMPTOMATIC DAVFS WITHOUT RLVD

Patients with minimally symptomatic DAVF and without RLVD can be safely managed conservatively, given the benign natural history of these lesions. However, patients with disabling symptoms associated with high-flow DAVF in the absence of RLVD may benefit from treatment. In such instances, the goal is symptom resolution/improvement without the need to achieve immediate cure of the fistula. Polyvinyl alcohol particles with a size greater than 150 μm (to prevent passage through "dangerous" anastomoses) are used for transarterial embolization via external carotid artery branches. This approach is safe and effective in resolving or significantly improving patients' symptoms. Endovascular treatment may be complemented by stereotactic radiosurgery, and this combination is effective in achieving complete obliteration, often within the first year after treatment, especially in the case of transverse/sigmoid and cavernous DAVF.[39] Friedman and coworkers[40] treated 25 patients with DAVF of the transverse/sigmoid sinus with stereotactic radiosurgery and embolization. With this staged combined approach, 96% of patients had either complete resolution or significant improvement in pulsatile tinnitus over a period of 50 months, despite the persistence of 59% of treated DAVF on follow-up angiography. There were no radiation-induced injuries and only one patient developed a temporary ischemic deficit.

SUMMARY

Endovascular embolization has become the mainstay of treatment of most intracranial DAVF. Transarterial, transvenous, combined, or direct percutaneous approaches can be used based on the angioarchitecture, clinical presentation, location, and operator preference. With individualized treatment, effective obliteration can be achieved in most cases with an acceptably low complication rate.

Tips and Pearls

Interpretation of pretreatment angiogram

- Differentiate normal brain versus DAVF venous drainage pathways
- Differentiate isolated versus functional involved dural venous sinus
- Scrutinize for the presence of dangerous anastomoses between external carotid and vertebral arteries

Transarterial treatment

- Use middle meningeal artery as the conduit of first choice for embolization
- Allow proximal Onyx reflux for up to a few centimeters above level of foramen spinosum when embolizing via the middle meningeal artery to avoid cranial nerve palsies
- Use low-concentration nBCA for optimal distal penetration in fistula

Transvenous treatment

- Assess for possible parallel venous pouch or compartmentalization of involved sinus
- Use gentle maneuvers when navigating through occluded venous tributaries
- Avoid excessive coil packing in the cavernous sinus

REFERENCES

1. Lanzino G, Fang S. Endovascular treatment of intracranial dural arteriovenous fistulas. World Neurosurg 2013. http://dx.doi.org/10.1016/j.wneu.2013.08.055. pii:S1878–8750(13)01086-3.

2. van Dijk JM, terBrugge KG, Willinsky RA, et al. Clinical course of cranial dural arteriovenous fistulas with long-term persistent cortical venous reflux. Stroke 2002;33:1233–6.
3. Strom RG, Botros JA, Refai D, et al. Cranial dural arteriovenous fistulae: asymptomatic cortical venous drainage portends less aggressive clinical course. Neurosurgery 2009;64:241–7 [discussion: 247–8].
4. Shi ZS, Loh Y, Gonzalez N, et al. Flow control techniques for Onyx embolization of intracranial dural arteriovenous fistulae. J Neurointerv Surg 2013;5: 311–6.
5. Abud TG, Nguyen A, Saint-Maurice JP, et al. The use of Onyx in different types of intracranial dural arteriovenous fistula. AJNR Am J Neuroradiol 2011;32: 2185–91.
6. Puffer RC, Daniels DJ, Kallmes DF, et al. Curative Onyx embolization of tentorial dural arteriovenous fistulas. Neurosurg Focus 2012;32:E4.
7. Lucas Cde P, Mounayer C, Spelle L, et al. Endoarterial management of dural arteriovenous malformations with isolated sinus using Onyx-18: technical case report. Neurosurgery 2007;61:E293–4 [discussion: E294].
8. Hu YC, Newman CB, Dashti SR, et al. Cranial dural arteriovenous fistula: transarterial Onyx embolization experience and technical nuances. J Neurointerv Surg 2011;3:5–13.
9. Cognard C, Januel AC, Silva NA Jr, et al. Endovascular treatment of intracranial dural arteriovenous fistulas with cortical venous drainage: new management using Onyx. AJNR Am J Neuroradiol 2008;29: 235–41.
10. van Rooij WJ, Sluzewski M. Curative embolization with Onyx of dural arteriovenous fistulas with cortical venous drainage. AJNR Am J Neuroradiol 2010;31: 1516–20.
11. Adamczyk P, Amar AP, Mack WJ, et al. Recurrence of "cured" dural arteriovenous fistulas after Onyx embolization. Neurosurg Focus 2012;32:E12.
12. Rangel-Castilla L, Barber SM, Klucznik R, et al. Mid and long term outcomes of dural arteriovenous fistula endovascular management with Onyx. Experience of a single tertiary center. J Neurointerv Surg 2013. [Epub ahead of print].
13. Maimon S, Nossek E, Strauss I, et al. Transarterial treatment with Onyx of intracranial dural arteriovenous fistula with cortical drainage in 17 patients. AJNR Am J Neuroradiol 2011;32:2180–4.
14. Lv X, Jiang C, Zhang J, et al. Complications related to percutaneous transarterial embolization of intracranial dural arteriovenous fistulas in 40 patients. AJNR Am J Neuroradiol 2009;30:462–8.
15. Nelson PK, Russell SM, Woo HH, et al. Use of a wedged microcatheter for curative transarterial embolization of complex intracranial dural arteriovenous fistulas: indications, endovascular technique, and outcome in 21 patients. J Neurosurg 2003;98: 498–506.
16. Kim DJ, Willinsky RA, Krings T, et al. Intracranial dural arteriovenous shunts: transarterial glue embolization–experience in 115 consecutive patients. Radiology 2011;258:554–61.
17. Guedin P, Gaillard S, Boulin A, et al. Therapeutic management of intracranial dural arteriovenous shunts with leptomeningeal venous drainage: report of 53 consecutive patients with emphasis on transarterial embolization with acrylic glue. J Neurosurg 2010;112:603–10.
18. Baltsavias G, Valavanis A. Endovascular treatment of 170 consecutive cranial dural arteriovenous fistulae: results and complications. Neurosurg Rev 2014;37(1):63–71.
19. Lanzino G, Meyer FB. Carotid-cavernous fistulas. In: Winn HR, editor. Youman's neurological surgery. 6th edition. Philadelphia: Elsevier Saunders; 2011. p. 4101–6.
20. Lekkhong E, Pongpech S, Ter Brugge K, et al. Transvenous embolization of intracranial dural arteriovenous shunts through occluded venous segments: experience in 51 Patients. AJNR Am J Neuroradiol 2011;32:1738–44.
21. Houdart E, Saint-Maurice JP, Chapot R, et al. Transcranial approach for venous embolization of dural arteriovenous fistulas. J Neurosurg 2002;97: 280–6.
22. Wakhloo AK, Perlow A, Linfante I, et al. Transvenous n-butyl-cyanoacrylate infusion for complex dural carotid cavernous fistulas: technical considerations and clinical outcome. AJNR Am J Neuroradiol 2005;26:1888–97.
23. Piske RL, Campos CM, Chaves JB, et al. Dural sinus compartment in dural arteriovenous shunts: a new angioarchitectural feature allowing superselective transvenous dural sinus occlusion treatment. AJNR Am J Neuroradiol 2005;26: 1715–22.
24. Nishino K, Ito Y, Hasegawa H, et al. Cranial nerve palsy following transvenous embolization for a cavernous sinus dural arteriovenous fistula: association with the volume and location of detachable coils. J Neurosurg 2008;109:208–14.
25. Caragine LP, Halbach VV, Dowd CF, et al. Parallel venous channel as the recipient pouch in transverse/sigmoid sinus dural fistulae. Neurosurgery 2003;53:1261–6 [discussion: 1266–7].
26. Satow T, Murao K, Matsushige T, et al. Superselective shunt occlusion for the treatment of cavernous sinus dural arteriovenous fistulae. Neurosurgery 2013;73:ons100–5.
27. Theaudin M, Saint-Maurice JP, Chapot R, et al. Diagnosis and treatment of dural carotid-cavernous fistulas: a consecutive series of 27 patients. J Neurol Neurosurg Psychiatr 2007;78:174–9.

28. Kirsch M, Henkes H, Liebig T, et al. Endovascular management of dural carotid-cavernous sinus fistulas in 141 patients. Neuroradiology 2006;48:486–90.
29. Liu HM, Wang YH, Chen YF, et al. Long-term clinical outcome of spontaneous carotid cavernous sinus fistulae supplied by dural branches of the internal carotid artery. Neuroradiology 2001;43:1007–14.
30. Bink A, Goller K, Luchtenberg M, et al. Long-term outcome after coil embolization of cavernous sinus arteriovenous fistulas. AJNR Am J Neuroradiol 2010;31:1216–21.
31. Kim DJ, Kim DI, Suh SH, et al. Results of transvenous embolization of cavernous dural arteriovenous fistula: a single-center experience with emphasis on complications and management. AJNR Am J Neuroradiol 2006;27:2078–82.
32. Yoshida K, Melake M, Oishi H, et al. Transvenous embolization of dural carotid cavernous fistulas: a series of 44 consecutive patients. AJNR Am J Neuroradiol 2010;31:651–5.
33. Chiu AH, Aw G, Wenderoth JD. Double-lumen arterial balloon catheter technique for Onyx embolization of dural arteriovenous fistulas: initial experience. J Neurointerv Surg 2014;6:400–3.
34. Jagadeesan BD, Grigoryan M, Hassan AE, et al. Endovascular balloon-assisted embolization of intracranial and cervical arteriovenous malformations using dual lumen co-axial balloon microcatheters and Onyx: initial experience. Neurosurgery 2013;73(2 Suppl Operative):238–43.
35. Shi ZS, Loh Y, Duckwiler GR, et al. Balloon-assisted transarterial embolization of intracranial dural arteriovenous fistulas. J Neurosurg 2009;110:921–8.
36. White JB, Layton KF, Evans AJ, et al. Transorbital puncture for the treatment of cavernous sinus dural arteriovenous fistulas. AJNR Am J Neuroradiol 2007;28:1415–7.
37. Chapot R, Saint-Maurice JP, Narata AP, et al. Transcranial puncture through the parietal and mastoid foramina for the treatment of dural fistulas. Report of four cases. J Neurosurg 2007;106:912–5.
38. Saura P, Saura J, Perez-Higueras A, et al. Direct transforaminal Onyx embolization of intracranial dural arteriovenous fistulas: technical note and report of five cases. J Neurointerv Surg 2013. [Epub ahead of print].
39. Yen CP, Lanzino G, Sheehan JP. Stereotactic radiosurgery of intracranial dural arteriovenous fistulas. Neurosurg Clin N Am 2013;24:591–6.
40. Friedman JA, Pollock BE, Nichols DA, et al. Results of combined stereotactic radiosurgery and transarterial embolization for dural arteriovenous fistulas of the transverse and sigmoid sinuses. J Neurosurg 2001;94:886–91.

Endovascular Treatment of Carotid-Cavernous Fistulas

Mario Zanaty, MD[a], Nohra Chalouhi, MD[a], Stavropaula I. Tjoumakaris, MD[a], David Hasan, MD[b], Robert H. Rosenwasser, MD[a], Pascal Jabbour, MD[a,c,*]

KEYWORDS

• Cavernous sinus • Carotid-cavernous fistulas • Endovascular treatment • Direct • Indirect

KEY POINTS

- The diagnosis of carotid-cavernous fistulas (CCFs) requires a high index of suspicion; a delay in treatment may lead to irreversible damage.
- Angiography remains the gold standard for diagnosing CCFs.
- The endovascular approach is the first-line treatment given the low complication rate and the favorable long-term outcome.
- The agents used for the endovascular management are balloons, coils, liquid embolic substances, and stents.
- Certain fistulas may require multiple agents or multiple sessions for complete closure.

INTRODUCTION

CCFs are arteriovenous malformations that result in shunting of the blood from the carotid artery to the cavernous sinus (CS). The pressure inside the CS increases, the draining vessels engorge, and the flow may get reversed leading to a myriad of clinical manifestation and mimicking many head and neck diseases. The management for most CCFs has shifted from open surgery to endovascular treatment. This novel therapy is still evolving in its approach, technique, and agents. The agents vary from balloons, to coils, to different liquid embolic substances, and recently, stents. The decision on the treatment modality is tailored to suit each patient depending on the risk factors and the characteristics of the fistula. This article reviews many aspects of the CCF while focusing on the endovascular management, which is the preferred treatment modality.

RELEVANT ANATOMY

The CS is located lateral to the sella turcica, expanding from the superior orbital fissure to the apex of the petrous bone. The CS is neither a sinus nor cavernous per se, rather it is a reticulated structure, formed by an assembly of multiple

Disclosure: Dr P. Jabbour is a consultant at Covidien.
Conflict of Interest: The authors declare no conflict of interest.

[a] Department of Neurosurgery, Jefferson Hospital for Neuroscience, Thomas Jefferson University, 909 Walnut Street, Philadelphia, PA 19107, USA; [b] Department of Neurosurgery, University of Iowa, 200 Hawkins Drive, Iowa City, IA 52242, USA; [c] Division of Neurovascular Surgery and Endovascular Neurosurgery, Department of Neurological Surgery, Thomas Jefferson University Hospital, 909 Walnut Street, 2nd Floor, Philadelphia, PA 19107, USA

* Corresponding author. Division of Neurovascular Surgery and Endovascular Neurosurgery, Department of Neurological Surgery, Thomas Jefferson University Hospital, 909 Walnut Street, 2nd Floor, Philadelphia, PA 19107.
E-mail address: pascal.jabbour@jefferson.edu

Neurosurg Clin N Am 25 (2014) 551–563
http://dx.doi.org/10.1016/j.nec.2014.04.011

thin-walled veins, as demonstrated by Parkinson and later by Hashimoto and colleagues.[1,2] Therefore, the name lateral sellar compartment was proposed to be more accurate and to avoid any misinterpretation.[2,3] The importance that this distinction brought has modified the CCF surgery (clipping a fistulous point) and more notably, the choice of embolic agent used to avoid compartmentalization, as discussed below (see Endovascular Treatment). The CS encloses important neurovascular structures responsible for the compliance of patients with fistula. The CS is divided into 4 compartments by the internal carotid artery (ICA), namely, medial, lateral, anteroinferior, and posterosuperior, in relation to the intracavernous portion of the ICA.[4] The CS receives:

- Anteriorly: the superior and inferior ophthalmic veins
- Laterally: the superficial middle (sylvian) cerebral vein, the deep middle cerebral vein, and the sphenoparietal sinus
- Posteriorly: the superior and inferior petrosal veins drain the CS
- The basilary plexus, which is posterior in location, and the intercavernous sinus are examples of venous anastomoses that join the 2 CS.

The connection between the multiple pathways represents alternative routes for drainage when the CS becomes obstructed and also serves as multiple ports of entry to the CS when endovascular treatment is being performed.

FISTULA CLASSIFICATION AND CHARACTERISTICS

CCF is sorted according to its cause, hemodynamic behavior, and angioarchitecture. Barrow and colleagues[5] classified the CCFs in to 4 distinct types (A, B, C, and D) depending on the arterial supply. This classification is preferred because it encompasses indirectly the cause and the hemodynamic features; it also has a therapeutic implication.

Direct CCF

Type A or direct CCF is the most common type accounting for up to 80% of all CCFs.[6] This type is a direct connection between the cavernous ICA and the CCF, mostly because of a tear in the carotid wall after trauma.[6] Rupture could be due to the collision of the vessel against a bony fracture, shearing forces that act on the vessel wall, or increased intraluminal pressure after the distal compression of the vessel.[7] Traumatic CCF can be bilateral in 2% of cases.[6] If so, it is usually more deadly and more severe at presentation.[6] The carotid disruption can result from blunt as well as penetrating head trauma, which explains the higher prevalence in young males. Direct CCF can be iatrogenic, following transsphenoidal surgery,[8] endovascular procedures, and percutaneous trigeminal rhizotomy.[6] This type of CCF can also be spontaneous in 20% cases,[9] which happens when an ICA aneurysm spontaneously ruptures in the CS or when the patient has any disease that weakens the carotid wall predisposing it to rupture.[9] It is important to be prudent when such diseases are present because of the increased risk of angiographic complications. Most Type A CCFs are high-flow lesions with minimal chance of spontaneous resolution.[6,7]

Indirect CCF

Type B, C, and D CCFs are indirect fistulas that arise from meningeal branches of the ICA or the external carotid artery (ECA). Type B is the least frequent; it arises from the meningeal branches of the ICA. Type C arises from the meningeal branches of the ECA, and Type D arises from meningeal branches of both the ICA and the ECA; it is the most frequent indirect type of CCF.[6] The indirect fistulas, also named dural fistulas, most commonly arise spontaneously but can occur after trauma. These fistulas are frequently nourished by the internal maxillary artery, the middle meningeal artery, the meningohypophyseal trunks, and the capsular arteries.[10] The underlying mechanism that leads to the formation of these fistulas remains unknown. It has been postulated that thrombosis of the microscopic venous vessels or partial thrombosis of the sinus leads to high pressure and rupture of the thin-walled dural vessel that traverses the sinus.[5,7,11] Reported predisposing factors are pregnancy, diabetes mellitus, collagen vascular disease, arterial hypertension, and phlebitis.[12–15] As with spontaneous direct CCF, arterial wall defect may also lead to spontaneous indirect CCF formation after minor strains.[7] Indirect fistulas occur in postmenopausal women most frequently, but can occur at any age including infancy.[9,11,16] Some reported indirect CCFs were considered to be congenital.[6,17] A subset type of indirect CCF is the posttraumatic CCF, and it differs from the spontaneous ones by having a single vessel for blood supply.[18] Unlike direct fistulas, indirect fistulas can have contralateral feeders and require bilateral angiography of the ICA and ECA.[19,20] Dural fistulas are low-flow lesions, have gradual onset, and may resolve spontaneously or by manual carotid compression in up to 30% to 50% of cases.[21,22] **Table 1** highlights the main difference between direct and indirect fistulas. Indirect fistulas, when fed by ICA branches, are hazardous and less amenable to transarterial embolization.[20]

PATHOPHYSIOLOGY AND CLINICAL PRESENTATION

The short-circuiting of the arterial blood increases the pressure in the CS leading to flow reversal. The flow then may follow any draining pattern producing venous hypertension and/or thrombosis. The signs and symptoms depend on the drainage pathway, the presence of collaterals, and finally the size and location of the CCF.[6] **Table 2** lists the symptoms with their underlying physiopathology. The most frequent complains are in the orbital region.[6,7] Anterior drainage leads to orbital vein congestion and transudation of fluids, increased intraocular pressure, impaired retinal perfusion, and rupture of dilated veins.[6] The patient may present with symptoms ranging from subconjunctival hemorrhage to visual loss. Whether the vision loss improves or not is difficult to predict, but as a general rule, minor defects improve with better chance than severe ones.[23] Chances of recovery decrease if the superior ophthalmic vein (SOV) is already thrombosed or the central retinal vein has been damaged by the time of the diagnosis.[24] Lateral drainage in the sphenoparietal sinus leads to cortical venous hypertension, which is associated with intracranial hemorrhage and neurologic deficits.[9,11] The risk is lower in posttraumatic young patients in whom the venous system is still resilient.[24] Posterior drainage can have cranial nerve palsies as the only ocular finding.[20,25] External hemorrhage such as epistaxis is rare but fatal; it has been reported in 2% of CCF cases, sometimes requiring emergent carotid sacrifice.[6,26] The clinical presentation of direct and indirect CCF overlaps; however, the onset of symptoms and the severity differ. Direct fistulas are high-flow lesions and present classically with proptosis, chemosis, orbital bruits, and headache. Vision loss has been reported in up to 50% of cases.[11] Less common presentations include intracerebral or subarachnoid hemorrhage in 5% of patients[9,11,27,28] and exteriorized bleeding in 3% of cases.[29] Indirect CCFs have relapsing and remitting symptoms often with an insidious course that tends to delay the diagnosis.[7,9,10] Proptosis, chemosis, and glaucoma are the most notable findings.[6,10] An important feature of the disease is the dynamicity of the venous drainage. When venous pathways become thrombosed, the outflow changes in direction, which may account for the relapsing and remitting symptoms of the indirect CCF, or sometimes for the spontaneous resolution of symptoms. Hence the need to follow patients with angiography when curative treatment was not achieved; clinical resolution might be due to the change in course of the venous circulation perhaps to a more risky location.[10,11]

WORKUP

The best initial tests used when CCF fistula is suspected for the reasons mentioned above are computed tomography (CT) or magnetic resonance

Table 1
Differences between direct and indirect CCFs

	Direct CCF	Indirect CCF
Type	A	B, C, D
Arterial source	Cavernous ICA Single feeder	ICA/ECA meningeal branches Multiple feeders[a]
Etiology	Traumatic>spontaneous	Spontaneous>traumatic
Epidemiology	Young individuals 75%–80% of fistulas	Elderly women 15%–20% of fistulas
Hemodynamic features	High flow	Low flow
Presentation	Abrupt onset	Gradual onset
Resolution	Spontaneous uncommon	Spontaneous common
Diagnostic angiography	Unilateral is enough	Bilateral to exclude contralateral
Treatment route	Intra-arterial: favored[b]	Intravenous: favored
Cure rate	80%–99%	80%–90%[c]

[a] Can be single in case of trauma.
[b] Some favor the transvenous route because of easier manipulation of the coil catheter.
[c] More than 90% cure for indirect CCF has been reported when combined treatment is used.

Table 2
The symptom presentation, physiopathology, and frequency

Clinical Symptoms	Underlying Physiopathology	Frequency (%)
Orbital findings	Proptosis/corneal damage: increased orbital pressure Pain: impaired aqueous humor return, increased IOP (glaucoma) Impaired vision: ischemic retinopathy, ischemic optic neuropathy Diplopia: cranial nerve palsies Chemosis: venous congestion[a] Subconjunctival hemorrhage: rupture arterialized veins	Very frequent >50
External bleeding	Otorrhagia: ruptured ear canal veins Epistaxis: drainage in the sphenoid sinus with consequent rupture	3
Intracranial bleeding Subarachnoid bleeding	Cerebral cortical venous hypertension	5
Headache	Bleeding, venous hypertension, trigeminal dysfunction	>30

Abbreviation: IOP, intraocular pressure.
[a] The tortuosity of the vessels suggests CCF as the cause rather than conjunctivitis, episcleritis, or thyroid disorder.

(MR). These tests can confirm the clinical symptoms by visualizing the proptosis, the cerebral edema, and the cerebral hemorrhage. Signs and symptoms that suggest CCF are the following: enlargement of the extraocular muscles; engorgement of the SOV; dilatation of the facial vein; expansion of the ipsilateral CS, which can be described as pseudoaneurysmal (bulging) or sinusoidal (less bulging); presence of venous aneurysm; and enlargement of pial and cortical veins.[9,11,30] CT adds the benefit of detecting bone fracture, whereas MR offers the advantage of detecting flow voids in the CS as well as the orbital edema when present. CT angiography (CTA) and MR angiography (MRA) are considered similar in accuracy, but in a recent study, CTA outperformed MRA in detecting the fistula when it was located in segment 4 or 5 of the ICA.[31] Doppler flow can assist in the diagnosis by looking for increased flow, decreased resistance, and the presence of orbital bruits. Digital subtraction angiography (DSA) remains the gold standard in the diagnosis of CCF, because many diseases might be confused with CCF on the CT scan. Recently, in a case report, a prominent bulging of the SOV on the CT scan was diagnosed as a CCF before the DSA revealed a direct fistula between the ICA and the SOV bypassing the CCF.[32] The DSA is required to evaluate the angioarchitecture of the fistula, assess the feeding arteries, and plan the intervention. DSA can provide information on flow velocity, steel phenomenon, associated vascular injuries, collaterals, and high-risk pathways[9–11]; it can also reveal small dural feeding arteries missed on the CTA.[33] To better evaluate the high-flow lesion, the Mehringer-Hieshima maneuver is used to control the flow by slowly injecting the ipsilateral ICA while gentle manual compression is applied to the artery.[34] Following the occlusion, the results should be carefully interpreted because a worsening of the steel phenomenon is possible; this may give the impression of a false-negative balloon occlusion test (BOT).[35] Another well-known maneuver is the Huber maneuver, which helps in identifying the distal extent of the fistula by manually compressing the ICA while injecting the ipsilateral vertebral artery.[36] The retrograde flow through the posterior communicating artery fills the fistula distally. Before initiating treatment, tolerance of carotid occlusion should be assessed. This assessment is usually done via the BOT or the single-photon emission computed tomography. The latter seems to be more sensitive because it can predict major stroke after carotid occlusion in patients with positive result of BOT.[11] The diagnosis of CCF in the setting of a patient with trauma can be challenging and even more problematic when the patient is comatose. To allow early diagnosis, Schiavi and colleagues[37] suggested monitoring the increase in the jugular venous oxygen saturation. Finally based on certain angiographic or clinical findings the fistula can be considered as lethal and an emergent aggressive treatment can be lifesaving and necessary to improve the outcome.[6,10,29] These indications are detailed in **Table 3**.

Table 3
Angiographic and clinical indication of emergent treatment

Angiographic Indications	
Findings	**Future Risk**
Pseudoaneurysm	SAH
Large varix of the cavernous sinus	SAH
Venous drainage to cortical veins	Hemorrhagic venous infarction
Thrombosis of distant venous outflow pathways	Hemorrhagic venous infarction
Clinical Indicators	
Presentation	**Mechanism**
Epistaxis/Otorrhagia	External bleeding due to venous hypertension or pseudoaneurysmal varix
Headache, diplopia	Increased intracranial pressure from cortical venous hypertension
Rapidly progressive proptosis Diminished visual acuity	Obstruction of venous outflow pathway to the orbit
TIA/stroke	Cerebral ischemia: Dysregulation of blood flow *or* Chronic steel

Abbreviations: SAH, subarachnoid hemorrhage; TIA, transient ischemic attack.

TREATMENT

The goal of the treatment of CCF is to restore the normal flow and occlude the fistula. The different options are conservative management, open surgery, stereotactic radiosurgery, and endovascular surgery. As discussed previously, the treatment depends on the patient's risk factor and the fistula characteristics. The lower risk of the endovascular approach when compared with surgery and the growing advances in this domain rendered the endovascular approach the treatment of choice for CCF management.[20]

Conservative Management

Conservative management consists of external manual compression several times each hour, using the contralateral hand. It is prudent therefore to start with Doppler imaging before therapy. Conservative management is reserved for low-flow indirect CCF with no indication for emergent treatment. The compression decreases arterial flow and increases venous drainage favoring spontaneous thrombosis. The response in the literature varies between 20% and 60% for indirect fistulas.[9,38] It is important to monitor the patient clinically and by imaging in search of ominous signs that require immediate intervention. Adjunctive treatment should be administrated while waiting for resolution. Failure of conservative management requires alternative treatment.

Radiosurgery

Radiosurgery can be used alone or in combination with endovascular surgery. Radiosurgery performs well on indirect CCF with low flow, but poorly on direct ones.[7] The reported successful treatment when used alone varied between 75% and 91%, and was higher when used in combination.[7] Radiosurgery is effective and safe but less favored, given the time delay of 8 to 22 months between treatment and clinical resolution.[6,30] This major limitation makes radiosurgery of limited use.

Surgery

Open surgery is reserved for cases in which endovascular surgery was unsuccessful or not possible. Surgical techniques include clipping the fistula point, suturing or trapping of the fistula, packing the CS when caused by diffuse indirect CCF, sealing the fistula with fascia and glue, ligation of the ICA, and/or a combination of these techniques.[20] Reported complications are cranial nerve permanent or transient palsies, trigeminal hypoesthesia, and permanent or transient hemiparesis (**Table 4**).[7,39]

Table 4
The indications, contraindications, and complications for each type of treatment

Type of Treatment	Indications	Contraindications	Complications
Conservative	Indirect carotid-cavernous fistula with no ominous signs	Symptomatic bradycardia with carotid compression Significant cortical venous drainage Atherosclerotic stenosis/ulceration of the carotid artery/history of cerebral ischemia	Syncope Hemorrhagic venous infarction Thromboembolic disease
Surgery	Failed or unsuitable endovascular treatment	Patient characteristics	Permanent abducens palsy (<10%) Transient abducens palsy (20%–80%) Permanent hemiparesis (10%) Transient hemiparesis (10%) Permanent hemiparesis (10%) Trigeminal dysfunction

ENDOVASCULAR TREATMENT

As previously discussed, endovascular treatment is the modality of choice in both direct and indirect fistulas. This treatment can be used for emergency as well as elective treatment. The agents mostly used in endovascular treatment are detachable balloons, platinum detachable coils, liquid embolic materials, and recently, stents. These agents can be used alone or in combination. To gain access to the fistula, a transarterial (**Fig. 1**) or a transvenous (**Fig. 2**) approach can be used. Choosing the type of access and agent depends on several factors, most significantly, on the fistula type. **Tables 4** and **5** list the indications, advantages, limitations, solutions, complications, and success rate for each of the techniques used.

Detachable Balloons

After Serbinenko and colleagues[40] safely and successfully embolized a CCF using a detachable silicon balloon with preservation of the ICA, a new era of endovascular treatment has emerged; detachable balloons were accepted as the treatment of choice for Type A fistula.[6] The success rate reported ranged from 82% to 99%, although some required additional interventions.[41,42] The technique involves inserting a partially inflated balloon through the ICA into the fistula and then inflating the balloon to occlude the connection. The balloon, being guided in a flow-directed manner, is easily navigated within the arterial system.[20] Latex balloons are preferred over silicone ones by some investigators.[41,43] The transvenous approach is relatively contraindicated given the difficulty of directing the balloon in the venous systems, the compartmentalization of the CS, and the risk of the procedure.[20] Therefore, the indication of choice for this technique is the direct CCF, where there is an evident fistula branching directly from the ICA to the CS. The advantage of balloon embolization is the fast occlusion of the fistulas with the preservation of the ICA. Size is the most important limitation for this technique. The fistulas should be big enough to allow the passage of a partially inflated balloon but small enough to prevent the herniation of the inflated balloon. The CS should be adequately small to be fully occluded; if not, multiple balloons could solve this problem. Complications are the following: partial balloon deflation, which may lead to pseudoaneurysmal pouch; balloon rupture when overinflated or when it impacts against a bony spur, which may result in treatment failure; balloon detachment with consequential ICA occlusion and stroke.[41,42] Teng and colleagues[44] found a solution to prevent retraction of the balloon to the ICA by using the double balloon method. Another complication, infrequent though, is the migration of the balloon with compression of the cranial nerves.[5,11,30] For all the previously mentioned reasons, along with the limited variability in the balloon size and shape, detachable balloons

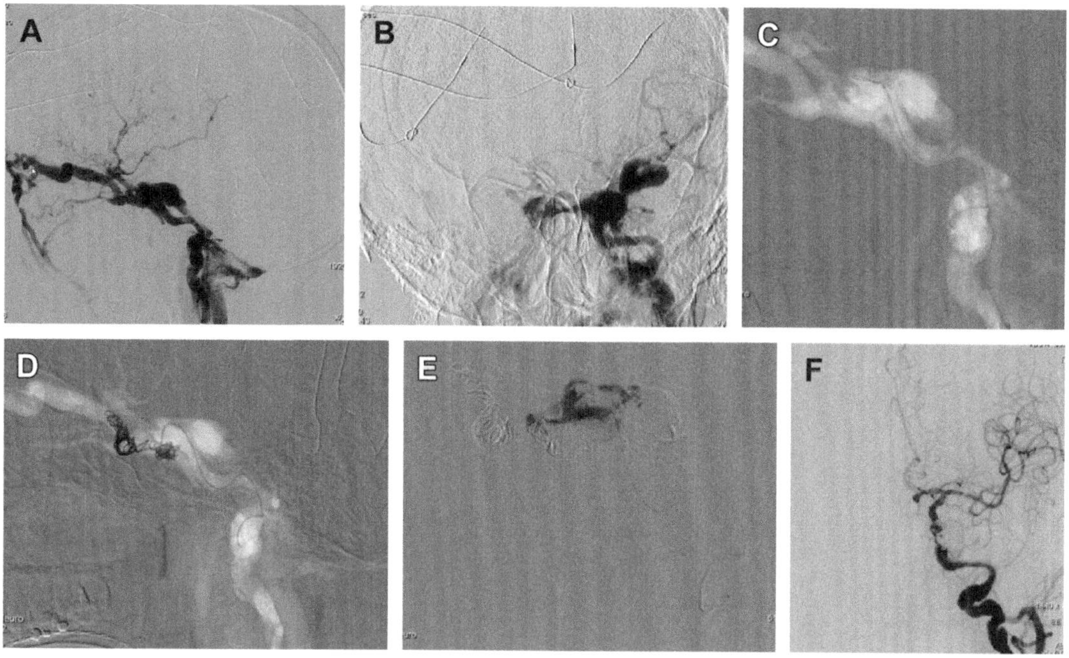

Fig. 1. (*A–F*) A transarterial approach. This 23-year-old patient with Ehler-Danlos syndrome was followed up for multiple intracranial aneurysms. The patient was found to have a left carotid-cavernous fistula (*A–C*). The patient was treated by onyx embolization and coiling via a transarterial approach (*D–F*).

gave away their place for liquid embolic agent, coils, and stents in the United States. Elsewhere, some investigators still use balloon detachment as the first-line treatment, although some cases require additional intervention.[24]

Coils

Coiling the CCF can be done in either transarterial or transvenous manner. This fact, along with the presence of coils in multiple sizes, makes this technique more advantageous than balloon embolization. The 2 types of coils that can be used are the detachable platinum coils and the thrombogenic fibered microcoils. Detachable coils are preferred to thrombogenic ones because they offer controllable adjustment after deployment. The former are easily manipulated and could be placed optimally in the sinus. Yet, full occlusion of the CS is rarely achievable using coils alone, primarily when the sinus is large or multiple fistula points are present. The septate nature of the CS poses another challenge to coiling, because the embolization may end up occluding one compartment resulting in suboptimal occlusion.[20] Even more, this approach necessitates more time to fully occlude the fistula with the risk of losing the arterial access and using the venous route to treat it gain.[11] The problem with partial occlusion is the potential redirection of venous flow toward more dangerous areas such as the cortical venous system with the risk of intracerebral hemorrhage, or the SOV with the risk of vision loss. The solution to these limitations is the use of coils in combination with liquid embolic agents to achieve complete occlusion, and the use of balloon-assisted technique or stent to prevent backward herniation with distal embolization.[10,11,30,45] In this setting, the use of a stent is preferred over the use of a balloon for better coverage and also because of the risk of balloon deflation.[46]

Liquid Embolic Agents

N-butyl cyanoacrylate (NBCA) and onyx are the main embolic agents used either alone or in combination with the coils to achieve denser packing and full occlusion. Onyx permits slow injection in the fistula so that monitoring with angiography is possible during embolization. NBCA has rapid polymerization that leads to successful treatment at the cost of heat production and risk of catheter retention because of the gluing property. Unlike with onyx, the adherent nature of NBCA does not permit slow injection and thus angiographic evaluation during the procedure. Nevertheless, difficult catheter retrieval is still present with onyx.[47] One solution would be the use of microcatheter with detachable tip.[47] Onyx has the advantage of overcoming trabeculation of the CS due its lavalike

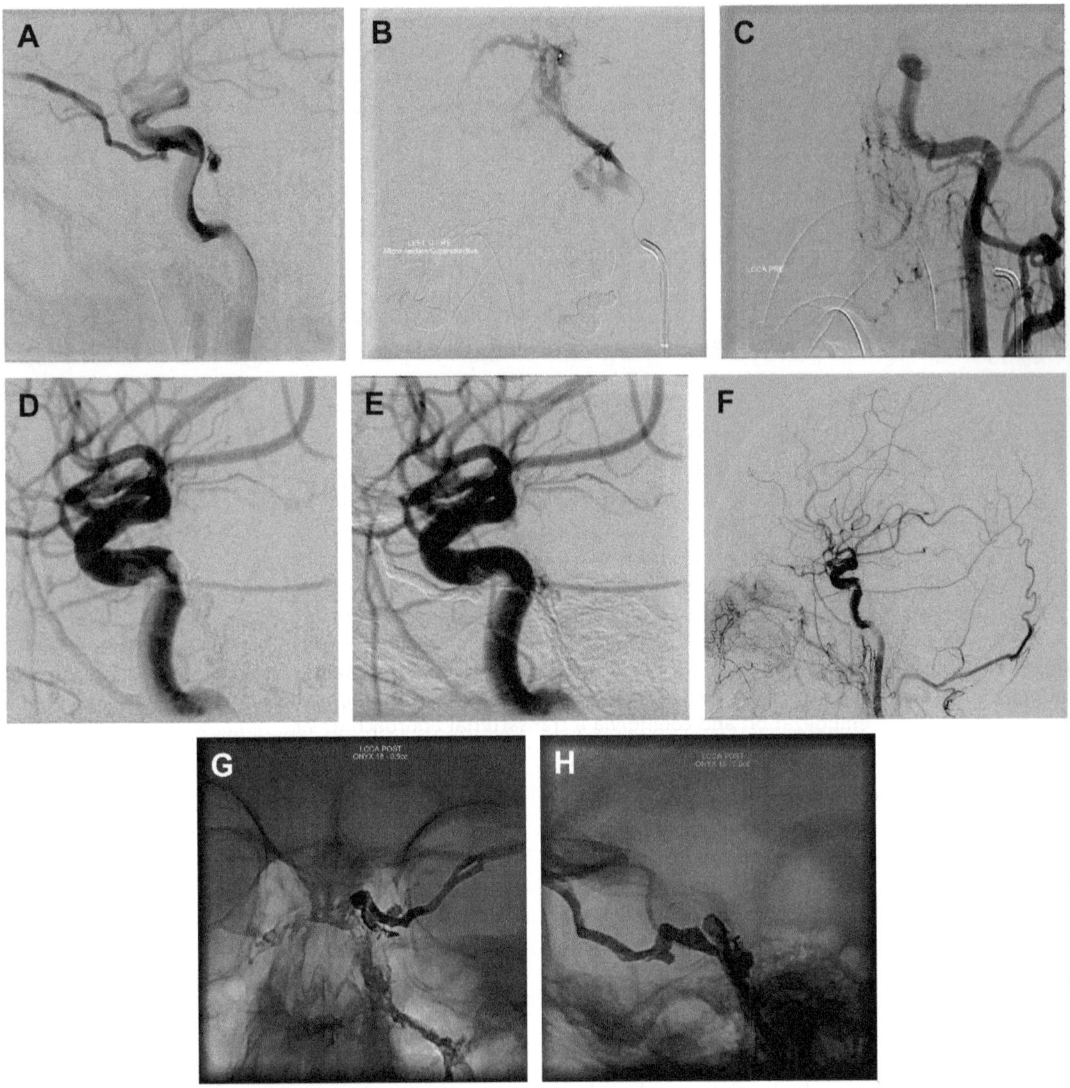

Fig. 2. (*A–H*) A 70-year-old patient with left Type D carotid-cavernous fistulas (*A–C*) fed by bilateral multiple internal and external feeders. A transfemoral transvenous approach was used, and the fistula was treated with onyx 18 embolization (*D–H*).

property.[20] This tendency to spread can cause major problem if onyx manages to penetrate the feeding arteries by backflow, or if it is spread down further to the SOV.[10,48,49] A suitable solution would be to coil the SOV before onyx injection. Overall, the embolic agents have a lesser risk of cranial nerve paresis than coiling, probably because of their smaller mass effect.[6]

Treatment Approach

For direct CCF, transarterial embolization is the mainstay of therapy. A guiding catheter is used first, followed by the advancement of a microcatheter into the CS through the fistula. The CS is then packed with coils, embolic agents, or both. As previously discussed, balloon assistance or stent assistance can be used to prevent the herniation of the coil into the ICA. Recently, balloon assistance has been used with onyx embolization to prevent its migration to the arterial system. In addition, it helped in visualizing better the ICA and served as an abutment for the coils placed in the CS.[50] Transarterial catheterization of the indirect CCF is hazardous, with lower cure rate. The small diameter of the feeder makes the fistula difficult to catheterize and increases the risk of distal ICA embolization. Dangerous ECA to ICA anastomosis and ECA branches feeding the cranial nerves can also make this method hazardous. However

Table 5
Pros and cons for different types of treatment

Type	Indication	Advantages	Limitations	Complications	Solutions	Success (%)
Detachable balloons	Direct carotid-cavernous fistula: medium to large	Rapid fistula obliteration ICA protection	Size of the cavernous sinus Size of the fistula Transvenous is not easily feasible Not present in the United States	Balloon rupture Balloon deflation Partial deflation (aneurysmal pouch) Cranial nerve compression ICA occlusion Stroke	Multiple balloon technique	82–99
Coils	Direct (small) or indirect carotid-cavernous fistula	Easy to manipulate	Partial occlusion if used alone Slow occlusion (loss of arterial access)	Cranial nerve deficits: Permanent (rare) Transient Thromboemboli ICA occlusion ICA dissection	Use combinations Balloon-assisted technique Stent	80–99
Embolic agent	Direct or indirect carotid-cavernous fistula	NBCA: Rapid polymerization and permanent occlusion Onyx: Slow injection (embolization can be evaluated) Penetrates interstices	Angionecrosis Microcatheter retention Cannot be monitored slowly Retrograde flow to other arterial feeders or to the ICA Distal spread to SOV Solvent's toxicity	Cranial nerve deficits: Transient (7%–17%) Permanent (8%) (arterial occlusion)	Use combinations Balloon protection of the ICA Coiling the SOV Using detachable microcatheter tip	
Stent	Direct or indirect carotid-cavernous fistula Trauma	No foreign body is introduced Allow ICA reconstruction	Tortuosity of intracranial vessels	Endoleak Vasospasm Dissection Rupture Exclusion of perforators Pseudoaneurysm	Balloon redilation Intra-arterial calcium channel blockers	

transarterial embolization is best used for Type C when only ECA feeders are present. The therapy is to obliterate the CS if accessible or the feeding branches when it is not. In the latter case, it is preferable to use NBCA to lessen the risk of dangerous distal vessel occlusion. Another subgroup of indirect CCF that can benefit from transarterial embolization is the one caused by trauma.[18] This subgroup usually has a single arterial feeder with a large-enough diameter for access.[18] With all these risks, the transvenous approach has become the mainstay mode for embolization of indirect CCF. Even more, with the shortage of detachable balloons, the transvenous approach is becoming the favorite approach for direct CCF as well, knowing that the catheter used for coiling and liquid embolic injection is more easily steerable in the venous pathway.[20] Yet, transarterial embolization using onyx is used in some centers as first-line treatment of dural CCF.[47] When using the transvenous route, the most common vein used to access the pathway is the inferior petrosal sinus, with a high success rate.[20] Once in the venous circulation, any of the venous pathways can be used, including the SOV, the lateral pterygoid, the contralateral Inferior Petrosal Sinus (IPS), and the contralateral intercavernous sinus. If the transfemoral approach fails, more aggressive alternatives are used (**Fig. 3**), such as direct catheterization of the SOV (**Fig. 4**). The use of onyx has not been well established in the SOV approach.[51] However, in a recent trial, onyx was successfully used to treat Type A, B, and D fistulas in one single session with complete obliteration. The treatment was combined with coils in 30% of the cases.[51] Finally, percutaneous access to the facial vein under sonography can also be done, followed by cannulation of the SOV.[6]

Carotid Sacrifice

The indication of carotid sacrifice is when CCF occlusion by endovascular means while preserving the ICA cannot be obtained, which is likely to happen in the setting of trauma with extensive damage to the ICA or in emergent situations such as active bleeding or expanding hematoma in the soft tissue. BOT is not performed if there is an immediate risk to the patient's life or if a complete steal without neurologic deficit is present.[30,35,42] The agents used for occluding the carotid are balloons, coils, and recently, the hydrocoil embolization system (HES). HES achieves a faster occlusion rate and volumetric expansion when compared with regular coils. When sacrificing the carotid, coils should be placed in a distal to proximal manner to avoid worsening the steal phenomenon.[6,9] Fistula entrapment can be done alternatively by using 2 balloons, one distal and one proximal, or by using a proximal balloon with distal coiling.[6]

Stents

A new technique in the endovascular management of CCF is the use of covered (polyfluorotetraethylene) or even noncovered stents. This technique relies on the principle of flow diversion to reconstruct the ICA and seal the fistula. The neointimal proliferation around the stent may also help in excluding the fistula out of the circulation.[46] Stent use brought an important solution to the case in which ICA sacrifice is required and the

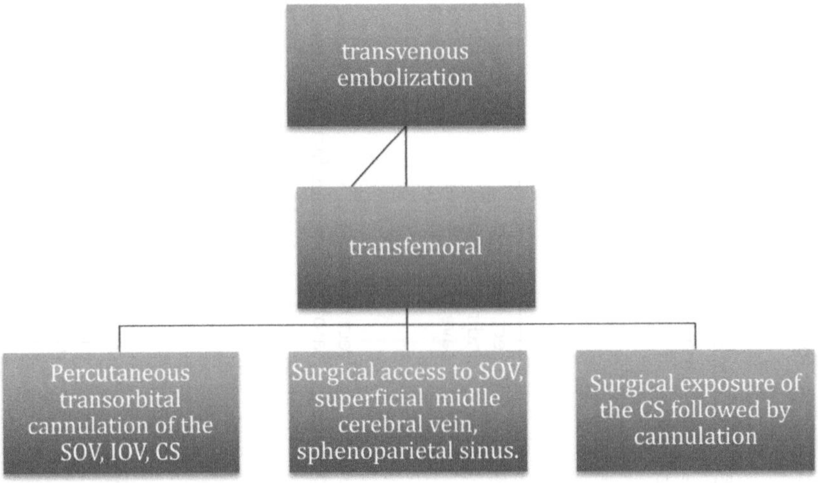

Fig. 3. Transvenous approach to CCF. When CCF access is not possible after the transfemoral route, more aggressive approaches are tried. IOV, inferior ophthalmic vein.

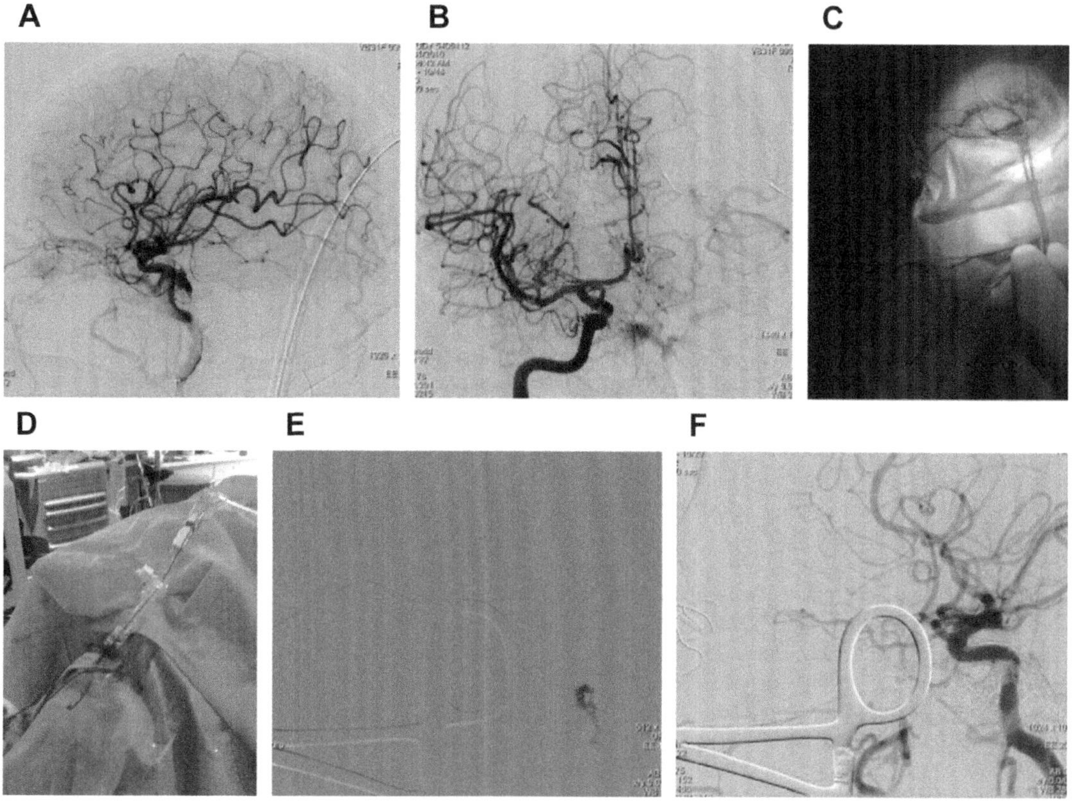

Fig. 4. (*A–F*) Superior ophthalmic vein approach. A 67-year-old woman presented with diplopia, retro-orbital pain, chemosis, and proptosis. Intraocular pressure measurement revealed a pressure of 34 mm Hg. The patient was found to have Type B carotid-cavernous fistulas (*A, B*). The superior ophthalmic vein was catheterized (*C, D*), and the fistulas was treated with onyx (*E, F*).

result of BOT is negative. Additional benefits are the avoidance of introducing a permanent foreign body in the fistula and the high rate of successful treatment. The complications include ICA dissection or rupture, covering of perforators, and endoleak. The limitations are difficult manipulation in tortuous intracranial vessels and the lack of adequate stent configuration.[6,9,52] Other problems include residual fistula filling, which may need further treatment using coils, and arterial vasospasm at the end of the stent, which can be treated and prevented by intra-arterial nifedipine or papaverine during the procedure.[53]

OUTCOME

Closure of the fistula has been reported in 80% to 99% of direct and indirect fistulas.[10,22] The treatment might require combination treatment and sometimes multiple sessions. Meyers and colleagues[10] managed to cure indirect CCF by transvenous embolization using coil and liquid embolic agents in 90% cases, of which 30% needed more than 2 procedures.[10] Clinical improvement needs hours to days, but complete resolution may take up to 6 months.[22] Notable complications are listed in **Tables 4** and **5**. Other complications include bleeding at the groin or in the orbit, local infection, sepsis, ophthalmic artery occlusion, and both transient and permanent neurologic deficits.[22]

SUMMARY

Endovascular treatment of CCF is an ever-advancing domain. This mode is the treatment of choice for direct and indirect CCF with a small complication and a high success rate. The multitude of agents used and the pathways leading to the CS offer a variety of treatments that can be tailored depending on the fistula type and the patient characteristics.

REFERENCES

1. Parkinson D. Lateral sellar compartment: history and anatomy. J Craniofac Surg 1995;6(1):55–68.
2. Hashimoto M, Yokota A, Yamada H, et al. Development of the cavernous sinus in the fetal period: a

morphological study. Neurol Med Chir (Tokyo) 2000;40(3):140–50.
3. Parkinson D. Lateral sellar compartment O.T. (cavernous sinus): history, anatomy, terminology. Anat Rec 1998;251(4):486–90.
4. Harris F, Rhoton A. Anatomy of the cavernous sinus. A microsurgical study. J Neurosurg 1976; 45(2):169–80.
5. Barrow D, Spector R, Braun I, et al. Classification and treatment of spontaneous carotid-cavernous sinus fistulas. J Neurosurg 1985;62(2):248–56.
6. Korkmazer B, Kocak B, Tureci E, et al. Endovascular treatment of carotid cavernous sinus fistula: a systematic review. World J Radiol 2013;5:143–55.
7. Ellis JA, Goldstein H, Connolly ES, et al. Carotid-cavernous fistulas. Neurosurg Focus 2012;32:E9.
8. Pigott TJ, Holland IM, Punt JA. Carotico-cavernous fistula after trans-sphenoidal hypophysectomy. Br J Neurosurg 1989;3(5):613–6.
9. Gemmete JJ, Ansari SA, Gandhi DM. Endovascular techniques for treatment of carotid-cavernous fistula. J Neuroophthalmol 2009;29(1):62–71.
10. Meyers PM, Halbach VV, Dowd CF, et al. Dural carotid cavernous fistula: definitive endovascular management and long-term follow-up. Am J Ophthalmol 2002;134(1):85–92.
11. Ringer AJ, Salud L, Tomsick TA. Carotid cavernous fistulas: anatomy, classification, and treatment. Neurosurg Clin N Am 2005;16(2):279–95.
12. Raskind R, Johnson N, Hance D. Carotid cavernous fistula in pregnancy. Angiology 1977; 28(10):671–6.
13. Lin TK, Chang CN, Wai YY. Spontaneous intracerebral hematoma from occult carotid-cavernous fistula during pregnancy and puerperium. Case report. J Neurosurg 1992;76(4):714–7.
14. Linskey ME, Sekhar LN, Hirsch W Jr, et al. Aneurysms of the intracavernous carotid artery: clinical presentation, radiographic features, and pathogenesis. Neurosurgery 1990;26(1):71–9.
15. Walker AE, Allegre GE. Carotid-cavernous fistulas. Surgery 1956;39(3):411–22.
16. Pang D, Kerber C, Biglan AW, et al. External carotid-cavernous fistula in infancy: case report and review of the literature. Neurosurgery 1981; 8(2):212–8.
17. Konishi Y, Hieshima GB, Hara M, et al. Congenital fistula of the dural carotid-cavernous sinus: case report and review of the literature. Neurosurgery 1990;27(1):120–6.
18. Luo CB, Teng MM, Chang FC, et al. Traumatic indirect carotid cavernous fistulas: angioarchitectures and results of transarterial embolization by liquid adhesives in 11 patients. Surg Neurol 2009;71(2): 216–22.
19. Dabus G, Batjer HH, Hurley MC, et al. Endovascular treatment of a bilateral dural carotid-cavernous fistula using an unusual unilateral approach through the basilar plexus. World Neurosurg 2012;77(1):201.e5–8.
20. Ashour R, Elhammady MS, Aziz-Sultan MA. Carotid-cavernous fistula. In: Jabbour PM, editor. Neurovascular surgical techniques. 1st edition. Philadelphia: Jaypee; 2013. p. 296–308.
21. Higashida RT, Hieshima GB, Halbach VV, et al. Closure of carotid cavernous sinus fistulae by external compression of the carotid artery and jugular vein. Acta Radiol Suppl 1986;369:580–3.
22. Miller NR. Dural carotid-cavernous fistulas: epidemiology, clinical presentation, and management Neurosurg Clin N Am 2012;23:179–92.
23. Yu SC, Cheng HK, Wong GK, et al. Transvenous embolization of dural carotid-cavernous fistulae with transfacial catheterization through the superior ophthalmic vein. Neurosurgery 2007;60(6):1037–8.
24. Malan J, Lefeuvre D, Mngomezulu V, et al. Angioarchitecture and treatment modalities in posttraumatic carotid cavernous fistulae. Interv Neuroradiol 2012;18:178–86.
25. Stiebel-Kalish H, Setton A, Nimii Y, et al. Cavernous sinus dural arteriovenous malformations: patterns of venous drainage are related to clinical signs and symptoms. Ophthalmology 2002;109(9):1685–91.
26. Wilson CB, Markesbery W. Traumatic carotid-cavernous fistula with fatal epistaxis. Report of a case. J Neurosurg 1966;24(1):111–3.
27. Gupta AK, Purkayastha S, Krishnamoorthy T, et al. Endovascular treatment of direct carotid cavernous fistulae: a pictorial review. Neuroradiology 2006;48: 831–9.
28. Huai RC, Yi CL, Ru LB, et al. Traumatic carotid cavernous fistula concomitant with pseudoaneurysm in the sphenoid sinus. Interv Neuroradiol 2008;14(1):59–68.
29. Halbach VV, Hieshima GB, Higashida RT, et al. Carotid cavernous fistulae: indications for urgent treatment. AJR Am J Roentgenol 1987;149(3): 587–93.
30. Tjoumakaris SI, Jabbour PM, Rosenwasser RH Neuroendovascular management of carotid cavernous fistulae. Neurosurg Clin N Am 2009 20(4):447–52.
31. Chen CC, Chang PC, Shy CG, et al. CT angiography and MR angiography in the evaluation of carotid cavernous sinus fistula prior to embolization: a comparison of techniques. AJNR Am J Neuroradiol 2005;26(9):2349–56.
32. Chalouhi N, Jabbour P, Bilyk JR, et al. Internal carotid artery to superior ophthalmic vein fistula: a case report. Clin Neurol Neurosurg 2013;115 833–5.
33. Coskun O, Hamon M, Catroux G, et al. Carotid cavernous fistulas: diagnosis with spiral CT angiography. AJNR Am J Neuroradiol 2000;21(4):712–6.

34. Mehringer CM, Hieshima GB, Grinnell VS, et al. Improved localization of carotid cavernous fistula during angiography. AJNR Am J Neuroradiol 1982;3(1):82–4.
35. Debrun GM. Angiographic workup of a carotid cavernous sinus fistula (CCF) or what information does the interventionalist need for treatment? Surg Neurol 1995;44(1):75–9.
36. Huber P. A technical contribution of the exact angiographic localization of carotid cavernous fistulas. Neuroradiology 1976;10(5):239–41.
37. Schiavi P, Picetti E, Donelli V, et al. Diagnosis and postoperative monitoring of a traumatic carotid-cavernous fistula by jugular venous oximetry: case report and literature review. Acta Neurochir 2013;155:1341–2.
38. Phelps CD, Thompson HS, Ossoinig KC. The diagnosis and prognosis of atypical carotid-cavernous fistula (red-eyed shunt syndrome). Am J Ophthalmol 1982;93(4):423–36.
39. Day JD, Fukushima T. Direct microsurgery of dural arteriovenous malformation type carotid-cavernous sinus fistulas: indications, technique, and results. Neurosurgery 1997;41(5):1119–24.
40. Serbinenko FA. Balloon catheterization and occlusion of major cerebral vessels. J Neurosurg 1974; 41(2):125–45.
41. Debrun G, Lacour P, Vinuela F, et al. Treatment of 54 traumatic carotid-cavernous fistulas. J Neurosurg 1981;55(5):678–92.
42. Higashida RT, Halbach VV, Tsai FY, et al. Interventional neurovascular treatment of traumatic carotid and vertebral artery lesions: results in 234 cases. AJR Am J Roentgenol 1989;153(3):577–82.
43. Lewis AI, Tomsick TA, Tew JM Jr. Management of 100 consecutive direct carotid-cavernous fistulas: results of treatment with detachable balloons. Neurosurgery 1995;36(2):239–44.
44. Teng MM, Chang CY, Chiang JH, et al. Double-balloon technique for embolization of carotid cavernous fistulas. AJNR Am J Neuroradiol 2000; 21(9):1753–6.
45. Wakhloo A, Perlow A, Linfante I, et al. Transvenous n-butyl-cyanoacrylate infusion for complex dural carotid cavernous fistulas: technical considerations and clinical outcome. AJNR Am J Neuroradiol 2005;26(8):1888–97.
46. Eddleman CS, Surdell D, Miller J, et al. Endovascular management of a ruptured cavernous carotid artery aneurysm associated with a carotid cavernous fistula with an intracranial self-expanding microstent and hydrogel-coated coil embolization: case report and review of the literature. Surg Neurol 2007;68:562–7 [discussion: 7].
47. Natarajan SK, Ghodke B, Kim LJ, et al. Multimodality treatment of intracranial dural arteriovenous fistulas in the onyx era: a single center experience. World Neurosurg 2010;73:365–79.
48. Suzuki S, Lee DW, Jahan R, et al. Transvenous treatment of spontaneous dural carotid-cavernous fistulas using a combination of detachable coils and onyx. AJNR Am J Neuroradiol 2006;27(6): 1346–9.
49. Morón FE, Klucznik RP, Mawad ME, et al. Endovascular treatment of high-flow carotid cavernous fistulas by stent-assisted coil placement. AJNR Am J Neuroradiol 2005;26(6):1399–404.
50. Gonzalez LF, Chalouhi N, Tjoumakaris S, et al. Treatment of carotid-cavernous fistulas using intra-arterial balloon assistance: case series and technical note. Neurosurg Focus 2012;32:E14.
51. Chalouhi N, Dumont AS, Tjoumakaris S, et al. The superior ophthalmic vein approach for the treatment of carotid-cavernous fistulas: a novel technique using onyx. Neurosurg Focus 2012;32:E13.
52. Kocer N, Kizilkilic O, Albayram S, et al. Treatment of iatrogenic internal carotid artery laceration and carotid cavernous fistula with endovascular stent-graft placement. AJNR Am J Neuroradiol 2002; 23(3):442–6.
53. Gomez F, Escobar W, Gomez AM, et al. Treatment of carotid cavernous fistulas using covered stents: midterm results in seven patients. AJNR Am J Neuroradiol 2007;28(9):1762–8.

Endovascular Treatment of Carotid Stenosis

Jorge L. Eller, MD[a,b,c], Kenneth V. Snyder, MD, PhD[a,b,d,e,f], Adnan H. Siddiqui, MD, PhD[a,b,e,f,g], Elad I. Levy, MD, MBA[a,b,e,f], L. Nelson Hopkins, MD[a,b,e,f,g,*]

KEYWORDS

- Carotid artery stenosis • Carotid revascularization • Carotid angioplasty and stenting
- Carotid endarterectomy • Atherosclerotic carotid disease

KEY POINTS

- Carotid artery stenosis is responsible for 15% to 25% of ischemic strokes, emphasizing the importance of carotid revascularization for stroke prevention.
- Carotid artery angioplasty and stenting (CAS) has become the treatment of choice for high-risk surgical patients with symptomatic carotid stenosis.
- Embolic protection devices and new stent technology have been the two most significant technical advances that have made CAS a viable alternative to carotid endarterectomy (CEA) in the treatment of carotid stenosis.
- CAS and CEA are currently equally effective and their risk profiles are evenly matched for patients with symptomatic carotid stenosis with standard surgical risk.

INTRODUCTION

Ischemic strokes remain the third leading cause of death and the major cause of adult disability in the United States, with an annual incidence of approximately 795,000 new or recurrent strokes (80% of which are ischemic).[1] Atherosclerotic occlusive disease of the carotid artery (carotid stenosis) is thought to be responsible for approximately 15% to 25% of such ischemic strokes,[2,3] with a prevalence that varies from approximately 0.5% at 60 years of age to approximately 10% at 80 years of age.[4] These statistics make carotid revascularization the most important surgical tool in the prevention of new ischemic strokes.

Carotid endarterectomy (CEA), first introduced in the 1950s,[5,6] has stood the test of time and was eventually established as the gold standard treatment of stroke prevention in patients with carotid stenosis by several landmark trials in the 1990s (**Table 1**).[7–10] Class I evidence in favor of CEA is divided between patients with symptomatic and asymptomatic carotid stenosis; symptomatic patients are defined as patients who experienced a transient ischemic attack (TIA) or a nondisabling stroke in the appropriate carotid vascular distribution in the preceding 6 months.

In symptomatic patients, the North American Symptomatic Carotid Endarterectomy Trial (NASCET),[7] completed in 1991, demonstrated a

Disclosure: See last page of article.
[a] Department of Neurosurgery, University at Buffalo, State University of New York, Buffalo, NY, USA; [b] Department of Neurosurgery, Gates Vascular Institute, Kaleida Health, Buffalo, NY, USA; [c] Cerebrovascular Neurosurgery, PeaceHealth Sacred Heart Medical Center, 333 Riverbend Drive, Springfield, OR 97477, USA; [d] Department of Neurology, University at Buffalo, State University of New York, Buffalo, NY, USA; [e] Department of Radiology, University at Buffalo, State University of New York, Buffalo, NY, USA; [f] School of Medicine and Biomedical Sciences, Toshiba Stroke and Vascular Research Center, University at Buffalo, State University of New York, Buffalo, NY, USA; [g] Jacobs Institute, Buffalo, NY, USA
* Corresponding author. Department of Neurosurgery, Jacobs Institute, University at Buffalo, 875 Ellicott Street, 5th Floor, Buffalo, NY 14203.
E-mail addresses: lnhbuffns@aol.com; dzbuffns@aol.com

Neurosurg Clin N Am 25 (2014) 565–582
http://dx.doi.org/10.1016/j.nec.2014.04.012
1042-3680/14/$ – see front matter

Abbreviations	
ACAS	Asymptomatic Carotid Atherosclerosis Study
ACST	Asymptomatic Carotid Surgery Trial
ACT	Activated coagulation time
CAS	Carotid artery angioplasty and stenting
CCA	Common carotid artery
CEA	Carotid endarterectomy
CMS	Centers for Medicare and Medicaid Services
CREST	Carotid Revascularization Endarterectomy versus Stenting Trial
CTA	Computed tomographic angiography
DSA	Digital subtraction angiography
ECA	External carotid artery
ECST	European Carotid Surgery Trial
EVA-3S	Endarterectomy versus Stenting in Patients with Symptomatic Severe Carotid Stenosis
FDA	Food and Drug Administration
ICA	Internal carotid artery
ICSS	International Carotid Stenting Study
MI	Myocardial infarction
MR	Magnetic resonance
MRA	Magnetic resonance angiography
NASCET	North American Symptomatic Carotid Endarterectomy Trial
SAPPHIRE	Stenting and Angioplasty with Protection in Patients at High Risk for Endarterectomy
SPACE	Stent-Supported Percutaneous Angioplasty of the Carotid Artery versus Endarterectomy
TIA	Transient ischemic attack

significant reduction in the 2-year stroke risk (from 26% to 9%; 17% absolute stroke risk reduction) among symptomatic patients with 70% or greater carotid stenosis treated by CEA when compared with the best medical management. Similarly, the European Carotid Surgery Trial (ECST),[8] completed in 1998, demonstrated that CEA reduced the stroke risk from 26.5% (medical management group) to 14.9% (surgical group) for patients with 0% or greater carotid stenosis. A pooled data analysis of the NASCET, ECST, and the Veterans Affairs Cooperative Trial of Symptomatic Carotid Disease,[11] which included 6092 patients with 35,000 patient-years of follow-up, showed that CEA increased the 5-year risk of ipsilateral ischemic stroke in patients with less than 30% stenosis, had no effect in patients with 30% to 49% stenosis, had marginal benefit in those with 50% to 69% stenosis, and was highly beneficial in patients with 70% or more stenosis but without near occlusion. In patients with near occlusion, there was a trend toward benefit from surgery at 2 years but none at 5 years of follow-up. Moreover, performing the surgery within 2 weeks of the ischemic event increased the effectiveness of the surgery; the number needed to treat in order to prevent one ipsilateral stroke in 5 years was 5 when treated within 2 weeks of the event and 125 when treated after 12 weeks.[12]

Similarly, the Asymptomatic Carotid Atherosclerosis Study (ACAS)[9] and the Asymptomatic Carotid Surgery Trial (ACST)[10] demonstrated that for asymptomatic patients with greater than 60% carotid stenosis, the aggregate risk for ipsilateral stroke or perioperative stroke over 5 years was 5.1% for patients undergoing surgery and 11% for patients treated medically with aspirin (325 mg daily) and risk factor management. This benefit of surgery could not be demonstrated in

Table 1
Landmark CEA trials for patients with symptomatic (NASCET and ECST) and asymptomatic (ACAS and ACST) carotid stenosis

			Stroke Rate (%)[a]		
Trial	CEA/Medical (No. of Patients)	Stenosis (%)	CEA	Medical	*P* Value
NASCET	328/331	≥70	9.0	26.0	<.001
ECST	586/389	≥80	14.9	26.5	<.001
ACAS	825/834	≥60	5.1	11.0	.004
ACST	1560/1560	≥60	6.4	11.8	.001

Abbreviations: ACAS, Asymptomatic Carotid Atherosclerosis Study; ACST, Asymptomatic Carotid Surgery Trial; ECST, European Carotid Surgery Trial; NASCET, North American Symptomatic Carotid Endarterectomy Trial.
[a] Stroke rate according to treatment modality.
Adapted from Siddiqui AH, Natarajan SK, Hopkins LN, et al. Carotid artery stenting for primary and secondary stroke prevention. World Neurosurg 2011;76:S40–59.

women in the ACAS. In the ACST, the number need to treat in order to prevent one ipsilateral stroke was 12 for men and 24 for women over the 5-year follow-up.

In these landmark trials (NASCET, ECAS, ACAS, and ACST), highly experienced surgeons treated carefully selected, low-surgical-risk patients only. To achieve the benefit described in these trials, the perioperative complication rate must be 6% or less for symptomatic patients and 3% or less for asymptomatic patients. However, in the general population, studies have demonstrated perioperative stroke and death rates as high as 11.1% for symptomatic patients and 5.5% for asymptomatic patients.[13] Moreover, there are several clinical and anatomic features that are considered high risk for surgery and have a profound negative impact on the final surgical outcome (**Box 1**). As a result of these limitations of open surgery, a minimally invasive endovascular approach alternative to CEA, carotid artery angioplasty and stenting (CAS), has evolved in the last 2 decades and has experienced an astonishing rate of improvement and technical development in the last few years. Endovascular CAS has now become an accepted alternative for carotid revascularization, especially in high-surgical-risk patients.

Box 1
Anatomic and clinical high-risk features for CEA

Anatomic

- Recurrent carotid stenosis
- Previous cervical surgery
- Contralateral laryngeal palsy
- Presence of tracheostomy
- Following cervical radiation therapy
- Carotid lesion above C2 vertebra
- Contralateral carotid occlusion
- Presence of tandem carotid stenosis
- Presence of intraluminal thrombus
- Carotid lesion below clavicle

Clinical

- Recent or evolving myocardial infarction
- Preoperative coronary artery bypass graft
- Presence of congestive heart failure
- Renal failure
- Angina pectoris
- Recurrent cerebrovascular attack
- Crescendo transient ischemic attacks
- Fluctuating neurologic deficit
- Stroke in evolution

RELEVANT ANATOMY AND PATHOPHYSIOLOGY OF CAROTID STENOSIS

Relevant Anatomy

The paired internal carotid arteries (ICAs) are the major conduits for blood flow to the brain. An understanding of their anatomy, including the origin of the common carotid arteries (CCAs) in the aortic arch, is fundamental in assessing the feasibility of any endovascular intervention.

The most proximal large vessel off the aortic arch is the brachiocephalic (or innominate) artery, which divides into the right CCA and the right subclavian artery. The left CCA is the next major branch off the aortic arch, followed by the left subclavian artery. Both the right and left CCAs bifurcate into internal and external carotid arteries at the level of the mid to upper cervical region. The CCA bifurcation and most proximal cervical ICA segment are the most common sites for carotid stenosis.

A very important consideration is the relative position of the origin of the great vessels (brachiocephalic, left CCA, and left subclavian arteries) and the apex of the aortic arch itself. As people age, the aortic arch becomes elongated, calcified, and less compliant, causing the takeoff of the brachiocephalic artery to be more proximal relative to the apex of the arch itself. A classification system has been developed to describe this relationship (**Fig. 1**). A so-called type I arch is one in which all 3 great vessels arise from the apex of the arch; A type II arch is one in which the takeoff of the brachiocephalic artery is between the 2 horizontal planes delineated by the apices of the outer and inner curves of the aortic arch, at the level of the arch apex; a type III arch is one in which the origin of the brachiocephalic artery lies below the horizontal plane delineated by the apex of the inner curve of the aortic arch at the level of the arch apex. This aortic arch classification is important because it correlates with increasing difficulty in catheterizing the great vessels and an increase in risk of complications during endovascular interventions.[14–16] Another important anatomic aspect to keep in mind is the development of progressive great vessel elongation with aging, which leads to increased vessel tortuosity, mostly at the proximal segments of these vessels. This factor creates great difficulty in obtaining stable endovascular access and is also related to increased risk of embolic complications.

Aortic arch anatomic variations are also relevant. One of the most common anatomic

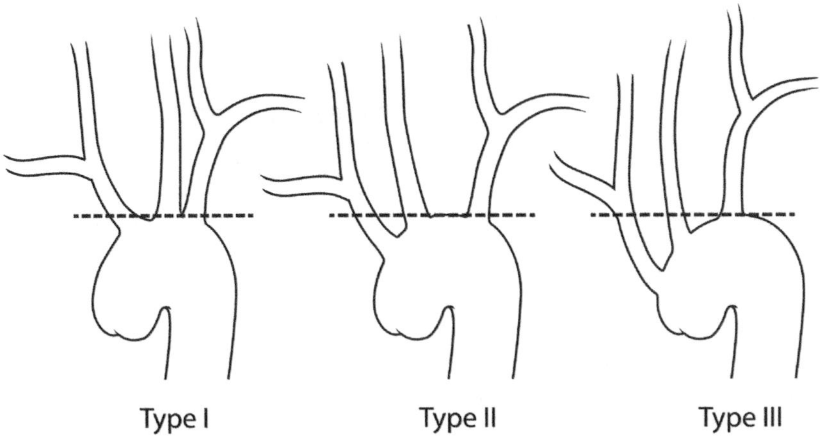

Fig. 1. Aortic arch classification according to the takeoff of the brachiocephalic artery in relationship to the apex of the arch. Types I, II, and III reflect a progressively more difficult arch to navigate, with type III being most difficult (see text). (*From* Eller JL, Siddiqui AH. Stent design choice based on anatomy (chapter 39). In: Gonzalez F, et al, editors. Neurointerventional surgery, tricks of the trade. Thieme, in press.)

variations is the so-called bovine arch, where the left CCA and the brachiocephalic artery share a common origin or the left CCA originates from the brachiocephalic artery itself. The angle created by the left CCA and the aortic arch in these cases makes access difficult for standard endovascular catheters. One has to be aware of such variations to successfully gain vascular access. In these circumstances, as well as in situations whereby there is significant tortuosity, elongation of vessels, and/or other kinds of anatomic variations in the takeoff of great vessels from the arch, the ability to safely and successfully navigate the arch anatomy becomes the greatest challenge to successful completion of an endovascular procedure and may be a contraindication for the procedure altogether.

Pathophysiology and Natural History of Carotid Atherosclerosis

Histopathologically, carotid stenosis is a narrowing of the native carotid lumen, with deposition of plaque material of either soft, atheromatous or hard, calcified consistency. Clinical factors associated with the development of atheromatous plaque in the carotid arteries include hypercholesterolemia, hypertension, diabetes mellitus, obesity, and cigarette smoking.[17,18] The role of systemic and/or local inflammation has also been described; an inflammatory process may lead to plaque formation, rupture, or hemorrhage.[19–21]

The natural history of carotid atherosclerosis depends on the presence or absence of symptoms. In asymptomatic patients, the degree of stenosis may worsen over time; this progression correlates with an increased risk of ipsilateral stroke.[22] Two studies[23,24] have demonstrated that patients with asymptomatic carotid bruits are at an increased risk for neurologic and/or cardiac events; however, these events are not necessarily related to the territory of the affected carotid artery. Another study[25] described a higher incidence of silent infarcts ipsilaterally to high-grade (>75%) carotid stenosis when compared with lower grades of stenosis.

The medical management of carotid stenosis has evolved significantly. The incidence of ipsilateral stroke in patients with stenosis treated medically in the ACAS (where medical management consisted of aspirin alone) was approximately 2.2% annually.[9] In the ACST (where medical management consisted of aspirin plus angiotensin inhibitors and statins), the incidence of ipsilateral ischemic stroke diminished to approximately 1.7% annually.[10] More recent studies show a less than 1% annual incidence of ipsilateral strokes in asymptomatic carotid stenosis treated medically.[26,27]

The natural history of symptomatic carotid stenosis has also been well described. Previous studies have demonstrated that the risk of stroke following a first-time carotid TIA is close to 5% annually,[28,29] with more than 50% of such strokes happening in the first year and 21% of them happening in the first month after such an event.[30] The natural history of carotid stenosis is also influenced by plaque morphology; the presence of ulceration or intraplaque hemorrhage may be associated with a higher likelihood of ischemic events.[31–33] Carotid revascularization has become the standard of care for patients with symptomatic carotid stenosis because of the dramatic stroke risk reduction shown in NASCET and ECAS.

CLINICAL PRESENTATION AND DIAGNOSIS

Patients with asymptomatic carotid stenosis are usually diagnosed after carotid bruits are noticed or during routine carotid Doppler screening. It is estimated that carotid bruits are heard in approximately 3% to 4% of the US population greater than 45 years of age and present in 10% to 23% of patients with symptomatic atherosclerosis in other arterial distributions.[23,24] Screening ultrasonography is frequently performed in patients with risk factors for carotid disease, a family history of carotid disease, or evidence of peripheral vasculopathy. If 60% or greater carotid stenosis is suspected, further imaging, such as computed tomographic angiography (CTA) or magnetic resonance angiography (MRA), is indicated.

Symptomatic patients may present with a single-episode TIA, crescendo TIAs, or a full stroke. These patients need to be evaluated promptly for a possible cardioembolic source of their symptoms as well as for carotid stenosis, with carotid Doppler and noninvasive neurovascular imaging, such as CTA or MRA. If any of these modalities is suggestive of carotid stenosis in excess of 50% by NASCET criteria, digital subtraction angiography (DSA) should be considered in preparation for carotid revascularization.

Many centers have adopted the practice of proceeding with CEA from neurovascular imaging alone. Although many surgeons have accepted CTA and/or MRA alone as sufficient, there is no doubt that DSA provides much better anatomic detail and more accurate estimation of the degree of stenosis. Despite the small amount of risk involved in angiography, there is some evidence that noninvasive neurovascular studies are inferior to DSA for preoperative assessment and decision making.[34]

ENDOVASCULAR CONSIDERATIONS

Background and Historical Perspectives

The stroke risk reduction attributed to CEA in the classic landmark trials of surgical versus medical management of carotid stenosis is achieved only under the condition of surgical complication rates kept below a very specific threshold. As mentioned earlier, in the NASCET, the 17% absolute stroke risk reduction in patients with 70% or greater stenosis treated surgically was obtained assuming a 30-day rate of perioperative complication (nonfatal strokes, myocardial infarction [MI], or death) of 6% or less.[7] For patients with asymptomatic carotid stenosis enrolled in the ACAS, the benefit of surgery assumed a perioperative complication rate of 3% or less.[9] In addition, the very strict inclusion criteria in both the NASCET and ACAS limited the benefit of CEA to patients considered low risk for surgical intervention.

The search for a minimally invasive endovascular approach for the treatment of carotid stenosis began as early as the 1980s. Interventional neuroradiologists began using balloons in the treatment of several intracranial vascular diseases following the pioneering work of Serbinenko in the late 1960s and early 1970s.[35] Working independently, Mathias and colleagues,[36] Kerber and colleagues,[37] and Theron,[38] were the first to consider balloon angioplasty of the extracranial carotid artery. Theron and colleagues[39] published the first series of 38 carotid balloon angioplasties in 1987, with an 8% embolic complication rate and a 5% carotid dissection rate. This high rate of distal embolic complications prompted the search for ways to protect the brain during these procedures.

Theron[38] developed a triple coaxial catheter system with an occlusive balloon at the tip to be used for embolic protection. This balloon was attached to a microcatheter and inflated within the distal cervical ICA during angioplasty of the stenotic carotid segment. The embolic particles obtained during angioplasty were subsequently aspirated through the guiding catheter before deflating the distal occlusive balloon. This technique led to a reduction in the rate of distal embolic complications to 0% in a series of 43 patients treated by carotid angioplasty and distal balloon protection.[40]

The next major step in the evolution of the endovascular management of carotid stenosis was the introduction of stents. The cardiology literature demonstrated that better clinical and angiographic outcomes were obtained in patients who received a coronary stent than those treated by coronary angioplasty alone, with lower rates of restenosis in those receiving stents.[41,42] Several researchers began applying this technique in the management of extracranial carotid stenosis in the mid-1990s, with similar improved outcomes, including lower rates of restenosis and avoidance of disastrous carotid dissections.[43–45]

Stents and embolic protection devices were undoubtedly the 2 major milestones that made CAS a promising and viable alternative to CEA for the treatment of extracranial carotid stenosis. In the following paragraphs, the authors discuss the historical evolution and technical aspects of current embolic protection devices and stents in greater detail, culminating with a description of modern endovascular technique for CAS.

Evolution of Embolic Protection

The first embolic protection device was the aforementioned balloon catheter system developed by

Theron and colleagues[40] to occlude the distal cervical ICA during angioplasty procedures. A direct evolution of the original Theron device is the PercuSurge GuideWire (Medtronic, Sunnyvale, CA, USA). This distal embolic protection device consists of a 0.014-in shapeable wire attached to a polyurethane occlusion balloon with a low crossing profile (0.036 in when deflated). Once the wire and balloon are advanced beyond the proximal ICA lesion, the balloon is inflated, occluding flow through the ICA. The stenotic segment is then treated by stenting and angioplasty as deemed necessary. After the stenting procedure is finished, an aspiration catheter is introduced over the wire up to the level of the distal occlusion balloon and used to aspirate the column of blood and debris proximal to the balloon. The aspiration catheter is subsequently removed and the balloon is deflated, thus restoring flow. The main disadvantages of distal balloon occlusion as an embolic protection device include the complete interruption of blood flow to the brain, which is occasionally not tolerated by patients with an inadequate circle of Willis, and the inability to obtain angiographic assessment of the lesion (and the stenting procedure itself) until the balloon is deflated.

To overcome the drawbacks of balloon occlusion devices, filter devices were subsequently developed as a suitable alternative. Filter devices function as an umbrella or windsock deployed between the stenotic carotid lesion and the brain to capture debris released during the stenting procedure, while allowing uninterrupted blood flow and continuous radiographic assessment during the entire procedure. The filter is subsequently recaptured and removed at the end of the procedure. There are different kinds of filter devices; but they all essentially consist of an expandable nitinol frame covered with a porous polyurethane membrane, with the pore size ranging from 36 to 140 μm.[46] They can be divided in 2 main groups: filters *built into* a microwire, so that they can be moved either proximally or distally by moving the microwire, like the FilterWire EZ filter (Boston Scientific, Mountainview, CA, USA), or filters *placed on* the microwire but able to move proximally or distally independently of the microwire movements, such as the Emboshield NAV-6 (Abbott Vascular, Santa Clara, CA, USA) (**Fig. 2**). Once the filter is deployed in the distal ICA beyond the stenotic segment, the filter wire is then used as a delivery wire for stents and angioplasty balloons as needed. Finally, at the end of the procedure, a retrieval catheter recaptures the filter and any trapped debris. The debris can also be aspirated through an aspiration catheter immediately before filter recapture, as is done with distal occlusion balloons, particularly if the debris burden is large and has occluded the filter. The pore size of the

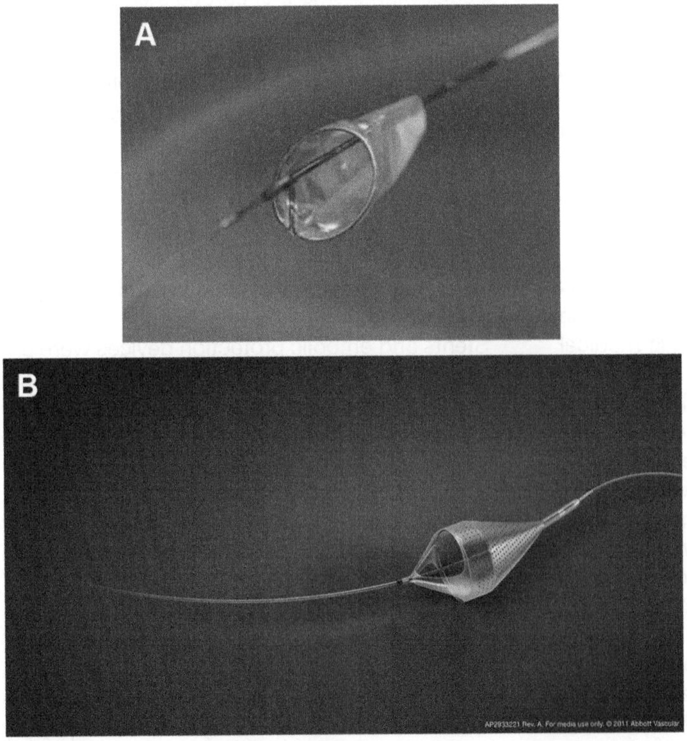

Fig. 2. Examples of different types of distal embolic protection filters. (*A*) FilterWire EZ filter: filter built into the microwire, moves proximally or distally according to the movements of the microwire. (*B*) Emboshield NAV-6 filter: filter built on the microwire, moves independently of the microwire. ([*A*] *Courtesy of* Boston Scientific Corporation or its affiliates, Maple Grove, MN, © 2013. All rights reserved, with permission; and [*B*] *Courtesy of* Abbott, Abbott Park, Il.)

filter is related to the risk of filter thrombosis. Smaller pore sizes increase the risk of filter thrombosis as a result of trapping too many particles; conversely, the larger the pore size, the higher the risk of microembolization, even with the filter. As a result of this dilemma, most filters have pore sizes ranging from 100 to 150 μm; although in one study of embolic particles recovered during 75 CAS procedures performed with the PercuSurge device, 50% of the particles were less than 100 μm.[47]

Despite the popularity of filter devices and the widespread use of distal embolic protection, an inherent shortcoming of this technique is the need for the device, either filter or balloon, to cross the stenotic lesion before its deployment and the establishment of effective embolic protection. The risk of embolic debris being released during the crossing process stimulated the search for a way to protect the brain before the lesion was crossed. As mentioned, Theron,[38] who used balloons to occlude the CCA, entertained this concept in the late 1980s; however, he realized that inversion of flow through the external carotid artery (ECA) would maintain flow in the ICA. Eventually, this concept of proximal embolic protection was further refined by Parodi to include a main balloon guide catheter positioned in the distal CCA and a smaller balloon positioned in the proximal ECA (at the level of the superior thyroid artery).[46] When both balloons are inflated, there is flow arrest (or flow reversal) in the ICA, with effective prevention of distal migration of embolic debris into the intracranial circulation (**Fig. 3**).

There are currently 2 main proximal protection devices available for sale in the United States: the Mo.Ma device (Invatec, Roncadelle, Italy) and the Gore Flow Reversal System (W.L. Gore, Flagstaff, AZ, USA), previously known as the Parodi Anti-Embolic System. The Mo.Ma device has 2 low-pressure compliant balloons mounted on a single catheter, the larger one placed in the distal CCA and the smaller one in the proximal ECA. Once the balloons are inflated, there is flow arrest in the ICA and the working channel of the main catheter is used to deliver stents and balloons as needed to treat the ICA stenosis.[48,49] The Gore Flow Reversal System also consists of 2 balloons, one positioned in the distal CCA and one in the proximal ECA; the main differences in comparison with the Mo.Ma device are that with the Gore device, the ECA balloon is mounted on a separate 0.015-in wire (navigated into the ECA independently of the main guide catheter) and the proximal hub of the main catheter is connected to the contralateral femoral vein (through a filter), allowing retrograde flow through the ICA. The guide-

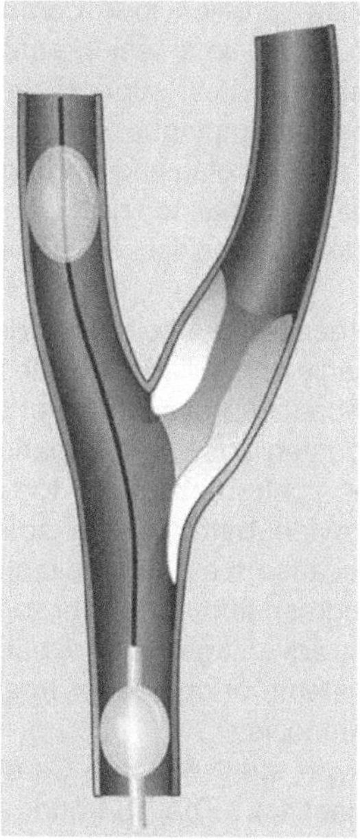

Fig. 3. Proximal embolic protection. The balloons occlude both the common carotid and external carotid arteries. Flow through the internal carotid artery can then be arrested or reversed to prevent embolic debris from reaching the intracranial circulation. (*From* Dumont TM, Kan P, Jahshan S, et al. Unyielding progress: carotid stenting cases from Millard Fillmore Gates Circle Hospital in Buffalo, New York. Clin Neurosurg 2012;59:50–8.)

catheter working channel of the Gore device is then used to deliver stents and balloons as needed to complete the procedure. The effectiveness of distal versus proximal embolic protection in reducing cerebral microembolization was assessed by transcranial Doppler and diffusion-weighted MR imaging. These preliminary trials demonstrated a significant reduction in cerebral embolization when using proximal protection compared with distal protection devices.[50,51]

Evolution of Stent Technology

Following developments in interventional cardiology,[41,42] the first stents used in the treatment of extracranial carotid artery stenosis were balloon-expandable coronary stents. However, these devices were susceptible to external compression, collapse, and dislodgment caused by cervical motion, leading to cerebral blood flow impairment.[52] Because they were inflated with a single-size balloon, these stents could not attain different sizes in their proximal and distal aspects; therefore, they poorly apposed the natural taper that exists between the CCA and the ICA diameters. Other disadvantages of these stents included a larger crossing profile; low conformability to tortuous lesions; minimal lesion scaffolding (pertaining to the amount of support the stents give to the atherosclerotic plaque, which prevents plaque debris from prolapsing through the stent tines); and the risk of balloon rupture and air embolism if deployed against a jagged, calcified lesion.[52,53]

The emergence of self-expandable stents, derived primarily from biliary stent designs, constituted a significant improvement over their balloon-mounted counterparts. Self-expandable stents have greater conformability to tortuous carotid anatomy, provide better lesion scaffolding and coverage (because they are available in different sizes and lengths), and are easier to deploy. As a result of these advantages, self-expandable stents became the stents of choice for treatment of carotid artery stenosis.

The first such stent was the Carotid Wallstent (Boston Scientific). The Carotid Wallstent is composed of a monofilament wire, braided in a tubular mesh configuration, and made of Elgiloy (a cobalt-chromium-iron-nickel-molybdenum alloy) enhanced with a radiopaque tantalum core.[52] This stent is fairly compressible and flexible and designed as a closed-cell stent, which means that all the adjacent bridges (or struts or tines) of the stent structure are connected at every possible junction, allowing excellent scaffolding properties. Once the stent is outside of its delivery sheath, a springlike action allows the device to expand; a partially delivered stent (up to 50% of its length) may be recaptured into its delivery sheath and repositioned if needed.

The introduction of nitinol stents represented another milestone in stent development. Nitinol stents are made from shape-memory alloys (nickel and titanium) that return to their preformed shape when exposed to normal body temperature (37°C). These stents can be designed as closed-cell stents (like the Wallstent) or open-cell stents, which means that some of the connecting bridges (or stent struts) are missing; therefore, open-cell stents are more flexible and conformable to tortuous anatomy, albeit provide less vessel wall support. Nitinol stents can have a cylindrical or tapered shape and, thus, are potentially better suited for the mismatch between CCA and ICA diameters. These various stent designs and materials allow great flexibility in tailoring the appropriate stent to a specific carotid lesion and greatly enhance the likelihood of successful endovascular treatment (**Fig. 4**).

Finally, hybrid stent technologies represent the latest step forward in the evolution of carotid stenting. These stents combine both open-cell and closed-cell designs. The Cristallo Ideale carotid stent (Medtronic Vascular, Minneapolis, MN, USA) has a closed-cell design in its center and an open-cell design at its edges, and the sinus-Carotid-RX stent (OptiMed, Ettlingen, Germany) has an open-cell design in its center and a closed-cell design at its edges. These devices attempt to provide better lesion scaffolding with more flexibility. There are also stents that combine open- and closed-cell designs throughout the length of the stent; however, they have yet to enter clinical trials. Another recent concept is the covered endoluminal stents, in which a layer of polytetrafluoroethylene lining is added to an external nitinol support to prevent plaque prolapse through the stents tines. These devices are also available with a bioactive surface of recombinant human thrombomodulin, which was found to inhibit neointimal hyperplasia in a porcine model of injured carotid artery.[54]

Modern CAS Techniques

One of the fundamental aspects for the success of CAS is the need to understand vascular access and carotid lesion anatomy and to select devices accordingly. For each specific case, angiographic runs and other noninvasive vascular images (CTA and/or MRA if available) should be studied carefully to determine the feasibility of endovascular access to the common and internal carotid arteries and the appropriateness of specific stents, embolic protection devices, and angioplasty balloons according to the carotid lesion. Careful selection of devices is important for successful and safe placement of a carotid artery stent and is detailed in the later sections. The technique of CAS involves angioplasty of the ICA for vascular lumen expansion and stent deployment over the plaque to prevent vessel recoil and restrain plaque debris from entering the stent lumen and migrating distally. A rapid-exchange over-the-wire system is preferred for the delivery of all devices used in this procedure because of its simplicity and speed.

Before the procedure, patients are placed on dual antiplatelet therapy with aspirin (325 mg daily) and clopidogrel (75 mg daily) for at least 5 days to obtain a proper therapeutic level of these medications and prevent intrastent and intraluminal thrombus buildup after stent placement. If antiplatelet therapy cannot be started in advance, a loading dose of aspirin (650 mg orally, one dose) and clopidogrel (600 mg orally, one dose) should be given immediately before the procedure. Alternatively, prasugrel may be given to patients with intolerance or resistance to clopidogrel. Dual antiplatelet therapy is continued for at least 1 month

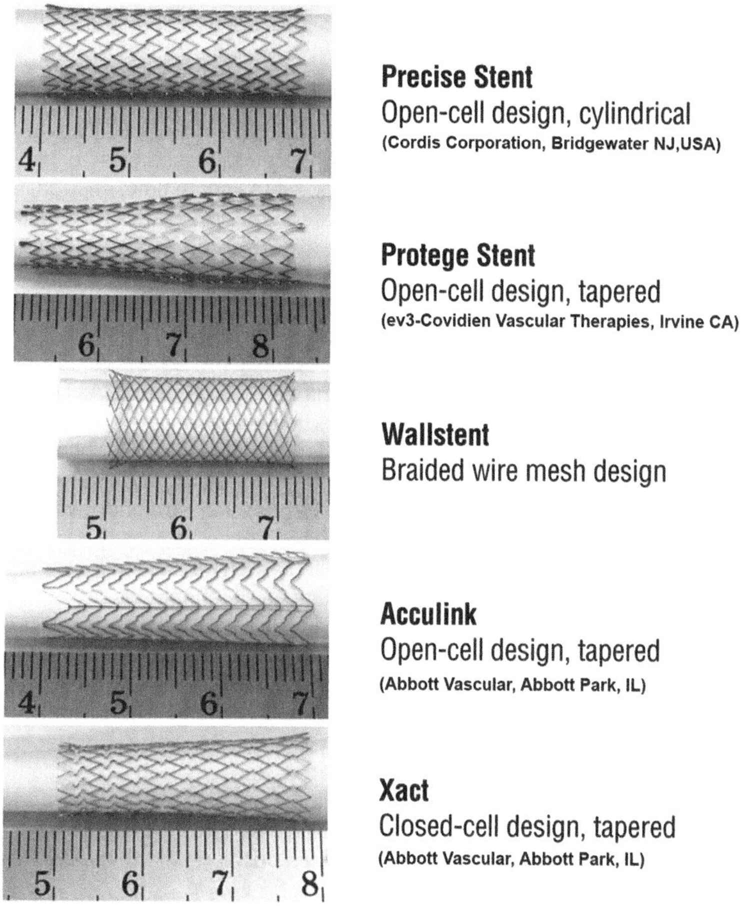

Fig. 4. Examples of different stent designs according to their mechanical structure and shape. (*From* Eller JL, Siddiqui AH. Stent design choice based on anatomy (chapter 39). In: Gonzalez F, et al, editors. NeuroInterventional surgery, tricks of the trade. Thieme, in press.)

after stent placement, after which time clopidogrel can usually be safely discontinued. Patients are kept on aspirin for life.

At the authors' institution, CAS is usually performed under conscious sedation and local anesthetic agents. Midazolam and fentanyl are administered and titrated to the patients' comfort, allowing patients to be easily aroused for a neurologic examination as needed throughout the procedure. Lidocaine is used as a local anesthetic at the site of arterial puncture. Glycopyrrolate is used to prevent the possibility of symptomatic bradycardia, especially during the angioplasty portion of the procedure. Dopamine is typically used as a vasopressor for treatment of intraprocedural or postprocedural hypotension. A weight-based bolus of heparin (between 50 and 70 units per kilogram of bodyweight) is given intravenously to achieve an activated coagulation time (ACT) between 250 and 300 seconds before crossing the ICA lesion in order to prevent thrombus formation during the procedure.

Device Selection

Embolic protection devices

Embolic protection has become the standard of care in all endovascular CAS procedures. The choice of which kind of embolic protection is based primarily on anatomic considerations. Distal embolic protection with filter devices is preferred in most cases because it has been reliably proven to reduce perioperative strokes and is easier to deploy than proximal protection balloons. Conversely, stenting with proximal protection is ideally performed in cases of symptomatic lesions with a high likelihood of distal embolization during filter crossing, such as very high-grade (>90%) stenosis, presence of ulcerations and/or "fresh thrombus" associated with the atheromatous plaque or severe vessel tortuosity distal to the stenotic segment with no "landing zone" for the filter to be deployed. However, the presence of stenosis or tortuosity in the proximal CCA or ECA may render proximal protection impossible. Another option (albeit an uncommon approach) is to deploy both proximal and distal protection devices concomitantly. To optimize embolic protection, the guide catheter hub may be opened for back bleeding during lesion crossing, stent deployment, and balloon angioplasty maneuvers, thereby diverting embolic debris away from the intracranial circulation.

Stents

Stent choice is also based primarily on anatomic considerations, although a closed-cell stent with a small free-cell area (the uncovered area between stent tines) is preferred in most cases. As mentioned, such stents have better scaffolding and are more likely to trap plaque debris between the stent and the vessel wall, thereby limiting the risk of acute or delayed thromboembolism. Also, closed-cell stents can be recaptured and repositioned before they are fully deployed, maximizing optimal device positioning. On the other hand, in cases of severe vessel tortuosity at the site of stenosis, open-cell stents may be the best choice to allow optimal conformability of the stent to the vessel anatomy and minimize the chance of stent kinking or malpositioning. The balance between conformability and scaffolding properties lies at the heart of choosing a specific carotid stent. Finally, a stent of sufficient length to cover the stenotic segment and bridge the ICA to the CCA should be chosen.

Angioplasty balloons

Balloon angioplasty is usually performed after stent deployment to maximize vessel lumen expansion and proper resolution of residual stenosis. In situations of severe stenosis, when the stent may not safely cross the lesion before its deployment, prestent angioplasty may also be performed. The angioplasty balloon catheter should be slightly undersized to the diameter of the nondiseased ICA. Given the high risk of distal embolization of plaque debris during angioplasty, this portion of the procedure should be done as few times as possible (preferably only once) and with the guide catheter hub left opened for passive back bleeding or active aspiration. Angioplasty balloon catheters are available in a wide range of diameters and lengths to conform to the anatomy of the vessel being treated.

Guide catheters

The choice of guide catheter is directed by the principle of using the smallest-diameter guide catheter that allows deployment of embolic devices, stents, and balloons without losing stable anchoring in the proximal CCA. For most carotid stenting procedures, the 6F Cook Shuttle (Cook Medical, Bloomington, IN, USA) is ideal because it has enough stiffness to be used as a sheath and, at the same time, enough flexibility to be navigated up to the distal CCA, functioning as a stable guide for carotid stenting. All distal filter devices, stents, and balloons can be safely delivered through the Cook Shuttle. Smaller stents, such as a 6- or 8-mm Wallstent, can also be delivered through a 6F Envoy guide catheter (Codman & Shartleff, Raynham, MA, USA), which is smaller and easier to navigate than the Cook Shuttle but offers relatively less stability and a higher risk of herniating down into the aortic arch. Therefore, only cases of straightforward arch anatomy and limited vessel tortuosity are amenable to stenting using an Envoy as a guide catheter. The Envoy requires a 6F sheath placed in the femoral artery.

Finally, for cases requiring proximal protection, both the Mo.Ma and Gore catheters are used as guide catheters and have a working channel for delivery of stents and balloons once the proximal CCA and ECA embolic protection balloons are inflated. Because both are 9F catheters, they require placement of a 9F femoral artery sheath and are navigated into the distal CCA over stiffer guidewires positioned in the distal ECA.

Technique Pearls and Pitfalls

Groin access and sheath placement

A micropuncture needle is used to gain access to the common femoral artery, usually on the right side. A modified Seldinger technique with a succession of vessel dilators is then used to exchange the microneedle for a 6F sheath. A groin angiographic run is performed to exclude any vessel injury, dissection, or contrast extravasation and confirm the safety of percutaneous closure of the arteriotomy site at the end of the procedure. Patients with a history of peripheral vascular disease or previous femoral artery surgery should be evaluated preoperatively for the feasibility of femoral artery access; in rare situations, brachial artery access may be required. As discussed earlier, in most cases, the 6F sheath is exchanged for a 6F Cook Shuttle, which works as a guide catheter as well as a femoral sheath; otherwise the 6F sheath may be all that is necessary if a 6F Envoy guide catheter is chosen, or the 6F sheath may need to be exchanged for a 9F sheath in cases of proximal embolic protection.

All devices are prepared and flushed with saline as described by the manufacturer's instructions and placed in order of use at the end of the table for easy and fast access by the operator during the procedure. Full heparinization is also performed at the time of femoral artery access, so that the ACT can reach a therapeutic level by the time of carotid artery access to minimize the risk of embolic complications.

Guide catheter placement

The guide catheter is firmly anchored in the distal CCA so as not to herniate back into the aortic arch during delivery of the embolic protection devices, stents, and balloons. The 6F Envoy catheter is flexible and navigable enough to be brought up into the distal CCA over a 0.035-in guidewire, without the need of further catheters. The guidewire is usually brought up into the distal ECA to allow enough wire purchase for the Envoy to climb over it without disturbing the atheromatous plaque in the ICA. Biplane fluoroscopy is of great importance. The view of the aortic arch provided by the anteroposterior plane and the view of the CCA bifurcation provided by the lateral plane ensure that the wire will not enter the ICA, potentially leading to distal embolic complications, during advancement of the guide catheter. Road map guidance is also used during this maneuver.

Placement of the 6F Cook Shuttle is a bit more challenging. Because the 6F Cook Shuttle is larger and stiffer than the 6F Envoy catheter, an intermediate 5F catheter is needed to provide more stable purchase of the proximal CCA and allow the Cook Shuttle to climb over it. A 5F Vitek catheter (Cook Medical) is typically used for this purpose. A 0.035-in exchange length guidewire is brought up to the aortic arch and used to exchange the original 6F sheath for the Cook Shuttle, which is brought up to the proximal descending aorta. The 5F Vitek catheter is then introduced through the Cook Shuttle and over the guidewire and used to selectively catheterize either the right or left proximal CCA. The exchange guidewire is advanced into the distal ECA for a more stable wire purchase. The Cook Shuttle is then advanced over the Vitek catheter and over the guidewire, up to the distal CCA. A 5F Slip-Cath (Cook Medical) can also be used as an intermediate catheter for purchase into the right CCA. In cases whereby the exchange length guidewire cannot enter the ECA owing to severe ECA stenosis or even distal CCA lesions, a stiffer guidewire, such as the Amplatz Super Stiff guidewire (Boston Scientific), may be placed in the proximal CCA and the Cook Shuttle advanced over it into its desired position.

In the case of using a proximal protection device, the 6F sheath is initially increased to a 9F sheath. As both the Mo.Ma and Gore catheters are fairly stiff, a stiffer wire is needed to allow these catheters to climb into the distal CCA. A Supra Core wire (Abbott Vascular, Abbott Park, IL, USA) is routinely used for this purpose. A 5F diagnostic catheter, such as the Sim-2 catheter (Terumo Medical Corporation, Ann Arbor, MI, USA), is used initially to catheterize the proximal CCA. Under fluoroscopy road map guidance, an exchange-length 0.035-in guidewire is then navigated into the distal ECA, after which the Sim-2 catheter is advanced over the guidewire until the tip of the Sim-2 catheter is located in the distal ECA. The 0.035-in guidewire is removed, and the Supra Core wire is then introduced into the Sim-2 catheter and positioned in the distal ECA. Finally, the Sim-2 catheter is removed; the Mo.Ma (or Gore) catheter is then advanced over the Supra Core wire, up to the distal CCA. This indirect technique is frequently used to position large, stiffer catheters (such as the Mo.Ma or Gore catheter) into the CCA. If the catheter starts herniating down into the aortic arch, a slightly softer guidewire, such as a 0.038-in guidewire, may be used.

Embolic protection device deployment

For most cases, distal embolic filters are used. These devices come with their own steerable 0.014-in microwire, which is used to cross the stenotic lesion and deliver the filter to the distal cervical ICA. This part is potentially the most dangerous aspect of the whole case because it has to be accomplished before embolic protection is established and, therefore, can lead to embolization of plaque debris and perioperative stroke events. It is very important that the lesion crossing be performed swiftly and gently to avoid disturbing the plaque. The tip of the 0.014-in microwire should be shaped by the operator in a way to facilitate its maneuvering through the carotid bifurcation and the proximal ICA plaque and minimize the likelihood of distal embolism. Once the 0.014-in microwire is beyond the lesion, its tip is positioned and maintained in the petrous segment of the carotid artery. The filter is then brought over this microwire and deployed in a straight segment of the cervical ICA, distal to the stenotic segment. The filter's delivery catheter is then exchanged out of the 0.014-in microwire for the stent and subsequently the angioplasty balloon. A rapid exchange technique is preferred for faster and easier device delivery.

In case of the use of proximal protection, the distal CCA and proximal ECA balloons are properly positioned in their respective vessels and inflated immediately before crossing the lesion with a steerable 0.014-in microwire, such as a

Spartacore wire (Abbott Vascular). The balloons are inflated with a 50:50 solution of saline and contrast material in order to be easily visualized during the procedure. Stasis of flow can be confirmed by injecting a small amount of contrast material into the vessel lumen. Road map guidance is obtained before inflating the balloons, as no further angiographic runs are possible until the balloons are deflated. Once proximal protection is established, the Spartacore wire is used to cross the lesion in the same fashion as the distal filter microwires and advanced up to the proximal petrous carotid artery. The stent and subsequent angioplasty balloon are brought over the Spartacore wire. It may be difficult to exit the guide catheter (between the CCA and ECA balloons) with the Spartacore wire. In this situation, a multipurpose angled catheter may be used to redirect the Spartacore away from the guide catheter and into the ICA.

In cases of very severe or critical ICA stenosis, it may not be possible to cross the lesion with a 0.014-in microwire. In these situations, using a stiffer wire, such as a 0.035-in guidewire, to cross the lesion, followed by advancing a multipurpose guide catheter over the wire beyond the lesion is an option. The 0.035-in guidewire is then exchanged for a 0.014-in microwire, which is advanced up to the petrous segment of the carotid artery. The multipurpose angled catheter is exchanged for the stent. This technique carries a higher risk of disrupting the carotid plaque and distal embolization of plaque debris; therefore, proximal protection is advised before lesion crossing in these situations.

Stent deployment

Once embolic protection is established and the 0.014-in microwire is in position in the petrous segment of the carotid artery, the stent and the angioplasty balloon are brought up over the wire using a rapid-exchange technique. During the exchange, it is imperative that the wire be kept in a stable position to prevent vessel wall injury by untoward movement of the wire tip or the distal filter. It is also important to visualize the position of the guide catheter while advancing different devices to prevent herniation of the guide catheter down into the aortic arch. The final stent position should be determined in relationship to osseous landmarks (such as a cervical vertebra) in case patient movement makes the road map unreliable. Continuous fluoroscopic visualization is used during stent positioning and deployment. If the stent is unable to cross the stenotic lesion, a pathway is created by performing prestent angioplasty using an undersized (compared with the nondiseased ICA) balloon to minimize plaque trauma. The stent is then centered over the area of greatest stenosis (confirmed by its relationship to the predetermined osseous landmark) and deployed according to the manufacturer's instructions. In the case of closed-cell stents, a partially deployed stent (usually up to 50% of the stent length) may be recaptured and repositioned if necessary. There is usually a residual area of stenosis within the stent after its deployment, requiring poststenting angioplasty.

Poststent balloon angioplasty

The poststenting angioplasty balloon is also slightly undersized compared with the nondiseased ICA. Once the stent is deployed, the stent-delivery catheter is exchanged for the balloon catheter, and the balloon markers are then centered in the area of residual narrowing. Once in place, the angioplasty balloon is inflated to its nominal pressure and quickly deflated. Even if the residual narrowing is not completely resolved, one angioplasty is usually sufficient, especially considering the risk of distal embolism associated with potential plaque disruption by the inflated balloon.

Embolic protection device recapture

After stent deployment and poststenting angioplasty, cervical and intracranial angiographic runs are performed to confirm adequate carotid revascularization and absence of vessel injury or distal embolism. A neurologic examination is also performed to ensure the absence of any new neurologic deficits. In cases of proximal embolic protection, the balloons are deflated before the final angiographic runs; as long as no problem is identified, the 0.014-in microwire is removed under fluoroscopic visualization. In cases of distal embolic protection, a retrieval catheter is exchanged over the 0.014-in microwire and placed just proximal to the filter after crossing the stent under direct fluoroscopic visualization. The filter is then pulled back inside the retrieval catheter and both are removed together through the stent and guide catheter while the guide catheter hub is open for back bleeding. If there is too much debris within the filter (ie, enough to occlude the filter), an aspiration catheter is advanced over the wire first in order to aspirate the column of blood immediately proximal to the filter and minimize the risk of debris being released distally as the filter is recaptured. It is also possible that the retrieval catheter may get stuck within the stent tines especially in the case of open-cell stents. In this case, asking patients to turn their head in either direction or, alternatively, advancing the guide catheter into the stent may allow the retrieval catheter to pass through the stent.

Groin closure

Whenever possible, a closure device is used at the common femoral arteriotomy site to minimize the risk of groin or peritoneal hematoma and reduce the time the patient needs to remain immobile following CAS. If the use of a closure device is not feasible, the groin sheath is kept in place until the patient's partial thromboplastin time is normalized, after which the femoral artery sheath is removed and manual pressure is applied until hemostasis is achieved. The patient is kept on bed rest for 4 hours afterward to minimize the risk of hematoma formation.

Indications and Contraindications

The current Food and Drug Administration (FDA)–approved indications for CAS include patients with either symptomatic (>50% stenosis) or asymptomatic (>80% stenosis) carotid stenosis plus the presence of high-risk features for CEA. These high-risk features involve anatomic factors as well as medical comorbidities and are essentially the same features considered exclusion criteria for surgical intervention in the classic CEA trials (see **Table 1**). However, the Centers for Medicare and Medicaid Services (CMS) have adopted more stringent criteria for approving reimbursement for CAS. Besides the presence of high-risk surgical features, CAS reimbursement is considered for symptomatic patients with a minimal degree of stenosis of 70% and for asymptomatic patients with 80% or greater stenosis and within the context of participation in a clinical trial.[55] The position of the CMS has greatly limited the growth of CAS in the United States.

The contraindications for CAS are basically related to unfavorable vascular anatomy, such as severe vessel tortuosity, presence of acute bends or turns in the carotid artery preventing safe navigation of catheters and devices, presence of a type III aortic arch with severe arch elongation, or presence of atherosclerotic plaque within the aortic arch with a high risk of distal embolization during catheterization maneuvers. It is important to emphasize that CEA and CAS are truly complementary procedures, in which high-risk features for one procedure make the other a very attractive alternative and vice versa (**Fig. 5**).

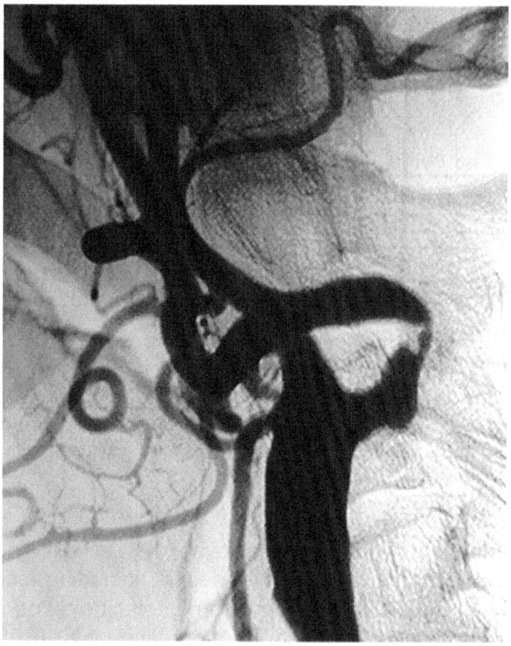

Fig. 5. Example of carotid stenosis not suitable for endovascular treatment. Digital subtraction angiogram, left carotid injection, lateral cervical view, demonstrating severe tortuosity of the cervical internal carotid artery with an ulcerated plaque and high-grade stenosis. The risk associated with carotid stenting in this scenario exceeds that associated with open carotid endarterectomy (see text).

CLINICAL OUTCOMES

The first clinical trial comparing surgical and endovascular treatments for carotid stenosis was the Carotid and Vertebral Transluminal Angioplasty Study, published in 2001.[56] In this trial, 504 patients were randomized to either CEA (n = 253) or endovascular treatment (n = 251, with 26% of patients treated with angioplasty and stent placement and 74% with angioplasty alone). No significant difference was found in the risk of stroke or death between surgical and endovascular treatment arms. The Stenting and Angioplasty with Protection in Patients at High Risk for Endarterectomy (SAPPHIRE) study, published in 2004, randomized 334 patients considered high risk for CEA to either CAS with embolic protection or CEA.[57] Symptomatic patients were required to have 50% or greater stenosis and asymptomatic patients 80% or greater stenosis. The 1-year rates of major adverse events (composite of death, stroke, or MI within 30 days of intervention or death or ipsilateral stroke between day 31 and 1 year) were 20.1% in the CEA group and 12.0% in the CAS group (**Table 2**). Because of these results, CAS performed with the use of an embolic protection device was considered noninferior to CEA and was granted FDA approval for use in high-surgical-risk patients in 2004.

Several European studies attempted to compare CAS with CEA in standard-surgical-risk patients (**Table 3**).[58–60] These trials failed to demonstrate the noninferiority of CAS when

Table 2
SAPPHIRE study: 1-year follow-up results

End Point	CAS (n = 159) (%)	CEA (n = 151) (%)	*P* Value
Death	7.0	12.9	.08
Stroke	5.8	7.7	.52
MI	2.5	8.1	.03
Cranial nerve palsy	0	5.3	.003
Major adverse event	12.0	20.1	.05

From Eller JL, Dumon TM, Sorkin GC, et al. Endovascular advances for extracranial carotid stenosis. Neurosurgery 2014;72:S92–101.

compared with CEA. However, they all suffered from serious limitations in design, including lack of embolic protection requirement, lack of experience by endovascular operators, and lack of statistical power. These trials were important to demonstrate unequivocally the importance of embolic protection and operator training and experience for successful performance of CAS.

The largest study comparing CAS versus CEA among standard-risk surgical patients was the Carotid Revascularization Endarterectomy versus Stenting Trial (CREST), carried out at 117 sites in the United States and Canada and published in 2010 (**Table 4**).[61] A total of 2502 patients was enrolled with both symptomatic (≥50% stenosis by angiography) and asymptomatic (≥60% stenosis by angiography) carotid artery disease and randomized to either CAS (n = 1271) or CEA (n = 1251). Unlike in the European studies described above, embolic protection was required in all cases in the endovascular arm. Furthermore more rigorous credentialing of the endovascular operators was required, with only 52% of interventionists who applied to participate in the study being selected.[62] There was no statistically significant difference between CAS and CEA for the primary end point of death, stroke, or MI, either periprocedurally or during the 4-year follow-up period (CAS 7.2%; CEA 6.8%). When examined separately, minor strokes were more frequent after CAS than CEA (4.1% vs 2.3%), whereas MI was more frequent after CEA than CAS (2.3% vs 1.1%). The impact of MI, either clinically or by biomarkers alone, was found to be more significant than stroke on increasing risk of subsequent mortality.[63] The CREST also demonstrated an association between age and outcome among patients with CAS, with an increased risk of stroke among patients greater than 70 years old undergoing CAS.[61] This trial represents the best estimate of periprocedural complications and long-term outcomes after CAS to date and definitively showed that CAS and CEA are equivalent procedures for standard-risk surgical patients.

Table 3
European trials comparing CAS with CEA in standard-risk surgical patients

Trial	Stroke Rate (CAS vs CEA) (%)	Major Criticism
EVA-3S	9.6 vs 3.9	Lack of interventionist experience, lack of consistent EP
SPACE	6.8 vs 6.3	Lack of consistent EP
ICSS	8.5 vs 5.2	Lack of consistent EP

These trials were considered negative CAS trials; however, they suffered from lack of operator experience, lack of consistent use of embolic protection, and lack of statistical power.

Abbreviations: EP, embolic protection; EVA-3S, Endarterectomy versus Stenting in Patients with Symptomatic Severe Carotid Stenosis; ICSS, International Carotid Stenting Study; SPACE, Stent-Supported Percutaneous Angioplasty of the Carotid Artery versus Endarterectomy.

From Eller JL, Dumon TM, Sorkin GC, et al. Endovascular advances for extracranial carotid stenosis. Neurosurgery 2014;72:S92–101.

Table 4
CREST results

Adverse Events	CAS (%)	CEA (%)	*P* Value
Perioperative stroke	4.1	2.3	.01
Perioperative MI	1.1	2.3	.03
Stroke at 4 y	2.0	2.4	.85

There was no statistical difference between CAS and CEA for the primary end points of death, stroke, and MI. When examined separately, minor strokes were more frequent after CAS and MI was more frequent after CEA.

From Eller JL, Dumon TM, Sorkin GC, et al. Endovascular advances for extracranial carotid stenosis. Neurosurgery 2014;72:S92–101.

COMPLICATIONS AND CONCERNS

Patient selection is the most important factor in minimizing complications associated with CAS.[6] The most feared complication is periprocedural embolic stroke. Our understanding of the importance of embolic protection and the specific risk associated with each step of the stenting procedure greatly minimizes this risk. As extensively discussed earlier, unfavorable anatomic features that are considered potential contraindications for CAS significantly increase the risk of distal cerebral embolization and stroke. Carotid plaque characteristics, such as the presence of soft thrombus, ulcerations, and plaque hemorrhages, may increase the risk of embolic events associated with crossing the lesion with the distal embolic protection microwire, making this a critical step during the procedure and possibly favoring the use of proximal protection instead.

Other potential complications include access site complications (hematomas and/or pseudoaneurysm formation, puncture site infection), acute carotid dissection and/or thrombosis, delayed strokes, and reperfusion hemorrhage. Systemic complications, such as MI, hemodynamic instability with acute postprocedural hypertension or hypotension, and bradycardia, are also possible and should be carefully monitored and treated aggressively.

FOLLOW-UP CONSIDERATIONS

Immediate follow-up after CAS requires neurovascular monitoring in a critical care unit or intermediate care setting for at least 12 to 24 hours. Patients may experience wide variations in their blood pressure and/or heart rate, potentially requiring infusion of vasopressors or antihypertensive agents. After carotid revascularization, especially in critical (>90%) stenosis situations, systolic blood pressure is kept at approximately 60% to 80% of normal to minimize the risk of reperfusion hemorrhage. Routine postprocedural electrocardiogram, complete blood count, electrolytes, and cardiac enzyme levels are checked to detect potential silent myocardial events.

Most patients are discharged home on the first or second postoperative day. Doppler ultrasonography of the stented carotid artery is obtained before discharge to serve as a new baseline for routine follow-up. Patients are subsequently monitored with carotid Doppler studies at 1 month, 6 months, and 1 year after the procedure; if the stent remains patent, yearly studies are performed henceforth. Severe carotid restenosis after successful carotid stenting is a rare phenomenon. Cernetti and colleagues[65] reported a 1.9% incidence of significant restenosis (≥70%) after 24 months of follow-up in 100 consecutive patients with CAS. The greater amount of wall coverage provided by closed-cell stents may be associated with greater potential for intimal hyperplasia and in-stent restenosis, although no clear benefit of one stent over another in terms of restenosis has been definitely established.[66]

SUMMARY

Carotid artery angioplasty and stenting has experienced an astonishing rate of development and technical improvement since its inception. The technique is now well developed, and its indications and potential shortcomings are clearly understood. The benefit of CAS for symptomatic patients considered high risk for surgical intervention is well established and unquestionable. For symptomatic patients with standard surgical risk, CAS and CEA are currently equally effective and their risk profiles are evenly matched, making these procedures complementary. For asymptomatic patients with carotid stenosis, there still remains the question of whether carotid revascularization adds any benefit to aggressive modern medical management. Further technological advances, clinical experience, and the benefit of a minimally invasive procedure are likely to expand the indications and reach of CAS.

DISCLOSURES

Dr J.L. Eller reports no financial relationships. Dr L.N. Hopkins receives grant/research support from Toshiba; serves as a consultant to Abbott, Boston Scientific, Cordis, Micrus, and Silk Road; holds financial interests in AccessClosure, Augmenix, Boston Scientific, Claret Medical, Endomation, Micrus, and Valor Medical; holds a board/trustee/officer position with Access Closure and Claret Medical; serves on Abbott Vascular's speakers' bureau; and has received honoraria from Bard, Boston Scientific, Cleveland Clinic, Complete Conference Management, Cordis, Memorial Health Care System, and the Society for Cardiovascular Angiography and Interventions (SCAI). Dr E.I. Levy receives research grant support, other research support (devices), and honoraria from Boston Scientific and research support from Codman & Shurtleff, Inc and ev3/Covidien Vascular Therapies; has ownership interests in Intratech Medical Ltd and Mynx/Access Closure; serves as a consultant on the board of Scientific Advisors to Codman & Shurtleff, Inc; serves as a consultant per project and/or per hour for Codman & Shurtleff, Inc, ev3/Covidien Vascular Therapies, and TheraSyn Sensors, Inc; and receives fees for carotid stent training from Abbott Vascular and ev3/Covidien Vascular Therapies. Dr E.I. Levy receives no consulting salary arrangements. All consulting is per project and/or per hour. Dr A.H. Siddiqui has received research grants from the National Institutes of Health (coinvestigator: National Institute of Neurological Disorders and Stroke 1R01NS064592-01A1) and the University at Buffalo (Research Development Award) (neither is related to the present submission); holds financial interests in Hotspur, Intratech Medical, StimSox, Valor Medical and Blockade Medical; serves as a consultant to Codman & Shurtleff, Inc, Concentric Medical, Covidien Vascular Therapies, GuidePoint Global Consulting, Penumbra, Inc, Stryker Neurovascular and Pulsar Vascular; belongs to the speakers' bureaus of Codman & Shurtleff, Inc and Genentech; serves on National Steering Committees for Penumbra, Inc 3D Separator Trial and Covidien SWIFT PRIME Trial; serves on an advisory board for Codman & Shurtleff and Covidien Vascular Therapies; and has received honoraria from American Association of Neurological Surgeons' courses, Annual Peripheral Angioplasty and All That Jazz Course, Penumbra, Inc, and from Abbott Vascular and Codman & Shurtleff, Inc for training other neurointerventionists in carotid stenting and for training physicians in endovascular stenting for aneurysms. Dr A.H. Siddiqui receives no consulting salary arrangements. All consulting is per project and/or per hour. Dr K.V. Snyder serves as a consultant and a member of the speakers' bureau for Toshiba and has received honoraria from Toshiba. He serves as a member of the speakers' bureau for and has received honoraria from ev3 and The Stroke Group.

REFERENCES

1. Go AS, Mozaffarian D, Roger VL, et al. Heart disease and stroke statistics–2013 update: a report from the American Heart Association. Circulation 2013;127:e6–245.
2. Kolominsky-Rabas PL, Weber M, Gefeller O, et al. Epidemiology of ischemic stroke subtypes according to TOAST criteria: incidence, recurrence, and long-term survival in ischemic stroke subtypes: a population-based study. Stroke 2001;32: 2735–40.
3. Liapis CD, Bell PR, Mikhailidis D, et al. ESVS guidelines. Invasive treatment for carotid stenosis: indications, techniques. Eur J Vasc Endovasc Surg 2009;37:1–19.
4. Prati P, Vanuzzo D, Casaroli M, et al. Prevalence and determinants of carotid atherosclerosis in a general population. Stroke 1992;23:1705–11.
5. Thompson JE. The evolution of surgery for the treatment and prevention of stroke. The Willis Lecture. Stroke 1996;27:1427–34.
6. DeBakey ME. Successful carotid endarterectomy for cerebrovascular insufficiency. Nineteen-year follow-up. JAMA 1975;233:1083–5.
7. North American Symptomatic Carotid Endarterectomy Trial Collaborators. Beneficial effect of carotid endarterectomy in symptomatic patients with high-grade carotid stenosis. N Engl J Med 1991;325: 445–53.
8. Randomised trial of endarterectomy for recently symptomatic carotid stenosis: final results of the MRC European Carotid Surgery Trial (ECST). Lancet 1998;351:1379–87.
9. Endarterectomy for asymptomatic carotid artery stenosis. Executive Committee for the Asymptomatic Carotid Atherosclerosis Study. JAMA 1995; 273:1421–8.
10. Halliday A, Mansfield A, Marro J, et al. Prevention of disabling and fatal strokes by successful carotid endarterectomy in patients without recent neurological symptoms: randomised controlled trial. Lancet 2004;363:1491–502.
11. Rothwell PM, Eliasziw M, Gutnikov SA, et al. Analysis of pooled data from the randomised controlled trials of endarterectomy for symptomatic carotid stenosis. Lancet 2003;361:107–16.
12. Rothwell PM, Eliasziw M, Gutnikov SA, et al. Endarterectomy for symptomatic carotid stenosis in relation to clinical subgroups and timing of surgery Lancet 2004;363:915–24.
13. Hartmann A, Hupp T, Koch HC, et al. Prospective study on the complication rate of carotid surgery Cerebrovasc Dis 1999;9:152–6.
14. Lin SC, Trocciola SM, Rhee J, et al. Analysis of anatomic factors and age in patients undergoing carotid angioplasty and stenting. Ann Vasc Surg 2005;19:798–804.
15. Lam RC, Lin SC, DeRubertis B, et al. The impact of increasing age on anatomic factors affecting carotid angioplasty and stenting. J Vasc Surg 2007 45:875–80.
16. Madhwal S, Rajagopal V, Bhatt DL, et al. Predictors of difficult carotid stenting as determined by aortic arch angiography. J Invasive Cardiol 2008;20 200–4.
17. Bogousslavsky J, Regli F, Van Melle G. Risk factors and concomitants of internal carotid artery occlusion or stenosis. A controlled study of 159 cases Arch Neurol 1985;42:864–7.
18. Duncan GW, Lees RS, Ojemann RG, et al. Concomitants of atherosclerotic carotid artery stenosis Stroke 1977;8:665–9.
19. Golledge J, Cuming R, Ellis M, et al. Carotid plaque characteristics and presenting symptom. Br J Surg 1997;84:1697–701.
20. Stoll G, Bendszus M. Inflammation and atherosclerosis: novel insights into plaque formation and destabilization. Stroke 2006;37:1923–32.
21. Redgrave JN, Lovett JK, Gallagher PJ, et al. Histological assessment of 526 symptomatic carotid plaques in relation to the nature and timing of ischemic symptoms: the Oxford plaque study. Circulation 2006;113:2320–8.

22. Hirt LS. Progression rate and ipsilateral neurological events in asymptomatic carotid stenosis (doi STROKEAHA.111.613711). Stroke 2014;45(3):702–6.
23. Cooperman M, Martin EW Jr, Evans WE. Significance of asymptomatic carotid bruits. Arch Surg 1978;113:1339–40.
24. Thompson JE, Patman RD, Talkington CM. Asymptomatic carotid bruit: long term outcome of patients having endarterectomy compared with unoperated controls. Ann Surg 1978;188:308–16.
25. Norris JW, Zhu CZ. Silent stroke and carotid stenosis. Stroke 1992;23:483–5.
26. Goessens BM, Visseren FL, Kappelle LJ, et al. Asymptomatic carotid artery stenosis and the risk of new vascular events in patients with manifest arterial disease: the SMART study. Stroke 2007; 38:1470–5.
27. Marquardt L, Geraghty OC, Mehta Z, et al. Low risk of ipsilateral stroke in patients with asymptomatic carotid stenosis on best medical treatment: a prospective, population-based study. Stroke 2010;41: e11–7.
28. Acheson J, Hutchinson EC. Observations on the natural history of transient cerebral ischaemia. Lancet 1964;2:871–4.
29. Baker RN, Ramseyer JC, Schwartz WS. Prognosis in patients with transient cerebral ischemic attacks. Neurology 1968;18:1157–65.
30. Whisnant JP. Epidemiology of stroke: emphasis on transient cerebral ischemia attacks and hypertension. Stroke 1974;5:68–70.
31. Altaf N, Daniels L, Morgan PS, et al. Detection of intraplaque hemorrhage by magnetic resonance imaging in symptomatic patients with mild to moderate carotid stenosis predicts recurrent neurological events. J Vasc Surg 2008;47:337–42.
32. Eliasziw M, Streifler JY, Fox AJ, et al. Significance of plaque ulceration in symptomatic patients with high-grade carotid stenosis. North American Symptomatic Carotid Endarterectomy Trial. Stroke 1994;25:304–8.
33. Altaf N, Goode SD, Beech A, et al. Plaque hemorrhage is a marker of thromboembolic activity in patients with symptomatic carotid disease. Radiology 2011;258:538–45.
34. Qureshi AI, Suri MF, Ali Z, et al. Role of conventional angiography in evaluation of patients with carotid artery stenosis demonstrated by Doppler ultrasound in general practice. Stroke 2001;32: 2287–91.
35. Teitelbaum GP, Larsen DW, Zelman V, et al. A tribute to Dr Fedor A. Serbinenko, founder of endovascular neurosurgery. Neurosurgery 2000;46: 462–70.
36. Mathias KD, Jaeger MJ, Sahl J. Internal carotid stents - PTA: 7-year experience. Cardiovasc Intervent Radiol (Suppl) 1997;20:S46.
37. Kerber CW, Cromwell LD, Loehden OL. Catheter dilatation of proximal carotid stenosis during distal bifurcation endarterectomy. AJNR Am J Neuroradiol 1980;1:348–9.
38. Theron J. My history of carotid angioplasty and stenting. J Invasive Cardiol 2008;20:E102–8.
39. Theron J, Raymond J, Casasco A, et al. Percutaneous angioplasty of atherosclerotic and postsurgical stenosis of carotid arteries. AJNR Am J Neuroradiol 1987;8:495–500.
40. Theron JG, Payelle GG, Coskun O, et al. Carotid artery stenosis: treatment with protected balloon angioplasty and stent placement. Radiology 1996;201:627–36.
41. Serruys PW, de Jaegere P, Kiemeneij F, et al. A comparison of balloon-expandable-stent implantation with balloon angioplasty in patients with coronary artery disease. Benestent Study Group. N Engl J Med 1994;331:489–95.
42. Serruys PW, van Hout B, Bonnier H, et al. Randomised comparison of implantation of heparin-coated stents with balloon angioplasty in selected patients with coronary artery disease (Benestent II). Lancet 1998;352:673–81.
43. Diethrich EB, Ndiaye M, Reid DB. Stenting in the carotid artery: initial experience in 110 patients. J Endovasc Surg 1996;3:42–62.
44. Wholey MH, Wholey M, Bergeron P, et al. Current global status of carotid artery stent placement. Cathet Cardiovasc Diagn 1998;44:1–6.
45. Yadav JS, Roubin GS, King P, et al. Angioplasty and stenting for restenosis after carotid endarterectomy. Initial experience. Stroke 1996;27:2075–9.
46. Eskandari MK. Cerebral embolic protection. Semin Vasc Surg 2005;18:95–100.
47. Whitlow PL, Lylyk P, Londero H, et al. Carotid artery stenting protected with an emboli containment system. Stroke 2002;33:1308–14.
48. Coppi G, Moratto R, Silingardi R, et al. Advancements in the Mo.Ma system procedure during carotid artery stenting. J Cardiovasc Surg (Torino) 2009;50:789–93.
49. Rabe K, Sugita J, Godel H, et al. Flow-reversal device for cerebral protection during carotid artery stenting–acute and long-term results. J Interv Cardiol 2006;19:55–62.
50. Bijuklic K, Wandler A, Hazizi F, et al. The PROFI study (Prevention of Cerebral Embolization by Proximal Balloon Occlusion Compared to Filter Protection During Carotid Artery Stenting): a prospective randomized trial. J Am Coll Cardiol 2012;59: 1383–9.
51. Montorsi P, Caputi L, Galli S, et al. Microembolization during carotid artery stenting in patients with high-risk, lipid-rich plaque. A randomized trial of proximal versus distal cerebral protection. J Am Coll Cardiol 2011;58:1656–63.

52. Nikas DN, Kompara G, Reimers B. Carotid stents: which is the best option? J Cardiovasc Surg (Torino) 2011;52:779–93.
53. Mathur A, Roubin GS, Iyer SS, et al. Predictors of stroke complicating carotid artery stenting. Circulation 1998;97:1239–45.
54. Wong G, Li JM, Hendricks G, et al. Inhibition of experimental neointimal hyperplasia by recombinant human thrombomodulin coated ePTFE stent grafts. J Vasc Surg 2008;47:608–15.
55. Siddiqui AH, Natarajan SK, Hopkins LN, et al. Carotid artery stenting for primary and secondary stroke prevention. World Neurosurgery 2011;76:S40–59.
56. Endovascular versus surgical treatment in patients with carotid stenosis in the Carotid and Vertebral Artery Transluminal Angioplasty Study (CAVATAS): a randomised trial. Lancet 2001;357:1729–37.
57. Yadav JS, Wholey MH, Kuntz RE, et al. Protected carotid-artery stenting versus endarterectomy in high-risk patients. N Engl J Med 2004;351:1493–501.
58. Mas JL, Chatellier G, Beyssen B, et al. Endarterectomy versus stenting in patients with symptomatic severe carotid stenosis. N Engl J Med 2006;355:1660–71.
59. Ringleb PA, Allenberg J, Bruckmann H, et al. 30 day results from the SPACE trial of stent-protected angioplasty versus carotid endarterectomy in symptomatic patients: a randomised non-inferiority trial. Lancet 2006;368:1239–47.
60. Ederle J, Dobson J, Featherstone RL, et al. Carotid artery stenting compared with endarterectomy in patients with symptomatic carotid stenosis (International Carotid Stenting Study): an interim analysis of a randomised controlled trial. Lancet 2010;375:985–97.
61. Brott TG, Hobson RW 2nd, Howard G, et al. Stenting versus endarterectomy for treatment of carotid-artery stenosis. N Engl J Med 2010;363:11–23.
62. Cutlip DE, Pinto DS. Extracranial carotid disease revascularization. Circulation 2012;126:2636–44.
63. Blackshear JL, Cutlip DE, Roubin GS, et al. Myocardial infarction after carotid stenting and endarterectomy: results from the carotid revascularization endarterectomy versus stenting trial. Circulation 2011;123:2571–8.
64. Goldstein LB, Samsa GP, Matchar DB, et al. Multicenter review of preoperative risk factors for endarterectomy for asymptomatic carotid artery stenosis. Stroke 1998;29:750–3.
65. Cernetti C, Reimers B, Picciolo A, et al. Carotid artery stenting with cerebral protection in 100 consecutive patients: immediate and two-year follow-up results. Ital Heart J 2003;4:695–700.
66. Muller-Hulsbeck S, Preuss H, Elhoft H. CAS: which stent for which lesion. J Cardiovasc Surg 2009;50:767–72.

Endovascular Management and Treatment of Acute Ischemic Stroke

Maxim Mokin, MD, PhD[a,b],
Kenneth V. Snyder, MD, PhD[a,b,c,d,e],
Adnan H. Siddiqui, MD, PhD[a,b,d,e,f],
L. Nelson Hopkins, MD[a,b,d,e,f], Elad I. Levy, MD, MBA[a,b,d,e,*]

KEYWORDS

• Acute ischemic stroke • Endovascular intervention • Intra-arterial therapy • Large vessel occlusion • Stentriever • Thrombectomy

KEY POINTS

- Endovascular therapy should be reserved for acute strokes with large vessel occlusion confirmed by noninvasive imaging (computed tomographic [CT] angiography or magnetic resonance angiography) or catheter angiography.
- Advanced perfusion imaging helps identify patients with a favorable penumbra/ischemic core mismatch irrespective of the time of onset of stroke symptom.
- Stentrievers lead to higher recanalization rates and improved long-term clinical outcomes in patients with stroke, compared with early mechanical thrombectomy approaches.
- Enrollment of eligible patients into clinical endovascular stroke trials is critical for better understanding of the role of endovascular interventions in the treatment of acute stroke.

Videos of Solitaire Deployment and Solitaire Withdrawal accompany this article at http://www.neurosurgery.theclinics.com/

INTRODUCTION

Each year approximately 795,000 Americans experience a new or recurrent stroke.[1] Ischemic stroke is by far the dominant stroke type, affecting 87% of all patients (the remaining 13% of strokes are caused by intracerebral and subarachnoid hemorrhages). At present, only 3% to 4% of patients with acute ischemic stroke are treated with systemic intravenous (IV) thrombolysis with recombinant tissue plasminogen activator (rt-PA).[2,3] Barriers to receiving IV thrombolysis

Disclosure Statement: See last page of article.

[a] Department of Neurosurgery, School of Medicine and Biomedical Sciences, University at Buffalo, State University of New York, Buffalo, NY, USA; [b] Department of Neurosurgery, Gates Vascular Institute, Kaleida Health, Buffalo, NY, USA; [c] Department of Neurology, School of Medicine and Biomedical Sciences, University at Buffalo, State University of New York, Buffalo, NY, USA; [d] Department of Radiology, School of Medicine and Biomedical Sciences, University at Buffalo, State University of New York, Buffalo, NY, USA; [e] Toshiba Stroke and Vascular Research Center, School of Medicine and Biomedical Sciences, University at Buffalo, State University of New York, Buffalo, NY, USA; [f] Jacobs Institute, Buffalo, NY, USA
* Corresponding author. University at Buffalo Neurosurgery, 100 High Street, Suite B4, Buffalo, NY 14203.
E-mail address: elevy@ubns.com

Neurosurg Clin N Am 25 (2014) 583–592
http://dx.doi.org/10.1016/j.nec.2014.04.013
1042-3680/14/$ – see front matter

Abbreviations and acronyms

ASPECTS	Alberta Stroke Program Early CT Score
CT	Computed tomography
IA	Intra-arterial
ICA	Internal carotid artery
IMS	Interventional Management of Stroke
IV	Intravenous
MCA	Middle cerebral artery
MR RESCUE	Mechanical Retrieval and Recanalization of Stroke Clots Using Embolectomy
NIHSS	National Institutes of Health Stroke Scale
Rt-PA	Recombinant tissue plasminogen activator
SWIFT	Solitaire with the Intention for Thrombectomy
SWIFT PRIME	Solitaire FR with the Intention for Thrombectomy as Primary Endovascular Treatment for Acute Ischemic Stroke
SYNTHESIS Expansion	Synthesis Expansion: A Randomized Controlled Trial on Intra-Arterial versus Intravenous Thrombolysis in Acute Ischemic Stroke
THERAPY	Assess the Penumbra System in the Treatment of Acute Stroke
TICI	Thrombolysis in cerebral infarction
TREVO 2	Thrombectomy Revascularization of Large Vessel Occlusions in Acute Ischemic Stroke

include the public's lack of knowledge of stroke symptoms; delay in recognizing stroke symptoms, seeking medical attention, and hospital arrival; as well as multiple contraindications to systemic administration of rt-PA.[2,4,5]

Endovascular intra-arterial (IA) therapy is reserved for strokes from large vessel occlusion. Data from academic medical centers in the United States and Canada show that large vessel occlusion is responsible for 29% to 46% of ischemic strokes and is associated with a higher National Institutes of Health Stroke Scale (NIHSS) score, 4-fold increase in mortality, and worse neurologic outcome than other types of ischemic strokes.[6–9]

According to previously published population- and epidemiology-based stroke studies, an estimated 4% to 14% of acute stroke cases (corresponding to 25,000–95,000 patients with stroke) may be eligible for endovascular stroke therapy.[8] At present, approximately 14,000 patients undergo IA stroke interventions in the United States.[8] The rapid evolution of endovascular stroke therapies has led to the ability to achieve successful recanalization with newer devices. The introduction of stent retriever (stentriever) technology to the arsenal of stroke neurointerventionists has led to improved clinical outcomes, making stentrievers the dominating modern thrombectomy device.[10,11]

Nevertheless, the efficacy of endovascular therapy against systemic thrombolysis or standard medical therapy has yet to be proved. In recent randomized trials of IA stroke interventions that included mostly early-generation thrombectomy devices, clinical outcomes were similar between endovascular and traditional approaches to stroke treatment.[12–14]

This article provides an overview of the current status of endovascular stroke interventions. The role of clot properties and advanced perfusion imaging in determining eligibility for endovascular treatment is discussed. Currently available revascularization devices and their technical characteristics are discussed. Finally, an update on ongoing and future trials of endovascular stroke therapies is provided.

SELECTION OF PATIENTS FOR ENDOVASCULAR THERAPY

Defining the Optimal Time Window for Intervention

At present, there are 4 thrombectomy devices approved by the Food and Drug Administration under 510(k) clearance for recanalization of cerebral vessels in patients with acute ischemic stroke – the Merci Retrieval System (Concentric Medical, Mountain View, CA, USA), the Penumbra system (Penumbra Inc, Alameda, CA, USA), the Solitaire FR stentriever (ev3/Covidien Vascular Therapies, Irvine, CA, USA), and the Trevo ProVue stentriever (Stryker, Kalamazoo, MI, USA). All these devices were tested in corresponding trials that enrolled patients presenting within 8 hours of symptom onset.

Widespread use of advanced physiologic perfusion imaging technology now challenges this strict time-based selection approach. A multicenter retrospective study of 247 patients treated with endovascular therapy based on CT perfusion imaging findings, regardless of the time from stroke symptom onset, showed that IA revascularization can be safe and effective beyond the 8-h time limit in a carefully selected population.[15] The rates of functional outcome and symptomatic intracerebral hemorrhage were similar in strokes within and beyond 8 hours from symptom onset to endovascular procedure.

Recent polling results of vascular neurologists and neurointerventionists showed a strong preference toward the use of advanced imaging in patient selection for endovascular therapy.[16] More than two-thirds (73%) of the responders supported IA stroke interventions beyond 8 hours, and there was unanimous agreement that time-based patient selection alone is no longer the accepted standard.

Role of Noncontrast CT and Magnetic Resonance Imaging

In the initial endovascular stroke trials, noncontrast CT and magnetic resonance imaging findings were used to identify patients with early extensive strokes who would be unlikely to benefit from revascularization. Key exclusion criteria were the presence of significant mass effect with midline shift, infarction in more than one-third of the middle cerebral artery (MCA) territory, or a large infarction (>100 mL of tissue) in other vascular territories (**Box 1**).[10,11,17,18]

The Alberta Stroke Program Early CT Score (ASPECTS) can be applied to identify early ischemic changes on noncontrast CT scans using a 10-point scoring system.[19] MCA areas with hypoattenuation or effacement of cortical sulci (10 areas total) are assigned a score of 0, and an overall low ASPECTS represents more extensive ischemia.

The application of ASPECTS to baseline noncontrast CT scans of patients enrolled in the Penumbra Pivotal Stroke Trial confirmed the validity of this score to identify patients who can benefit from endovascular therapy.[20] Patients with an ASPECTS less than or equal to 4 showed no benefit from aspiration thrombectomy with the Penumbra system, whereas an ASPECTS greater than 7 was associated with the most benefit from revascularization.

The prognostic value of ASPECTS in the Interventional Management of Stroke (IMS) III trial (which compared combined IV thrombolysis plus IA revascularization with IV thrombolysis alone) confirmed its strong prognostic value.[21] Patients with an ASPECTS of 8 to 10 were almost twice as likely to achieve a favorable outcome at 3 months than those with a lower score.

Box 1
Noncontrast CT- and magnetic resonance imaging-based exclusion criteria for endovascular therapy

- Intracranial hemorrhage
- Significant mass effect with midline shift
- Infarction in more than one-third of the middle cerebral artery territory
- Infarction of greater than 50 to 100 mL of tissue (threshold depends on clinical trial or operator decision)
- ASPECTS less than 8

Abbreviation: ASPECTS, Alberta Stroke Program Early CT Score.

Perfusion Imaging

Several CT and magnetic resonance perfusion techniques have been proposed to distinguish the infarct core from the penumbra (brain tissue at risk of infarction but potentially salvageable with restoration of blood flow), each using different algorithms and perfusion maps, definitions of perfusion mismatch, and processing software packages.[22–26] At present, there is no uniformly accepted perfusion protocol to quantify the extent of ischemic core and penumbra when screening potential candidates for endovascular therapy.

Perfusion-based patient selection is currently the subject of several ongoing stroke trials (**Table 1**). The Perfusion Imaging Selection of Ischemic Stroke Patients for Endovascular Therapy (POSITIVE) trial is testing the efficacy of modern endovascular thrombectomy devices within an extended time window (0–12 hours from stroke onset) by using advanced physiologic imaging. The Solitaire FR with the Intention for Thrombectomy as Primary Endovascular Treatment for Acute Ischemic Stroke (SWIFT PRIME) trial is currently testing the efficacy of IV rt-PA therapy plus Solitaire FR stentriever thrombectomy and uses CT perfusion or diffusion-weighted imaging/perfusion-weighted imaging as one of the selection criteria.

In the Mechanical Retrieval and Recanalization of Stroke Clots Using Embolectomy (MR RESCUE) trial, perfusion-based endovascular treatment with the Merci and Penumbra systems was compared with standard medical therapy.[13] Patients were randomized for treatment within 8 hours of stroke onset after a stratification process that was based on the presence of a favorable penumbral pattern (small core and large penumbra) or an unfavorable penumbral pattern (large core and small penumbra). The study was criticized for defining an infarct core as large as 90 mL as a favorable penumbra threshold.[27]

Other studies showed that higher infarct volume is associated with less-favorable outcomes and that an infarct core exceeding 70 mL is strongly predictive of poor neurologic outcome and an

Table 1
Endovascular clinical trials incorporating advanced perfusion imaging

Trial	Goal and Design	Key Perfusion-Based Selection Criteria
SWIFT PRIME Clinicaltrials.gov identifier: NCT01657461	Compares combined IV rt-PA and Solitaire FR thrombectomy approach to IV rt-PA thrombolysis alone in patients with MCA M1 or ICA terminus occlusion	CT- or MRI-assessed infarct core should be <50 mL Ischemic penumbra should be >15 mL and mismatch ratio ≥1.8 Treatment should be started within 90 min of obtaining the perfusion study
POSITIVE Clinicaltrials.gov identifier: NCT01852201	Compares IV rt-PA-ineligible patients presenting with either wake-up stroke or within 0–12 h of symptom onset and treated with traditional endovascular therapies (at the discretion of the neurointerventionist) vs medical therapy	CT or MR perfusion imaging per the institution standard At least 50% volume of tissue at risk and infarct core ≤35 mL
REVASCAT Clinicaltrials.gov identifier: NCT01692379	Compares thrombectomy with Solitaire FR stentriever to medical therapy (standard-of-care medical therapy, including IV rt-PA) in patients with ICA or MCA M1 occlusion in patients presenting within 0–8 h of symptom onset	If stroke onset is beyond 4.5 h, favorable ASPECTS must be evaluated by CT perfusion or DWI-MRI

Abbreviations: DWI, diffusion-weighted imaging; ICA, internal carotid artery; MR, magnetic resonance; MRI, magnetic resonance imaging; POSITIVE, Perfusion Imaging Selection of Ischemic Stroke Patients for Endovascular Therapy; REVASCAT, Randomized Trial of Revascularization with Solitaire FR Device versus Best Medical Therapy in the Treatment of Acute Stroke due to Anterior Circulation Large Vessel Occlusion Presenting Within 8 hours of Symptom Onset; SWIFT PRIME, Solitaire FR with the Intention for Thrombectomy as Primary Endovascular Treatment for Acute Ischemic Stroke.

increased chance of hemorrhagic transformation in patients treated with IV thrombolysis or IA revascularization.[28–30] In the MR RESCUE trial, near-complete or complete reperfusion (Thrombolysis in Cerebral Infarction [TICI] grade 2b–3) was achieved in only 27% of patients who received IA interventions and similar clinical outcomes were seen in patients irrespective of the penumbral pattern on perfusion imaging.[13]

Modern stentriever technology, which is discussed later in this article, allows higher rates of recanalization and reperfusion than were seen in MR RESCUE. In the ongoing SWIFT PRIME trial of the Solitaire FR stentriever in acute stroke, the core infarct threshold is set at 50 mL to ensure selection of patients who may receive maximal benefit from IA therapy.

Defining IV Thrombolysis Failure

IA interventions are often considered in patients with stroke with large vessel occlusion and high NIHSS score who are eligible for and receive IV rt-PA. It is still debatable whether one can reliably predict whether a patient with stroke will have a favorable clinical outcome after IV thrombolysis or become an rt-PA-nonresponder and remain with long-term neurologic deficits.[31] In the commonly cited National Institute of Neurological Disorders and Stroke IV rt-PA study, although no difference was seen in NIHSS score improvement between the control and IV thrombolysis arms in the first 24 hours, there was a clear benefit of IV rt-PA in lowering mortality and improving functional outcomes at 3 months.[32] However, this original study of IV thrombolysis included strokes due to different causes and its findings do not directly reflect the efficacy of IV rt-PA for large vessel occlusion. Location of the occlusion, clot characteristics on CT imaging and lack of immediate clinical improvement should all be taken into account when identifying patients who are unlikely to benefit from IV thrombolysis alone.[31]

Occlusion Location and IV Thrombolysis

When estimating the likelihood of thrombolysis success with IV rt-PA, determination of the presence and the anatomic location of the large vessel occlusion is extremely important (**Box 2**). In a multicenter study examining the likelihood of recanalization with IV rt-PA using transcranial Doppler imaging, dramatic recovery (measured as NIHSS score ≤2 at 24 hours) was seen in 33% of patients with M2 MCA occlusion and in 16% of patients with M1 MCA occlusion.[33] None of the patients with an occlusion located at the internal carotid artery (ICA) terminus demonstrated such rapid improvement in stroke symptoms.

Similarly, successful long-term recovery can be predicted by identifying an occlusion of a smaller-diameter intracranial vessel. In the same multicenter study, more than half of the patients (52%) with M2 MCA occlusion achieved a modified Rankin Scale score of 2 or less at 3 months, whereas only 25% with M1 MCA occlusion and 18% with ICA terminus occlusion had a good long-term recovery.

Clot Characteristics

A hyperdense MCA sign is a well-described marker of acute thrombotic occlusion, and thin-slice noncontrast CT reconstructions can be used to accurately measure the length of the MCA clot.[34–36] In acute MCA stroke, clot length exceeding 8 mm has a very low chance of successful recanalization with IV rt-PA alone.[37] This observation is the key selection criterion for the Assess the Penumbra System in the Treatment of Acute Stroke (THERAPY) trial, which is evaluating the Penumbra system in anterior circulation stroke with a clot length of 8 mm or longer (Clinicaltrials.gov identifier NCT01429350).

Another important clot characteristic is its density, which is reflective of its fibrin, erythrocyte, and white blood cell contents.[38] Clot density is measured on noncontrast CT with Hounsfield unit values and can also predict early revascularization with IV rt-PA.[39] At present, there are no consistent data regarding the value of Hounsfield unit as a marker of successful revascularization with endovascular therapies, and Hounsfield unit measurements are not a part of any current trial selection criteria (see **Box 2**). Lower clot density (measured by Hounsfield unit values) has been shown to predict failure of the Merci and Penumbra systems in achieving successful recanalization.[40,41] However, such predictive value for thrombus quantification was not confirmed in a different study in which cases were treated with the Penumbra system or first-generation stentrievers.[42] The authors' data from 41 patients with anterior circulation stroke treated with the Solitaire stent retriever as the primary treatment device demonstrate that higher thrombus Hounsfield unit values predict successful recanalization (Mokin and colleagues, unpublished communication, 2013).

Box 2
Important thrombus properties to consider in selecting patients for endovascular interventions

- Location of occlusion: proximal middle cerebral artery, intracranial internal carotid artery, basilar artery, vertebral artery
- Density: presence of hyperdense middle cerebral artery or internal carotid artery sign, Hounsfield unit value
- Thrombus length greater than 8 mm

AVAILABLE ENDOVASCULAR APPROACHES AND DEVICES

A wide range of endovascular devices specifically designed for the treatment of large vessel occlusion in stroke is currently available. In an analysis of 13 prospective trials of acute stroke therapy published since 1995, a progressive improvement in the ability of newer devices to achieve revascularization was demonstrated.[43] Stentrievers are recommended over the Merci retriever as the first-line mechanical thrombectomy approach based on the acute stroke management guidelines published by the American Heart Association-American Stroke Association in 2013.[44] The guidelines acknowledge that presently there are no data to directly compare the effectiveness of aspiration thrombectomy with the Penumbra system versus that with stentrievers.

Stentrievers

Two stentriever devices currently available on the US market are the Trevo ProVue stentriever and the Solitaire FR stentriever. The Trevo ProVue is the next-generation version of the original Trevo device with improved visibility of the stent struts under direct fluoroscopy (**Fig. 1**). This device comes in one standard size with a 4 × 20-mm active retrieval area and tapered ends. The Solitaire FR is available in various diameters (4 and 6 mm) and lengths (15, 20, and 30 mm), and the proper size is selected based on the extent of the clot and the diameter of the affected vessel.

Stentrievers act by crossing the thrombus in a constrained form while inside the microcatheter

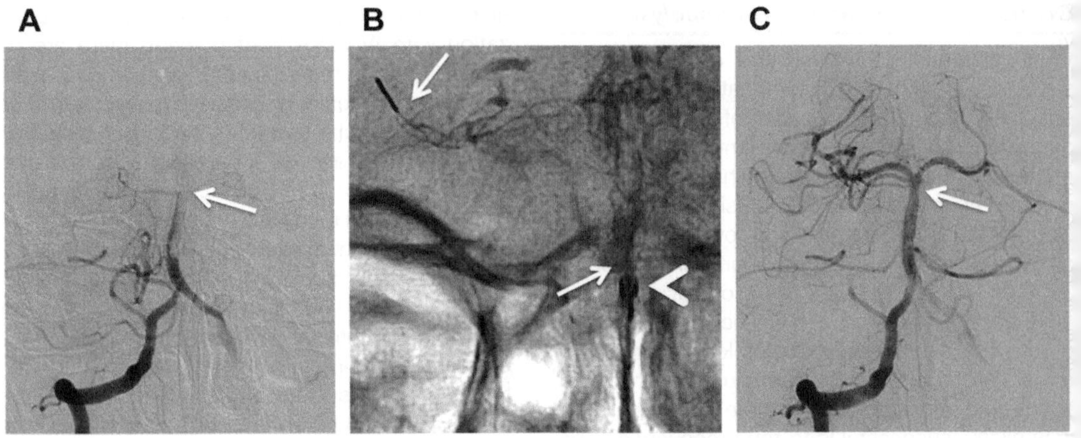

Fig. 1. Trevo. (*A*) Cerebral angiography, anteroposterior view; right vertebral artery injection showing occlusion of the basilar artery (*arrow*) in a patient with acute stroke. (*B*) Cerebral angiography, higher magnification, showing Trevo ProVue stentriever deployed within the proximal right posterior cerebral artery and the distal half of the basilar artery. Arrows point to the proximal and distal ends of the device. Arrowhead shows the location of a large-bore distal access catheter within the basilar artery. (*C*) After withdrawal of the stentriever under continuous aspiration through the intermediate catheter, complete revascularization is achieved. Arrow indicates the original location of the occlusion.

and then apposing the clot against the wall of the vessel when deployed (Video 1 available online at http://www.neurosurgery.theclinics.com/). This process causes the clot to become incorporated into the stent struts, and both the clot and the stentriever are withdrawn into the guide or intermediate catheter (Video 2 available online at http://www.neurosurgery.theclinics.com/).

Stentriever trials

The Solitaire with the Intention for Thrombectomy (SWIFT) trial evaluated the efficacy of the Solitaire FR stentriever, and the Thrombectomy Revascularization of Large Vessel Occlusions in Acute Ischemic Stroke (TREVO 2) trial tested the Trevo device.[10,11] Both trials had a similar design: they enrolled patients with confirmed large vessel occlusion strokes within 8 hours of symptom onset and randomized them in a 1:1 ratio to mechanical thrombectomy with the Merci device or to a stentriever. Three thrombectomy attempts were allowed in SWIFT, whereas up to 6 attempts could be performed in TREVO 2.

The main primary end point was Thrombolysis in Myocardial Infarction score 2 to 3 in the SWIFT trial and TICI score of 2 to 3 in the TREVO 2 trial, achieved without any rescue treatments. In both trials, significantly higher recanalization rates were seen with stentrievers than with the Merci – 86% of cases treated with the Trevo and 61% of cases in which the Solitaire FR was used reached the primary end point. Success rates with Merci thrombectomy were only 60% in TREVO 2 and 24% in SWIFT.

Both trials demonstrated greater ability of stentrievers to lead to favorable long-term clinical outcomes than early-generation thrombectomy devices, again confirming a strong association between angiographically confirmed recanalization and clinical outcomes in acute stroke.[45] The absolute difference in good functional outcome at 3 months was 18% in TREVO 2 and 25% in SWIFT, in favor of stentrievers.

Stentrievers in clinical practice

Several registries and retrospective studies conducted in Europe and North America tested the efficacy and safety of stentrievers in clinical practice outside the SWIFT and TREVO 2 trials.[46–50] Recanalization results and clinical outcomes achieved were similar to those seen in SWIFT and TREVO 2, supporting the value of stentrievers for acute stroke treatment. These studies showed that in modern clinical practice, a variety of adjunct devices are used in combination with stentrievers in an attempt to achieve maximal reperfusion and reduce the chance of distal embolization. Such a multimodal approach most commonly includes the use of balloon guide catheters and proximal aspiration through a distal access catheter while withdrawing a stentriever.[46,47,51]

In the IMS III trial, in which IV thrombolysis alone was compared with the combined bridging approach (IV thrombolysis plus IA intervention) stentrievers were used in only 5 of 334 patients who were randomized to the interventional arm.[12] In another recent randomized clinical trial of endovascular therapy, Synthesis Expansion: A

Randomized Controlled Trial on Intra-Arterial versus Intravenous Thrombolysis in Acute Ischemic Stroke (SYNTHESIS Expansion), of 181 cases treated with the IA approach stentrievers were used in only 23 cases.[14] These trials failed to show any significant benefit of the IA approach and were criticized by the neurointerventional community for not targeting the appropriate population of patients, for using outdated thrombectomy devices, and for failing to include rapidly evolving noninvasive stroke imaging and more successful novel revascularization technologies, such as stentrievers.[52–56]

Aspiration Thrombectomy

Aspiration thrombectomy is another popular approach to IA revascularization. This approach is used in clinical practice with several variations, ranging from primary aspiration thrombectomy alone to a combined aspiration plus stentriever approach. Aspiration thrombectomy with the Penumbra aspiration system in its traditional form uses a series of separators and continuous aspiration via a large-bore catheter, which was tested in the Penumbra Pivotal Stroke trial.[18]

A next-generation separator, the 3D separator (Penumbra Inc), has a unique design. Although it shares some properties with traditional stentrievers, it has a distinct geometry, with multiple connections of stent struts creating separate chambers within the device. The 3D separator is already approved in Europe for revascularization of large vessel occlusion in acute ischemic stroke and is being tested at present in the United States (Clinicaltrials.gov identifier NCT01584609).

In primary aspiration thrombectomy, a large-bore catheter is delivered directly next to the thrombus and continuous or pulse aspiration is applied to extract the clot.[57] Cost-effectiveness and simplicity of this approach have made this variation of aspiration thrombectomy quite popular among neurointerventionists.

SUMMARY

Endovascular stroke trials have advanced to a next step whereby a variety of available IA revascularization therapies labeled together as endovascular treatment are being compared with other treatment options, such as IV thrombolysis or medical management with antithrombotic medications. Accurate comparison of such treatments can and should be pursued to establish the value and role of IA interventions in acute stroke.

However, because the interventional stroke field evolves rapidly, with new devices emerging every year, this is a challenging task. Improved clinical outcomes are seen in strokes treated with next-generation devices, such as stentrievers. A clinical trial conducted over a 5-year or even a longer period might be acceptable in a more conservative medical field but is not acceptable to test technological advances, which are likely to become obsolete. Recent randomized trials of endovascular versus medical therapy for stroke are important milestones for the neurointerventional field and have provided us with valuable information about which patients should and, more importantly, which patients should *not* be considered for endovascular interventions. Lessons learned from these trials should be applied to continue advancing the field with the ultimate goal of discovering more effective ways to treat ischemic stroke.

DISCLOSURE STATEMENT

Dr L.N. Hopkins receives grant/research support from Toshiba; serves as a consultant to Abbott, Boston Scientific, Cordis, Micrus, and Silk Road; holds financial interests in AccessClosure, Augmenix, Boston Scientific, Claret Medical, Endomation, Micrus, and Valor Medical; holds a board/trustee/officer position with Access Closure and Claret Medical; serves on Abbott Vascular's speakers' bureau; and has received honoraria from BARD, Boston Scientific, Cleveland Center, Complete Conference Management, Cordis, Memorial Health Care System, and the Society for Cardiovascular Angiography and Interventions (SCAI). Dr E.I. Levy receives research grant support, other research support (devices), and honoraria from Boston Scientific and research support from Codman & Shurtleff, Inc and ev3/Covidien Vascular Therapies; has ownership interests in Intratech Medical Ltd and Mynx/Access Closure; serves as a consultant on the board of Scientific Advisors to Codman & Shurtleff, Inc; serves as a consultant per project and/or per hour for Codman & Shurtleff, Inc, ev3/Covidien Vascular Therapies, and TheraSyn Sensors, Inc; and receives fees for carotid stent training from Abbott Vascular and ev3/Covidien Vascular Therapies. Dr E.I. Levy receives no consulting salary arrangements. All consulting is per project and/or per hour. Dr M. Mokin has received an educational grant from Toshiba. Dr A.H. Siddiqui has received research grants from the National Institutes of Health (coinvestigator: NINDS 1R01NS064592-01A1) and the University at Buffalo (Research Development Award) (neither is related to the present submission); holds financial interests in Hotspur, Intratech Medical, StimSox, Valor Medical, and Blockade Medical; serves as a consultant to Codman &

Shurtleff, Inc, Concentric Medical, Covidien Vascular Therapies, GuidePoint Global Consulting, Penumbra, Inc, Stryker Neurovascular, and Pulsar Vascular; belongs to the speakers' bureaus of Codman & Shurtleff, Inc and Genentech; serves on National Steering Committees for Penumbra, Inc 3D Separator trial and Covidien SWIFT PRIME trial; serves on the advisory board for Codman & Shurtleff and Covidien Vascular Therapies; and has received honoraria from American Association of Neurologic Surgeons' courses, Annual Peripheral Angioplasty, and All That Jazz Course, Penumbra, Inc, and from Abbott Vascular and Codman & Shurtleff, Inc. for training other neurointerventionists in carotid stenting and for training physicians in endovascular stenting for aneurysms. Dr A.H. Siddiqui receives no consulting salary arrangements. All consulting is per project and/or per hour. Dr K.V. Snyder serves as a consultant and a member of the speakers' bureau for Toshiba and has received honoraria from Toshiba. He serves as a member of the speakers' bureau for and has received honoraria from ev3 and The Stroke Group.

SUPPLEMENTARY DATA

Supplementary data related to this article can be found online at http://dx.doi.org/10.1016/j.nec.2014.04.013.

REFERENCES

1. Go AS, Mozaffarian D, Roger VL, et al. Heart disease and stroke statistics–2014 update: a report from the American Heart Association. Circulation 2014;129(3):e28–292.
2. California Acute Stroke Pilot Registry Investigators. Prioritizing interventions to improve rates of thrombolysis for ischemic stroke. Neurology 2005;64:654–9.
3. Hassan AE, Chaudhry SA, Grigoryan M, et al. National trends in utilization and outcomes of endovascular treatment of acute ischemic stroke patients in the mechanical thrombectomy era. Stroke 2012;43:3012–7.
4. Centers for Disease Control Prevention (CDC). Prehospital and hospital delays after stroke onset–United States, 2005-2006. MMWR Morb Mortal Wkly Rep 2007;56:474–8.
5. Bouckaert M, Lemmens R, Thijs V. Reducing prehospital delay in acute stroke. Nat Rev Neurol 2009;5:477–83.
6. Smith WS, Lev MH, English JD, et al. Significance of large vessel intracranial occlusion causing acute ischemic stroke and TIA. Stroke 2009;40:3834–40.
7. Smith WS, Tsao JW, Billings ME, et al. Prognostic significance of angiographically confirmed large vessel intracranial occlusion in patients presenting with acute brain ischemia. Neurocrit Care 2006;4 14–7.
8. Zaidat OO, Lazzaro M, McGinley E, et al. Demand-supply of neurointerventionalists for endovascular ischemic stroke therapy. Neurology 2012;79:S35–41.
9. Bhatia R, Hill MD, Shobha N, et al. Low rates of acute recanalization with intravenous recombinant tissue plasminogen activator in ischemic stroke real-world experience and a call for action. Stroke 2010;41:2254–8.
10. Nogueira RG, Lutsep HL, Gupta R, et al. Trevo versus Merci retrievers for thrombectomy revascularisation of large vessel occlusions in acute ischaemic stroke (TREVO 2): a randomised trial Lancet 2012;380:1231–40.
11. Saver JL, Jahan R, Levy EI, et al. Solitaire flow restoration device versus the Merci Retriever in patients with acute ischaemic stroke (SWIFT): a randomised, parallel-group, non-inferiority trial. Lancet 2012;380:1241–9.
12. Broderick JP, Palesch YY, Demchuk AM, et al. Endovascular therapy after intravenous t-PA versus t-PA alone for stroke. N Engl J Med 2013;368 893–903.
13. Kidwell CS, Jahan R, Gornbein J, et al. A trial of imaging selection and endovascular treatment for ischemic stroke. N Engl J Med 2013;368:914–23.
14. Ciccone A, Valvassori L, Nichelatti M, et al. Endovascular treatment for acute ischemic stroke N Engl J Med 2013;368:904–13.
15. Turk AS, Magarick JA, Frei D, et al. CT perfusion guided patient selection for endovascular recanalization in acute ischemic stroke: a multicenter study. J Neurointerv Surg 2013;5:523–7.
16. Nguyen TN, Zaidat OO, Edgell RC, et al. Vascular neurologists and neurointerventionalists on endovascular stroke care: polling results. Neurology 2012;79:S5–15.
17. Smith WS, Sung G, Starkman S, et al. Safety and efficacy of mechanical embolectomy in acute ischemic stroke: results of the MERCI trial. Stroke 2005;36:1432–8.
18. Penumbra Pivotal Stroke Trial Investigators. The penumbra pivotal stroke trial: safety and effectiveness of a new generation of mechanical devices for clot removal in intracranial large vessel occlusive disease. Stroke 2009;40:2761–8.
19. Barber PA, Demchuk AM, Zhang J, et al. Validity and reliability of a quantitative computed tomography score in predicting outcome of hyperacute stroke before thrombolytic therapy. ASPECTS Study Group. Alberta Stroke Programme Early CT Score. Lancet 2000;355:1670–4.

20. Goyal M, Menon BK, Coutts SB, et al. Effect of baseline CT scan appearance and time to recanalization on clinical outcomes in endovascular thrombectomy of acute ischemic strokes. Stroke 2011;42:93–7.
21. Hill MD, Demchuk AM, Goyal M, et al. Alberta stroke program early computed tomography score to select patients for endovascular treatment: interventional management of stroke (IMS)-III trial. Stroke 2014;45(2):444–9.
22. Kidwell CS, Wintermark M, De Silva DA, et al. Multiparametric MRI and CT models of infarct core and favorable penumbral imaging patterns in acute ischemic stroke. Stroke 2013;44:73–9.
23. Fahmi F, Marquering HA, Streekstra GJ, et al. Differences in CT perfusion summary maps for patients with acute ischemic stroke generated by 2 software packages. AJNR Am J Neuroradiol 2012;33:2074–80.
24. Campbell BC, Christensen S, Levi CR, et al. Cerebral blood flow is the optimal CT perfusion parameter for assessing infarct core. Stroke 2011;42:3435–40.
25. Dani KA, Thomas RG, Chappell FM, et al. Computed tomography and magnetic resonance perfusion imaging in ischemic stroke: definitions and thresholds. Ann Neurol 2011;70:384–401.
26. Gonzalez RG. Current state of acute stroke imaging. Stroke 2013;44:3260–4.
27. Morais LT, Leslie-Mazwi TM, Lev MH, et al. Imaging-based selection for intra-arterial stroke therapies. J Neurointerv Surg 2013;5(Suppl 1):i13–20.
28. Sanak D, Nosal V, Horak D, et al. Impact of diffusion-weighted MRI-measured initial cerebral infarction volume on clinical outcome in acute stroke patients with middle cerebral artery occlusion treated by thrombolysis. Neuroradiology 2006;48:632–9.
29. Olivot JM, Mosimann PJ, Labreuche J, et al. Impact of diffusion-weighted imaging lesion volume on the success of endovascular reperfusion therapy. Stroke 2013;44:2205–11.
30. Yoo AJ, Verduzco LA, Schaefer PW, et al. MRI-based selection for intra-arterial stroke therapy: value of pretreatment diffusion-weighted imaging lesion volume in selecting patients with acute stroke who will benefit from early recanalization. Stroke 2009;40:2046–54.
31. Guerrero WR, Grotta JC. Defining intravenous recombinant tissue plasminogen activator failure. Stroke 2013;44:819–21.
32. National Institute of Neurological Disorders and Stroke rt-PA Stroke Study Group. Tissue plasminogen activator for acute ischemic stroke. N Engl J Med 1995;333:1581–7.
33. Saqqur M, Uchino K, Demchuk AM, et al. Site of arterial occlusion identified by transcranial Doppler predicts the response to intravenous thrombolysis for stroke. Stroke 2007;38:948–54.
34. Zorzon M, Mase G, Pozzi-Mucelli F, et al. Increased density in the middle cerebral artery by nonenhanced computed tomography. Prognostic value in acute cerebral infarction. Eur Neurol 1993;33:256–9.
35. Gacs G, Fox AJ, Barnett HJ, et al. CT visualization of intracranial arterial thromboembolism. Stroke 1983;14:756–62.
36. Riedel CH, Jensen U, Rohr A, et al. Assessment of thrombus in acute middle cerebral artery occlusion using thin-slice nonenhanced Computed Tomography reconstructions. Stroke 2010;41:1659–64.
37. Riedel CH, Zimmermann P, Jensen-Kondering U, et al. The importance of size: successful recanalization by intravenous thrombolysis in acute anterior stroke depends on thrombus length. Stroke 2011;42:1775–7.
38. Liebeskind DS, Sanossian N, Yong WH, et al. CT and MRI early vessel signs reflect clot composition in acute stroke. Stroke 2011;42:1237–43.
39. Puig J, Pedraza S, Demchuk A, et al. Quantification of thrombus Hounsfield units on noncontrast CT predicts stroke subtype and early recanalization after intravenous recombinant tissue plasminogen activator. AJNR Am J Neuroradiol 2012;33:90–6.
40. Moftakhar P, English JD, Cooke DL, et al. Density of thrombus on admission CT predicts revascularization efficacy in large vessel occlusion acute ischemic stroke. Stroke 2013;44:243–5.
41. Froehler MT, Tateshima S, Duckwiler G, et al. The hyperdense vessel sign on CT predicts successful recanalization with the Merci device in acute ischemic stroke. J Neurointerv Surg 2013;5:289–93.
42. Spiotta AM, Vargas J, Hawk H, et al. Hounsfield unit value and clot length in the acutely occluded vessel and time required to achieve thrombectomy, complications and outcome. J Neurointerv Surg 2013. [Epub ahead of print].
43. Fargen KM, Meyers PM, Khatri P, et al. Improvements in recanalization with modern stroke therapy: a review of prospective ischemic stroke trials during the last two decades. J Neurointerv Surg 2013;5:506–11.
44. Jauch EC, Saver JL, Adams HP Jr, et al. Guidelines for the early management of patients with acute ischemic stroke: a guideline for healthcare professionals from the American Heart Association/American Stroke Association. Stroke 2013;44:870–947.
45. Rha JH, Saver JL. The impact of recanalization on ischemic stroke outcome: a meta-analysis. Stroke 2007;38:967–73.
46. Dorn F, Stehle S, Lockau H, et al. Endovascular treatment of acute intracerebral artery occlusions

with the Solitaire stent: single-centre experience with 108 recanalization procedures. Cerebrovasc Dis 2012;34:70–7.
47. Mokin M, Dumont TM, Veznedaroglu E, et al. Solitaire flow restoration thrombectomy for acute ischemic stroke: retrospective multicenter analysis of early postmarket experience after FDA approval. Neurosurgery 2013;73:19–26.
48. Davalos A, Pereira VM, Chapot R, et al. Retrospective multicenter study of Solitaire FR for revascularization in the treatment of acute ischemic stroke. Stroke 2012;43:2699–705.
49. Zaidat OO, Castonguay AC, Gupta R, et al. North American solitaire stent retriever acute stroke registry: post-marketing revascularization and clinical outcome results. J Neurointerv Surg 2013. [Epub ahead of print].
50. Broussalis E, Trinka E, Wallner A, et al. Thrombectomy in patients with large cerebral artery occlusion: A single-center experience with a new stent retriever. Vasc Endovascular Surg 2014;48(2):144–52.
51. Nguyen TN, Malisch T, Castonguay AC, et al. Balloon guide catheter improves revascularization and clinical outcomes with the Solitaire device: analysis of the North American Solitaire Acute Stroke Registry. Stroke 2014;45:141–5.
52. Nogueira RG, Gupta R, Davalos A. IMS-III and SYNTHESIS expansion trials of endovascular therapy in acute ischemic stroke: how can we improve? Stroke 2013;44:3272–4.
53. Khalessi AA, Fargen KM, Lavine S, et al. Commentary: societal statement on recent acute stroke intervention trials: results and implications. Neurosurgery 2013;73:E375–9.
54. Zaidat OO, Lazzaro MA, Gupta R, et al. Interventional Management of Stroke III trial: establishing the foundation. J Neurointerv Surg 2012;4:235–7.
55. Yoo AJ, Leslie-Mazwi TM, Jovin TG. Future directions in IAT: better studies, better selection, better timing and better techniques. J Neurointerv Surg 2013;5(Suppl 1):i1–6.
56. Saver JL, Jovin TG, Smith WS, et al. Stroke treatment academic industry roundtable: research priorities in the assessment of neurothrombectomy devices. Stroke 2013;44:3596–601.
57. Turk AS, Spiotta A, Frei D, et al. Initial clinical experience with the ADAPT technique: a direct aspiration first pass technique for stroke thrombectomy. J Neurointerv Surg 2014;6(3):231–7.

Endovascular Management of Intracranial Atherosclerosis

Mohamed S. Teleb, MD, Kaiz Asif, MD,
Alicia C. Castonguay, PhD, Osama O. Zaidat, MD, MS*

KEYWORDS

- Intracranial atherosclerotic disease • Endovascular • Stroke • Stenosis • Angioplasty • Stenting
- Percutaneous transluminal angioplasty and stenting

KEY POINTS

- Intracranial atherosclerotic disease (ICAD) is responsible for a considerable proportion of ischemic strokes worldwide.
- The clinical presentation of ICAD is heterogeneous and may involve more than 1 mechanism.
- Delineating the mechanism of ischemia requires careful clinical analysis, and usually necessitates multimodal imaging.
- Conservative medical management is the appropriate first step in the treatment of ICAD.
- An endovascular treatment approach based on the mechanism of stroke may be beneficial for select patients.
- Patient selection will be a critical factor in the design of future ICAD clinical trials.

INTRODUCTION

Epidemiology and Natural History

A common cause of stroke worldwide, intracranial atherosclerotic disease (ICAD) is most prevalent in Black, Asian, and Hispanic populations.[1] In the United States, ICAD was found in an estimated 10% of stroke patients, whereas in Asia ICAD accounts for approximately 30% to 50% of all strokes.[2] Risk factors for ICAD include age, hypertension, smoking, diabetes mellitus, hypercholesterolemia, and metabolic syndrome.[3] Although the high rate of certain uncontrolled risk factors, such as diabetes mellitus, hypertension, and hyperlipidemia, may partially account for the increased incidence of ICAD in African Americans,[4,5] the rates of these risk factors do not differ significantly in the Chinese population in comparison with Caucasians, and thus do not account for the significant burden of ICAD in this population.[6]

Data from the randomized, double-blind, controlled trial Warfarin versus Aspirin for Symptomatic Intracranial Disease (WASID) revealed that patients with symptomatic ICAD carry a high risk of subsequent stroke.[7] Despite the use of aspirin and management of risk factors, patients with a recent transient ischemic attack (TIA) or stroke and a stenosis of 70% or greater had a 23% risk of stroke at 1 year.[7,8]

Clinical Manifestations

Intracranial atherosclerotic disease presents with ischemic stroke or TIA, which may be single or recurrent.[9] Depending on the stroke location, there

Funding Sources: None.
Conflict of Interest: None.
Division of Neurointervention, Department of Neurology, Froedtert Hospital and Medical College of Wisconsin, 9200 West Wisconsin Ave, Milwaukee, WI 53226, USA
* Corresponding author.
E-mail address: szaidat@mcw.edu

Neurosurg Clin N Am 25 (2014) 593–605
http://dx.doi.org/10.1016/j.nec.2014.04.014
1042-3680/14/$ – see front matter

can be various clinical presentations including isolated motor or sensory involvement and/or cortical function impairments.[10–12] In addition, cognitive deficits, such as impairment of executive function and anterograde amnesia, can occur especially with infarcts involving the anterior-medial thalamus, caudate nucleus, or areas of cerebral cortical or white matter.[13,14] White matter degeneration, hypoperfusion, and hypometabolism can lead to cognitive changes in the absence of infarcts.[15]

Mechanisms of Ischemia

Downstream ischemia from ICAD can be due to hypoperfusion, in situ thromboembolism, perforator orifice occlusion, or a combination of these mechanisms.[16,17] In situ thrombosis followed by distal arterial embolism, in addition to delayed washout of emboli resulting from hypoperfusion, can be present at the same time. Similarly, a combination of local branch occlusion and embolism, with or without hemodynamic compromise, can occur concurrently.[10,18]

Neuroimaging may aid in delineating the stroke mechanisms, although sometimes one imaging pattern can be produced by a combination of mechanisms. In general, border-zone infarcts are suggestive of hypoperfusion, territorial infarcts point to peripheral embolism, and deep subcortical infarcts indicate perforator artery orifice occlusion.[19,20] In a study investigating lesion patterns on diffusion-weighted imaging (DWI) for middle cerebral artery atherosclerotic disease, 15 (83.3%) of 18 patients with border-zone infarcts had concomitant infarcts suggestive of either peripheral embolism (territorial infarcts) or perforator artery involvement (subcortical infarcts), indicating the coexistence of multiple mechanisms.[10] Inferring the initial stroke mechanism is important as it could be predictive of the risk of recurrent stroke or the mechanism of the next ischemic event. In an analysis of patients presenting with an index stroke in the WASID trial, the risk of recurrent stroke was similar in patients who presented with lacunar and nonlacunar strokes, and recurrent strokes in patients presenting with lacunar stroke were typically nonlacunar.[21]

DIAGNOSIS

The goals of imaging are: to detect intracranial stenosis with high sensitivity; to ascertain the degree and length of stenosis; to differentiate the atherosclerotic stenosis from mimics such as a recanalized partial thrombus, intracranial dissection, or nonatherosclerotic vasculopathy; and to assess the state of collateral circulation.

Detection and Quantification of Stenosis

Digital subtraction angiography (DSA) is considered the reference standard for the evaluation of intracranial stenosis. The high resolution of DSA allows for excellent quantification of luminal stenosis. Calculation of the degree of stenosis on DSA uses the equation $[1 - (D_{stenosis}/D_{normal})] \times 100$ where $D_{stenosis}$ is the diameter of the artery at the site of most severe degree of stenosis and D_{normal} is the diameter of the proximal normal artery (**Fig. 1**).[22]

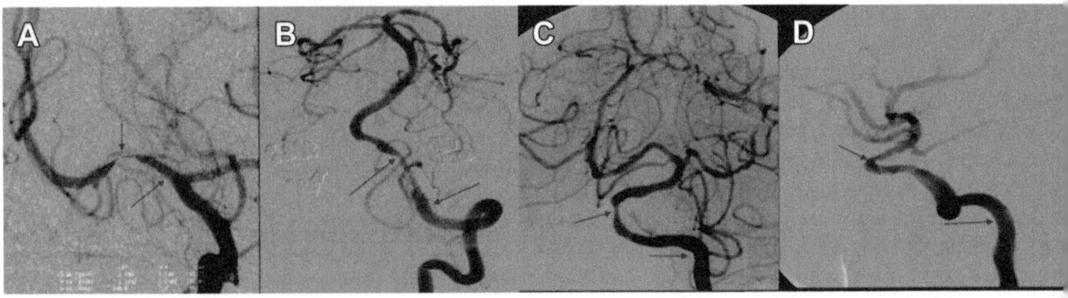

Fig. 1. Measurement of intracranial stenosis using the Warfarin versus Aspirin for Symptomatic Intracranial Disease (WASID) method. The diameter of the proximal part of the artery at its widest, nontortuous, normal segment is chosen (first choice), as shown in *A* and *B* (proximal *arrows* reference the normal vessel diameter; distal *arrows* reference the area of stenosis). If the proximal artery is diseased, the diameter of the distal portion of the artery at its widest, parallel, nontortuous normal segment is substituted (second choice; not shown). If the entire intracranial artery is diseased, the most distal, parallel, nontortuous normal segment of the feeding artery is measured (third choice), as in *C* (the proximal *arrow* denote the normal vessel diameter to compare the stenotic diameter to). For internal carotid artery disease involving the precavernous, cavernous, and postcavernous segments, the petrous carotid segment with parallel margins is measured at its widest, nontortuous, normal portion as shown in *D* as the reference diameter (the proximal *arrow* in *D*). If the entire petrous carotid is diseased, the most distal, parallel part of the extracranial internal carotid artery is substituted (second choice; not shown). The distal most *arrows* in all figures denote the area of maximum narrowing.

Among the noninvasive modalities for evaluating ICAD, a study assessing the accuracy of transcranial Doppler sonography (TCD) and magnetic resonance angiography (MRA) in comparison with DSA showed TCD and MRA to have good negative predictive values of 86% to 91% but low positive predictive values of 36% to 59%.[23] In another study comparing computed tomographic angiography (CTA) with MRA, using DSA as the reference standard, CTA was shown to have higher sensitivity, specificity, and positive predictive value.[24] The higher sensitivity and specificity of CTA has been observed especially for stenosis, which is 50% or higher.[25] As far as the evaluation of small intracranial arteries, a study comparing multidetector-row computed tomography (MDCT) angiography with DSA concluded that MDCT depicted 90% or more of all examined small intracranial arteries, and the smallest arterial size reliably detected with CTA was 0.7 mm, versus 0.4 mm for DSA.

Differentiation from Mimics

Radiographic mimics of intracranial atherosclerotic disease continue to pose a challenge in assigning an etiology for the anatomic arterial narrowing detected on imaging studies. Mimics include partially recanalized thrombus, intracranial dissection, vasculitis, and vasospasm; a careful analysis of the clinical scenario is require, which could potentially warrant repeat or multimodal imaging to distinguish between these mimics. Detailed history regarding prior diagnosis of coronary or peripheral atherosclerotic disease or the presence of atherosclerotic risk factors can help in differentiating from nonatherosclerotic causes of stenosis.[26] Partially recanalized thrombus in the setting of an acute stroke mimics intracranial atherosclerosis, and resolution on repeat imaging, which is frequently seen in this scenario, can help to make this distinction.[27] Limited data exist on the radiopathologic correlation for intracranial arterial stenotic diseases, but studies of extracranial vessel imaging with pathologic correlation have shown inflammatory conditions to be associated with concentric, circumferential wall thickening and enhancement, whereas atherosclerotic disease is frequently eccentric.[28,29]

Assessment of Collaterals

Degree of collateral circulation is a powerful risk factor for recurrent stroke in the setting of medical therapy for symptomatic intracranial atherosclerosis.[16] Impaired distal territory perfusion can be compensated with good leptomeningeal collaterals, which can play a protective role in the future risk of stroke in patients with severe symptomatic atherosclerotic disease. The American Society of Interventional and Therapeutic Neuroradiology collateral scale (**Table 1**) is the most commonly used grading system.[30]

Vessel-Wall Imaging

Vessel-wall imaging includes high-resolution 3-T magnetic resonance imaging (MRI), intravascular ultrasonography, and T1-weighted fat-suppressed MRI. High-resolution MRI can identify the thickness and pattern of protrusion.[31,32] Plaque components such as calcium and lipid can potentially be identified with intravascular ultrasonography, but is invasive in nature.[33] Identification of recent intraplaque hemorrhage and inflammation can be made with fat-suppressed T1-weighted MRI, on which these plaques show an increase in signal and enhancement after contrast injection.[34,35]

MEDICAL TREATMENT OF INTRACRANIAL ATHEROSCLEROTIC DISEASE

The medical treatment of ICAD has evolved over the years. The first major trial to evaluate medical treatments was WASID trial, which compared aspirin with warfarin in patients with ICAD. The results revealed that overall risk was similar between warfarin and aspirin, with the primary end point of ischemic stroke, brain hemorrhage, or vascular death occurring in 22.1% of patients assigned aspirin versus 21.8% in the warfarin group. The warfarin cohort had significantly more adverse events defined as death, major hemorrhage, and myocardial infarction or sudden death.[7] The

Table 1
The American Society of Interventional and Therapeutic Neuroradiology collateral scale

Grade	Description
0	No collaterals visible to the ischemic site
1	Slow collaterals to the periphery of the ischemic site with persistence of some of the defect
2	Rapid collaterals to periphery of ischemic site with persistence of some of the defect and to only a portion of the ischemic territory
3	Collaterals with slow but complete angiographic blood flow of the ischemic bed by the late venous phase
4	Complete and rapid collateral blood flow to the vascular bed in the entire ischemic territory by retrograde perfusion

GESICA study demonstrated that despite medical treatment, the 2-year rate of ischemic events in the territory of the stenotic artery was 38.2%, with the highest risk of stroke in clinically significant hemodynamic stenosis.[36] More recently, a randomized trial from China of medical therapy versus endovascular treatment for middle cerebral artery stenosis, and the Stenting versus Aggressive Medical Therapy for Intracranial Arterial Stenosis (SAMMPRIS) trial revealed much better outcomes with medical treatment, showing an event rate of 17.6% and 12.2%, respectively, at 1 year. SAMMPRIS demonstrated a statistically significant reduced event rate in comparison with endovascular treatment while the study from China revealed a similar rate. The medical arm of SAMMPRIS is now considered the standard of care for first-time symptomatic ICAD patients. The regimen was aspirin 325 mg and clopidogrel (Plavix) 75 mg daily for 3 months, followed by aspirin only, in addition to statin use, blood-pressure control, and a lifestyle modification program. Goal systolic blood pressure was less than 140 mm Hg, and the level of low-density lipoprotein cholesterol was less than 70 mg/dL (1.81 mmol/L). In addition to this regimen, management of secondary risk factors (diabetes, elevated non–high-density lipoprotein cholesterol levels, smoking, excess weight, and insufficient exercise) was also included.

ENDOVASCULAR TREATMENT OF INTRACRANIAL ATHEROSCLEROTIC DISEASE

Endovascular treatment of intracranial stenosis can be divided into 3 possible treatments: balloon angioplasty alone, balloon-mounted stent (BMS) placement, or self-expanding stent (SES) placement. This section addresses indications for each procedure, outcomes from the literature, and example case presentations.

Intracranial Balloon Angioplasty Without Stenting

Intracranial angioplasty alone, without the use of a stent, has been advocated by some as possibly decreasing periprocedural complications.[37,38] Balloon angioplasty was first used in the coronary circulation. The goal of angioplasty is to reduce luminal stenosis and increase perfusion to downstream tissue. The proposed mechanisms include plaque redistribution and dilatation of the actual vessel diameter,[39] which was initially described with percutaneous transluminal angioplasty (PTA) of the coronary arteries.

Initially there was some enthusiasm for the use of balloon angioplasty in the intracranial circulation with the first reported cases in the 1980s.[40] There were cases of basilar followed by cavernous segment carotid, and then middle cerebral artery stenosis treated with angioplasty.[40–42] Unfortunately, because of higher rates of complications its use was limited until new techniques and technologies were developed and innovated.[43]

Dissections, emboli, and rupture were not uncommon, with a complication rate of up to 50% reported in one study.[43–45] These complications were attributed to the large size of balloons and their rate of inflation. Unlike coronary vessels, the intracranial circulation is surrounded by brain and cerebrospinal fluid in the subarachnoid space. A muscular myocardium and a pericardial sac surround the coronary arteries. A small rupture or dissection is usually not significant in the coronary circulation. On the other hand, a subarachnoid hemorrhage can be fatal, with morbidity and mortality reported in 40% to 50% of patients.[46] In addition, intraparenchymal hemorrhage also carries high morbidity and mortality.[47] Dissections can cause ischemic strokes which, depending on territory, can also lead to high morbidity. Stroke, largely ischemic stroke, today remains the principal cause of disability.[48] With slow inflation over minutes as opposed to seconds and undersizing the balloon, complication rates have been reported to be as low as 5%.[37,49,50] **Figs. 2** and **3** show examples of balloon angioplasty.

There have been multiple recent case reports of balloon angioplasty for intracranial stenosis with low complication rates and technical success rates exceeding 90%. Defining technical success as less than 50% stenosis, as was done by a Standard of Practice Guideline Committee from the Society of Neurointerventional Surgery, puts modern series at a technical success rate of 60% to more than 90%.[37,38,49–53] The largest of the studies was by Marks and colleagues,[37] with 120 patients. Some studies have suggested that restenosis and outcomes in balloon angioplasty without stenting are similar to those with stenting, as was demonstrated by a comparison study of angioplasty alone versus stenting by Siddiq and colleagues.[52]

Balloon types

Several intracranial balloons have been approved for use, but only one for intracranial angioplasty. These balloons include the Scepter (Microvention, Tustin, CA, USA), HyperForm (Covidien, Dublin, Ireland), and Transform (Stryker, Kalamazoo, MI, USA), to mention a few. Of the other intracranial balloons used for balloon-assisted coil embolization of aneurysms, the Gateway balloon (Stryker) is the only one approved by the Food and Drug Administration (FDA) for intracranial angioplasty

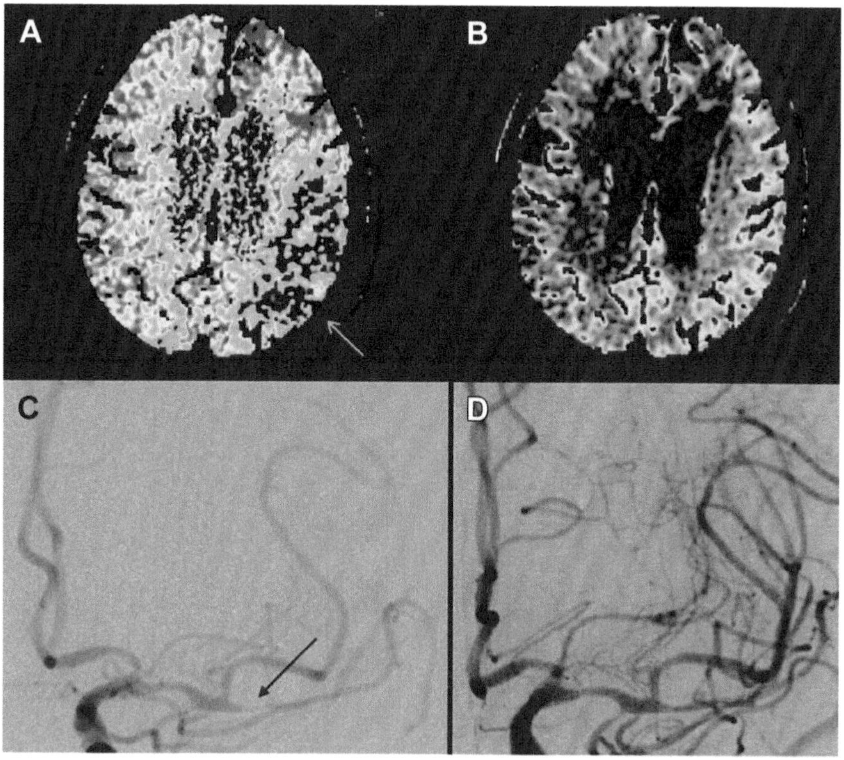

Fig. 2. A patient with severe left M2 middle cerebral artery (MCA) stenosis who is symptomatic when her blood pressure has dropped. (*A*) Cerebral blood flow decreased in the corresponding area of symptoms and stenosis as depicted by the blue color (*arrow*). (*B*) Cerebral blood volume increased in corresponding area. (*C*) Cerebral angiogram demonstrating the MCA inferior division stenosis before angioplasty (*arrow*). (*D*) Cerebral angiogram after angioplasty, with improved stenosis.

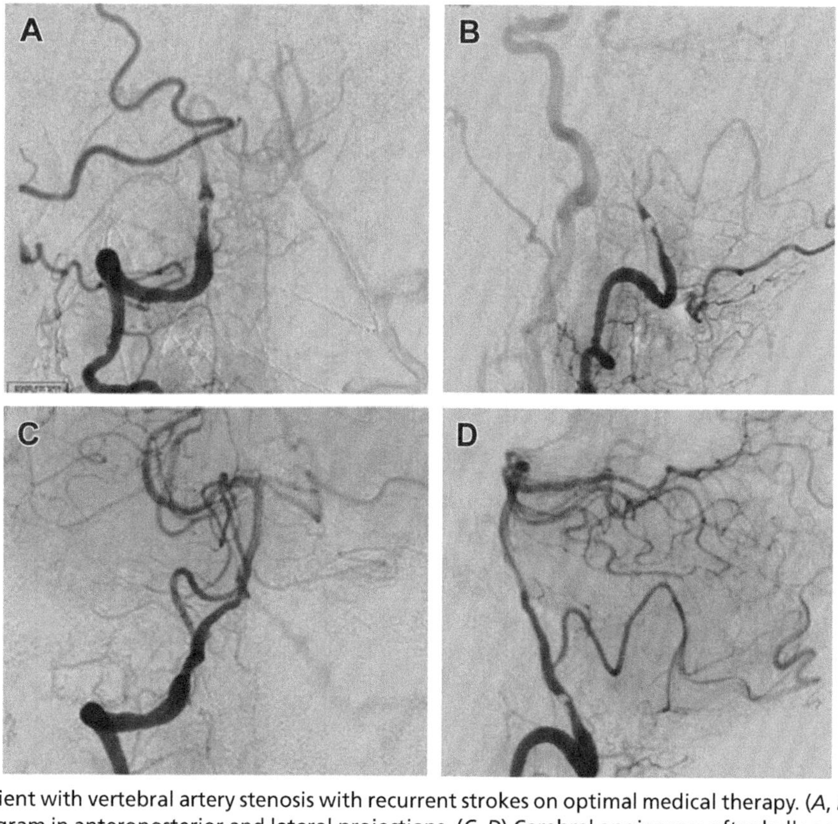

Fig. 3. A patient with vertebral artery stenosis with recurrent strokes on optimal medical therapy. (*A, B*) Before cerebral angiogram in anteroposterior and lateral projections. (*C, D*) Cerebral angiogram after balloon angioplasty.

Table 2
Major[a] studies on endovascular treatment of intracranial atherosclerotic disease

Authors,[Ref.] Year	Type of Study	Treatment Groups Compared	Endovascular Treatment, Location	Mean Pre- and Posttreatment Stenosis (%)	Restenosis Rate (>50%)	Periprocedural Complication Rate (%)	Outcome Stroke or Death (%)
Miao et al,[63] 2012	R, P	Medical	PTA, stent MCA	84→N/R	N/R	8.3	19.4 stent 17.6 med
SAMMPRIS,[26] 2011	R, P	Aggressive medical	SES A & P circulation	80→N/R	N/R	19.2	14.7 stent 5.8 med
Yu et al,[64] 2011	NR, Rt	MCA vs other locations	SES MCA, ICA, BA, VA	78→N/R	10	2.4 MCA 4 other	5.7 MCA 12 other
Nguyen et al,[50] 2011	NR, Rt	None	PTA ICA, MCA, ACA, BA, VA	79→34	N/R	5	8.5
Qureshi et al,[65] 2011	NR, Rt	None	PTA, SES, BMS, DES ICA, MCA, BA, VA	75→N/R	N/R	9.8	9.8
Tang et al,[66] 2011	NR, Rt	Medical therapy	BMS, SES ICA, MCA, BA, VA	80→N/R	4	17	22
Chamczuk et al,[67] 2010	NR, Rt	None	SES, BMS A & P circulation	76→22	N/R	6.6	6.1
INTRASTENT,[68] 2010	NR, P	None	Stenting (NR) ICA, MCA, BA, VA	N/R	N/R	N/R	12.4
Samaniego et al,[69] 2009	NR, Rt	Medical therapy	SES, BMS A & P circulation	N/R	N/R	5.6	7.5 13.8 med
Wolfe et al,[70] 2009	NR, Rt	None	SES	73→21	24	6	10
Miao et al,[71] 2009	NR, Rt	None	BMS MCA	N/R	9	N/R	4.4

Siddiq et al,[52] 2008	NR, Rt	PTA vs stent placement	PTA, stent (NR) A & P circulation	89→N/R 90→N/R	15 4	8 PTA 9 stent	8 PTA 11 stent
Mazighi et al,[53] 2008	NR, Rt	None	PTA, DES, BMS ICA, MCA, BA, VA	85→0	16	N/R	10.1
Suh et al,[72] 2008	NR, Rt	None	BMS ICA, MCA, BA, VA	70→25	0	N/R	10
Zaidat et al,[61] 2008	NR, P	None	SES ICA, MCA, BA, VA	82→20	25	6.2	14
Jiang et al,[73] 2007	NR, Rt	None	BMS ICA, MCA, BA, VA	N/R	N/R	N/R	11.8
Fiorella et al,[60] 2007	NR, P	None	SES ICA, MCA, BA, VA	75→27	N/R	15.3	6.1
Marks et al,[37] 2006	NR, Rt	None	PTA, Stent (NR) ICA, MCA, PCA, BA, VA	82→36	N/R	N/R	5.8
Wojak et al,[49] 2005	NR, Rt	None	PTA, BMS ICA, MCA, PCA, ACA, BA, VA	N/R	27	9.5	4.8
Lylyk et al,[74] 2005	NR, Rt	None	BMS, DES ICA, MCA, PCA, BA, VA	75→<30	13	10	9.5
SSYLVIA,[75] 2004	NR, P	None	BMS ICA, MCA, PCA, BA, VA	N/R	32	N/R	9.3

Abbreviations: ACA, anterior cerebral artery; BA, basilar artery; BMS, balloon-mounted stent; DES, drug-eluting stent; ICA, internal cerebral artery; MCA, middle cerebral artery; med, medical therapy; NR, nonrandomized; N/R, not reported; P, prospective; PTA, percutaneous transluminal angioplasty; R, randomized; Rt, retrospective; SES, self-expanding stent; VA, vertebral artery.

[a] Major study has been defined as randomized, highly referenced, or with more than 50 patients.

The other most commonly used balloons are coronary angioplasty balloons that are off label.[49]

Drug-Eluting Stents

Drug-eluting stents (DES) have been used off label in the intracranial circulation, and multiple reports have been published on its use. DES have been used in both anterior and posterior circulations, with periprocedural complication rates ranging from 0% to 25%.[54–56] An inherent problem with DES is that most are balloon mounted and are more difficult to track in the intracranial circulation. Other criticisms include the need for dual antiplatelet therapy for 6 months or longer, as suggested by some of the cardiac literature.[57] There is some literature on newer DES that may lead to fewer thrombosis events, but research is still ongoing.[58] Lack of long-term outcomes has also been a discouraging factor, although a recent publication with a mean follow-up period of 67 months has shown no patient with greater than 50% restenosis. However, there were only 11 patients in this report.[59]

Balloon-Mounted Stents

BMS have also been used in ICAD, with a success rate similar to that of balloon angioplasty. Most of the reported literature has used coronary BMS for the reported case series. The only intracranial system is the NeuroLink, which was used in the SSYLVIA trial. The difficulty with the current BMS systems is that they are stiff, and therefore may cause more complications and are more difficult to track in the tortuous intracranial circulation. The SSYLVIA trial did confirm a 35% restenosis rate, although 61% of patients were asymptomatic, which was very worrisome.

Self-Expanding Stents

SES have been the mainstay for intracranial stenting ever since the FDA approval of the Wingspan stent. This stent has had a high technical success rate ranging from 98.8% to 96.7% in the 2 large reported registries, and 94.6% (12 failures out of 224) in the SAMMPARIS randomized controlled trial, with 7 patients having the procedure aborted and 5 having only angioplasty because of technical reasons.[26,60,61] It has been argued that the use of this system is more appropriate for the intracranial circulation because of its small outward radial force (<0.1 atm). Because of its self-expanding design, it also does not need a balloon and can be delivered through a microcatheter, which in addition makes it easier to track through tortuous anatomy. Despite these advantages, the SAMMPRIS trial short-term and long-term outcomes data revealed better outcomes in long-term rates of stroke and death under medical treatment: at a median follow-up of 32.4 months, 34 (15%) of 227 patients in the medical group and 52 (23%) of 224 patients in the stenting group had a primary end-point event.[26,62]

TRIALS AND TRIBULATIONS OF ENDOVASCULAR TREATMENT OF ICAD

Despite having many options for the treatment of ICAD with endovascular techniques, none has been established as a primary treatment. In addition to the foregoing review on PTA, DES, BMS, and SES, **Table 2** outlines the major literature on these approaches.[26,37,49,50,52,53,60,61,63–75]

There have been positive results from nonrandomized registries and case series, but there have been no positive trials to indicate the endovascular approach as the primary treatment of symptomatic patients with ICAD. In fact, the SAMMPRIS trial argues that it is likely harmful as first-line treatment.[26] Despite this, many neurovascular practitioners and academics still believe that there is a role for endovascular treatment of ICAD, as evidenced by a survey at the International Stroke Conference.[76] In fact, subsequent analysis of SAMMPRIS periprocedural strokes revealed that perforator-rich areas, location (basilar) and close monitoring of hemorrhages from wire perforation, clopidogrel loading, and an activated clotting time higher than the target range might help clinicians to produce better results from endovascular treatment.[77,78] Although SAMMPRIS was a well-designed trial and some of the initial criticisms have been addressed, there are some concerns. These initial critiques included lack of inclusion of patients who failed best medical therapy once the time to treatment, and stenting in perforator-rich areas, which have been addressed well by the investigators in separate articles.[79] That being said, SAMMPRIS did not use perfusion or collateral imaging to assess patients. Hemodynamic patients were also excluded from the trial. There were no set criteria for hemodynamic or perioperative care in the intensive care unit. Given these limitations and patients who can potentially benefit from this treatment, it would be judicious to evaluate every patient individually for intracranial endovascular revascularization.

SURGICAL MANAGEMENT OF INTRACRANIAL STENOSIS

Surgical management has been used for more than 40 years in the treatment of intracranial stenosis. Multiple surgical treatments such as direct and ndirect bypass surgeries have been developed. The EC/IC Bypass Study, published in 1985, revealed no benefit of surgical bypass over medical therapy for the reduction of overall ipsilateral major strokes or death.[80] The surgical treatment used a direct bypass from the superficial temporal artery to the middle cerebral artery at one of the M2 branches. The medical arm was limited to single antiplatelet use (aspirin 325 mg, 4 times daily) and blood-pressure reduction, but no specific lifestyle modification regimen.[80]

More recently the Carotid Occlusion Surgery Study (COSS) evaluated patients with ipsilateral ischemic events within 120 days as a result of intracranial artery occlusion. Patients were randomized if they had increased oxygen extraction fraction. Patients were randomized to medical treatment versus extracranial to intracranial (EC/IC) bypass surgery. Overall stroke and death at 30 days and 2-year ipsilateral stroke rates were not statistically different between the surgical and medical group (21% vs 23%).[81] Interestingly the surgical group did experience decreased oxygen extraction fraction, but no cognitive outcomes testing was conducted. As a consequence of these studies, EC/IC bypass is not recommended. Bearing this in mind, none of these patients were pressure dependent and needed to be on pressure-augmenting medications to avoid strokes.

FUTURE DIRECTIONS

Although at present endovascular treatment is reserved for patients who have failed medical treatment, there will likely be further trials, as even medical treatment has a 12% stroke rate at 1 year and an increased number of strokes at further follow-up.[26,62] A recent survey done at the 2012 International Stroke Conference reveals that most neurovascular clinicians including neurologists, neurosurgeons, and interventionalists would enroll ICAD patients in endovascular trials.[76] Perhaps patients with poor collaterals, hemodynamic symptoms, and recurrence despite medical therapy will benefit from endovascular treatment. Other treatment options may include indirect bypass surgery, as recently proposed.[82] Lastly, the type of stenosis and location, whether in perforator-rich areas or not, may play a role in regard of which patients may be better treated with surgical rather than medical techniques.[64,77,78,83] **Box 1** lists the proposed treatments.

Box 1
Possible indications and Food and Drug Administration (FDA) indications for intracranial stenting/angioplasty

1. Hemodynamic symptoms
2. Poor collaterals
3. Large mismatch on imaging with signs of collateral failure
4. Recurrent symptoms despite best medical therapy
5. FDA Wingspan use criteria: (1) age 22 to 80 years; (2) two or more strokes despite aggressive medical management; (3) most recent stroke occurring more than 7 days before planned intervention; (4) 70% to 99% stenosis attributable to atherosclerosis of the related intracranial artery; and (5) good recovery from previous stroke and modified Rankin score of 3 or less before intervention.[76]

REFERENCES

1. Sacco RL, Kargman DE, Gu Q, et al. Race-ethnicity and determinants of intracranial atherosclerotic cerebral infarction. The Northern Manhattan Stroke Study. Stroke 1995;26(1):14–20.
2. Wong LK. Global burden of intracranial atherosclerosis. Int J Stroke 2006;1(3):158–9. http://dx.doi.org/10.1111/j.1747-4949.2006.00045.x.
3. Chaturvedi S, Turan TN, Lynn MJ, et al. Risk factor status and vascular events in patients with symptomatic intracranial stenosis. Neurology 2007;69(22):2063–8. http://dx.doi.org/10.1212/01.wnl.0000279338.18776.26.
4. Carson AP, Howard G, Burke GL, et al. Ethnic differences in hypertension incidence among middle-aged and older adults: the multi-ethnic study of atherosclerosis. Hypertension 2011;57(6):1101–7. http://dx.doi.org/10.1161/HYPERTENSIONAHA.110.168005.
5. Waddy SP, Cotsonis G, Lynn MJ, et al. Racial differences in vascular risk factors and outcomes of patients with intracranial atherosclerotic arterial stenosis. Stroke 2009;40(3):719–25. http://dx.doi.org/10.1161/STROKEAHA.108.526624.
6. Stevens J, Truesdale KP, Katz EG, et al. Impact of body mass index on incident hypertension and diabetes in Chinese Asians, American Whites, and American Blacks: the People's Republic of China Study and the Atherosclerosis Risk in Communities Study. Am J Epidemiol 2008;167(11):1365–74. http://dx.doi.org/10.1093/aje/kwn060.
7. Chimowitz MI, Lynn MJ, Howlett-Smith H, et al. Comparison of warfarin and aspirin for symptomatic intracranial arterial stenosis. N Engl J Med 2005;352(13):1305–16.
8. Kasner SE, Chimowitz MI, Lynn MJ, et al. Predictors of ischemic stroke in the territory of a symptomatic intracranial arterial stenosis. Circulation

2006;113(4):555–63. http://dx.doi.org/10.1161/CIRCULATIONAHA.105.578229.
9. Ois A, Gomis M, Rodriguez-Campello AR, et al. Factors associated with a high risk of recurrence in patients with transient ischemic attack or minor stroke. Stroke 2008;39(6):1717–21. http://dx.doi.org/10.1161/STROKEAHA.107.505438.
10. Lee DK, Kim JS, Kwon SU, et al. Lesion patterns and stroke mechanism in atherosclerotic middle cerebral artery disease: early diffusion-weighted imaging study. Stroke 2005;36(12):2583–8. http://dx.doi.org/10.1161/01.STR.0000189999.19948.14.
11. Kang DW, Kwon SU, Yoo SH, et al. Early recurrent ischemic lesions on diffusion-weighted imaging in symptomatic intracranial atherosclerosis. Arch Neurol 2007;64(1):50–4. http://dx.doi.org/10.1001/archneur.64.1.50.
12. Cho KH, Kang DW, Kwon SU, et al. Location of single subcortical infarction due to middle cerebral artery atherosclerosis: proximal versus distal arterial stenosis. J Neurol Neurosurg Psychiatry 2009;80(1):48–52. http://dx.doi.org/10.1136/jnnp.2007.143354.
13. Andrade SP, Brucki SM, Bueno OF, et al. Neuropsychological performance in patients with subcortical stroke. Arq Neuropsiquiatr 2012;70(5):341–7.
14. Saczynski JS, Sigurdsson S, Jonsdottir MK, et al. Cerebral infarcts and cognitive performance: importance of location and number of infarcts. Stroke 2009;40(3):677–82. http://dx.doi.org/10.1161/STROKEAHA.108.530212.
15. Lee JS, Im DS, An YS, et al. Chronic cerebral hypoperfusion in a mouse model of Alzheimer's disease: an additional contributing factor of cognitive impairment. Neurosci Lett 2011;489(2):84–8. http://dx.doi.org/10.1016/j.neulet.2010.11.071.
16. Liebeskind DS, Cotsonis GA, Saver JL, et al. Collaterals dramatically alter stroke risk in intracranial atherosclerosis. Ann Neurol 2011;69(6):963–74. http://dx.doi.org/10.1002/ana.22354.
17. Caplan LR. Intracranial branch atheromatous disease: a neglected, understudied, and underused concept. Neurology 1989;39(9):1246–50.
18. Caplan LR, Hennerici M. Impaired clearance of emboli (washout) is an important link between hypoperfusion, embolism, and ischemic stroke. Arch Neurol 1998;55(11):1475–82. http://dx.doi.org/10.1001/archneur.55.11.1475.
19. Ryoo S, Park JH, Kim SJ, et al. Branch occlusive disease: clinical and magnetic resonance angiography findings. Neurology 2012;78(12):888–96. http://dx.doi.org/10.1212/WNL.0b013e31824c4699.
20. Holmstedt CA, Turan TN, Chimowitz MI. Atherosclerotic intracranial arterial stenosis: risk factors, diagnosis, and treatment. Lancet Neurol 2013;12(11):1106–14. http://dx.doi.org/10.1016/S1474-4422(13)70195-9.
21. Khan A, Kasner SE, Lynn MJ, et al, for the Warfarin Aspirin Symptomatic Intracranial Disease (WASID) Trial Investigators. Risk factors and outcome of patients with symptomatic intracranial stenosis presenting with lacunar stroke. Stroke 2012;43(5):1230–3. http://dx.doi.org/10.1161/STROKEAHA.111.641696.
22. Samuels OB, Joseph GJ, Lynn MJ, et al. A standardized method for measuring intracranial arterial stenosis. AJNR Am J Neuroradiol 2000;21(4):643–6.
23. Feldmann EE, Wilterdink JL, Kosinski AA, et al. The Stroke Outcomes and Neuroimaging of Intracranial Atherosclerosis (SONIA) trial. Neurology 2007;68(24):2099–106. http://dx.doi.org/10.1212/01.wnl.0000261488.05906.c1.
24. Bash S, Villablanca JP, Jahan R, et al. Intracranial vascular stenosis and occlusive disease: evaluation with CT angiography, MR angiography, and digital subtraction angiography. AJNR Am J Neuroradiol 2005;26(5):1012–21.
25. Nguyen-Huynh MN, Wintermark M, English J, et al. How accurate is CT angiography in evaluating intracranial atherosclerotic disease? Stroke 2008;39(4):1184–8. http://dx.doi.org/10.1161/STROKEAHA.107.502906.
26. Chimowitz MI, Lynn MJ, Derdeyn CP, et al. Stenting versus aggressive medical therapy for intracranial arterial stenosis. N Engl J Med 2011;365(11):993–1003. http://dx.doi.org/10.1056/NEJMoa1105335.
27. Choi HY, Ye BS, Ahn SH, et al. Characteristics and the fate of intraluminal thrombus of the intracranial and extracranial cerebral arteries in acute ischemic stroke patients. Eur Neurol 2009;62(2):72–8.
28. Adams GJ, Greene JJ, Vick GW, et al. Tracking regression and progression of atherosclerosis in human carotid arteries using high-resolution magnetic resonance imaging. Magn Reson Imaging 2004;22(9):1249–58. http://dx.doi.org/10.1016/j.mri.2004.08.020.
29. Bley TA, Uhl M, Venhoff N, et al. 3-T MRI reveals cranial and thoracic inflammatory changes in giant cell arteritis. Clin Rheumatol 2007;26(3):448–50. http://dx.doi.org/10.1007/s10067-005-0160-7.
30. Higashida RT, Furlan AJ, Roberts H, et al. Trial design and reporting standards for intra-arterial cerebral thrombolysis for acute ischemic stroke. Stroke 2003;34(8):e109–37. http://dx.doi.org/10.1161/01.STR.0000082720.85129.0A.
31. Swartz RH, Bhuta SS, Farb RI, et al. Intracranial arterial wall imaging using high-resolution 3-tesla contrast-enhanced MRI. Neurology 2009;72(7):627–34. http://dx.doi.org/10.1212/01.wnl.0000342470.69739.b3.
32. Ryu CW, Jahng GH, Kim EJ, et al. High resolution wall and lumen MRI of the middle cerebral arteries at 3 tesla. Cerebrovasc Dis 2009;27(5):433–42.

33. Diethrich EB, Margolis MP, Reid DB, et al. Virtual histology intravascular ultrasound assessment of carotid artery disease: the Carotid Artery Plaque Virtual Histology Evaluation (CAPITAL) study. J Endovasc Ther 2007;14(5):676–86. http://dx.doi.org/10.1583/1545-1550(2007)14[676:VHIUAO]2.0.CO;2.
34. Xu WH, Li ML, Gao S, et al. Middle cerebral artery intraplaque hemorrhage: prevalence and clinical relevance. Ann Neurol 2012;71(2):195–8. http://dx.doi.org/10.1002/ana.22626.
35. Vergouwen MD, Silver FL, Mandell DM, et al. Eccentric narrowing and enhancement of symptomatic middle cerebral artery stenoses in patients with recent ischemic stroke. Arch Neurol 2011;68(3):338–42. http://dx.doi.org/10.1001/archneurol.2011.20.
36. Mazighi M, Tanasescu R, Ducrocq X, et al. Prospective study of symptomatic atherothrombotic intracranial stenoses: The GESICA Study. Neurology 2006;66(8):1187–91. http://dx.doi.org/10.1212/01.wnl.0000208404.94585.b2.
37. Marks MP, Wojak JC, Al-Ali F, et al. Angioplasty for symptomatic intracranial stenosis: clinical outcome. Stroke 2006;37(4):1016–20. http://dx.doi.org/10.1161/01.STR.0000206142.03677.c2.
38. Marks MP, Marcellus ML, Do HM, et al. Intracranial angioplasty without stenting for symptomatic atherosclerotic stenosis: long-term follow-up. AJNR Am J Neuroradiol 2005;26(3):525–30.
39. Castaneda-Zuniga WR, Formanek A, Tadavarthy M, et al. The mechanism of balloon angioplasty. Radiology 1980;135(3):565–71.
40. Sundt TM, Smith HC, Campbell JK, et al. Transluminal angioplasty for basilar artery stenosis. Mayo Clin Proc 1980;55(11):673–80.
41. O'Leary DH, Clouse ME. Percutaneous transluminal angioplasty of the cavernous carotid artery for recurrent ischemia. AJNR Am J Neuroradiol 1984;5(5):644–5.
42. Purdy PD, Devous MD, Unwin DH, et al. Angioplasty of an atherosclerotic middle cerebral artery associated with improvement in regional cerebral blood flow. AJNR Am J Neuroradiol 1990;11(5):878–80.
43. Takis C, Kwan ES, Pessin MS, et al. Intracranial angioplasty: experience and complications. AJNR Am J Neuroradiol 1997;18(9):1661–8.
44. Connors JJ, Wojak JC. Percutaneous transluminal angioplasty for intracranial atherosclerotic lesions: evolution of technique and short-term results. J Neurosurg 1999;91(3):415–23.
45. Terada T, Tsuura M, Matsumoto H, et al. Endovascular therapy for stenosis of the petrous or cavernous portion of the internal carotid artery: percutaneous transluminal angioplasty compared with stent placement. J Neurosurg 2003;98(3):491–7.
46. Johnston S, Selvin S. The burden, trends, and demographics of mortality from subarachnoid hemorrhage. Neurology 1998;50(5):1413–8.
47. Broderick J, Connolly S, Feldmann E, et al. Guidelines for the management of spontaneous intracerebral hemorrhage in adults: 2007 update: a guideline from the American Heart Association/American Stroke Association Stroke Council, High Blood Pressure Research Council, and the Quality of Care and Outcomes in Research Interdisciplinary Working Group: The American Academy of Neurology affirms the value of this guideline as an educational tool for neurologists. Stroke 2007;38(6):2001–23. http://dx.doi.org/10.1161/STROKEAHA.107.183689.
48. Go AS, Mozaffarian D, Roger VL, et al. Heart disease and stroke statistics–2013 update: a report from the American Heart Association. Circulation 2013;127(1):e6–245. http://dx.doi.org/10.1161/CIR.0b013e31828124ad.
49. Wojak JC, Dunlap DC, Hargrave KR, et al. Intracranial angioplasty and stenting: long-term results from a single center. AJNR Am J Neuroradiol 2006;27(9):1882–92.
50. Nguyen TN, Zaidat OO, Gupta R, et al. Balloon angioplasty for intracranial atherosclerotic disease: periprocedural risks and short-term outcomes in a multicenter study. Stroke 2011;42(1):107–11. http://dx.doi.org/10.1161/STROKEAHA.110.583245.
51. Hussain MS, Fraser JF, Abruzzo T, et al. Standard of practice: endovascular treatment of intracranial atherosclerosis. J Neurointerv Surg 2012;4(6):397–406. http://dx.doi.org/10.1136/neurintsurg-2012-010405.
52. Siddiq F, Vazquez G, Memon MZ, et al. Comparison of primary angioplasty with stent placement for treating symptomatic intracranial atherosclerotic diseases: a multicenter study. Stroke 2008;39(9):2505–10. http://dx.doi.org/10.1161/STROKEAHA.108.515361.
53. Mazighi M, Yadav JS, Abou-Chebl A. Durability of endovascular therapy for symptomatic intracranial atherosclerosis. Stroke 2008;39(6):1766–9. http://dx.doi.org/10.1161/STROKEAHA.107.500587.
54. Qureshi AI, Kirmani JF, Hussein HM, et al. Early and intermediate-term outcomes with drug-eluting stents in high-risk patients with symptomatic intracranial stenosis. Neurosurgery 2006;59(5):1044–51. http://dx.doi.org/10.1227/01.NEU.0000245593.54204.99 [discussion: 1051].
55. Abou-Chebl A, Bashir Q, Yadav JS. Drug-eluting stents for the treatment of intracranial atherosclerosis: initial experience and midterm angiographic follow-up. Stroke 2005;36(12):e165–8. http://dx.doi.org/10.1161/01.STR.0000190893.74268.fd.
56. Boulos AS, Agner C, Deshaies EM. Preliminary evidence supporting the safety of drug-eluting stents in neurovascular disease. Neurol Res

2005;27(Suppl 1):S95–102. http://dx.doi.org/10.1179/016164105X35459.
57. Roy PP, Bonello LL, Torguson RR, et al. Temporal relation between clopidogrel cessation and stent thrombosis after drug-eluting stent implantation. Am J Cardiol 2009;103(6):801–5. http://dx.doi.org/10.1016/j.amjcard.2008.11.038.
58. Palmerini T, Biondi-Zoccai G, Riva Della D, et al. Stent thrombosis with drug-eluting stents: is the paradigm shifting? J Am Coll Cardiol 2013;62(21):1915–21. http://dx.doi.org/10.1016/j.jacc.2013.08.725.
59. Park S, Lee DG, Chung WJ, et al. Long-term outcomes of drug-eluting stents in symptomatic intracranial stenosis. Neurointervention 2013;8(1):9–14. http://dx.doi.org/10.5469/neuroint.2013.8.1.9.
60. Fiorella D, Levy EI, Turk AS, et al. US multicenter experience with the wingspan stent system for the treatment of intracranial atheromatous disease: periprocedural results. Stroke 2007;38(3):881–7. http://dx.doi.org/10.1161/01.STR.0000257963.65728.e8.
61. Zaidat OO, Klucznik R, Alexander MJ, et al. The NIH registry on use of the Wingspan stent for symptomatic 70-99% intracranial arterial stenosis. Neurology 2008;70(17):1518–24. http://dx.doi.org/10.1212/01.wnl.0000306308.08229.a3.
62. Derdeyn CP, Chimowitz MI, Lynn MJ, et al. Aggressive medical treatment with or without stenting in high-risk patients with intracranial artery stenosis (SAMMPRIS): the final results of a randomised trial. Lancet 2014;383(9914):333–41. http://dx.doi.org/10.1016/S0140-6736(13)62038-3.
63. Miao Z, Jiang L, Wu H, et al. Randomized controlled trial of symptomatic middle cerebral artery stenosis: endovascular versus medical therapy in a Chinese population. Stroke 2012;43(12):3284–90. http://dx.doi.org/10.1161/STROKEAHA.112.662270.
64. Yu SC, Leung TW, Lee KT, et al. Angioplasty and stenting of atherosclerotic middle cerebral arteries with Wingspan: evaluation of clinical outcome, restenosis, and procedure outcome. AJNR Am J Neuroradiol 2011;32(4):753–8. http://dx.doi.org/10.3174/ajnr.A2363.
65. Qureshi AI, Tariq N, Hassan AE, et al. Predictors and timing of neurological complications following intracranial angioplasty and/or stent placement. Neurosurgery 2011;68(1):53–61. http://dx.doi.org/10.1227/NEU.0b013e3181fc5f0a.
66. Tang CW, Chang FC, Chern CM, et al. Stenting versus medical treatment for severe symptomatic intracranial stenosis. AJNR Am J Neuroradiol 2011;32(5):911–6. http://dx.doi.org/10.3174/ajnr.A2409.
67. Chamczuk AJ, Ogilvy CS, Snyder KV, et al. Elective stenting for intracranial stenosis under conscious sedation. Neurosurgery 2010;67(5):1189–94. http://dx.doi.org/10.1227/NEU.0b013e3181efbcac.
68. Kurre W, Berkefeld J, Brassel F, et al. In-hospital complication rates after stent treatment of 388 symptomatic intracranial stenoses: results from the INTRASTENT multicentric registry. Stroke 2010;41(3):494–8. http://dx.doi.org/10.1161/STROKEAHA.109.568063.
69. Samaniego EA, Hetzel S, Thirunarayanan S, et al. Outcome of symptomatic intracranial atherosclerotic disease. Stroke 2009;40(9):2983–7. http://dx.doi.org/10.1161/STROKEAHA.109.549972.
70. Wolfe TJ, Fitzsimmons BF, Hussain SI, et al. Long term clinical and angiographic outcomes with the Wingspan stent for treatment of symptomatic 50-99% intracranial atherosclerosis: single center experience in 51 cases. J Neurointerv Surg 2009;1(1):40–3. http://dx.doi.org/10.1136/jnis.2009.000331.
71. Miao ZR, Feng L, Li S, et al. Treatment of symptomatic middle cerebral artery stenosis with balloon-mounted stents: long-term follow-up at a single center. Neurosurgery 2009;64(1):79–84. http://dx.doi.org/10.1227/01.NEU.0000335648.31874.37 [discussion: 84–5].
72. Suh DC, Kim JK, Choi JW, et al. Intracranial stenting of severe symptomatic intracranial stenosis: results of 100 consecutive patients. AJNR Am J Neuroradiol 2008;29(4):781–5. http://dx.doi.org/10.3174/ajnr.A0922.
73. Jiang WJ, Du B, Leung TW, et al. Symptomatic intracranial stenosis: cerebrovascular complications from elective stent placement 1. Radiology 2007;243(1):188–97. http://dx.doi.org/10.1148/radiol.2431060139.
74. Lylyk P, Vila JF, Miranda C, et al. Partial aortic obstruction improves cerebral perfusion and clinical symptoms in patients with symptomatic vasospasm. Neurol Res 2005;27(Suppl 1):S129–35 http://dx.doi.org/10.1179/016164105X35512.
75. The SSYLVIA Study Investigators. Stenting of symptomatic atherosclerotic lesions in the vertebral or intracranial arteries (SSYLVIA): study results. Stroke 2004;35(6):1388–92. http://dx.doi.org/10.1161/01.STR.0000128708.86762.d6.
76. Zaidat OO, Castonguay AC, Nguyen TN, et al. Impact of SAMMPRIS on the future of intracranial atherosclerotic disease management: polling results from the ICAD symposium at the International Stroke Conference. J Neurointerv Surg 2014;6(3):225–30 http://dx.doi.org/10.1136/neurintsurg-2013-010667.
77. Derdeyn CP, Fiorella D, Lynn MJ, et al. Mechanisms of stroke after intracranial angioplasty and stenting in the SAMMPRIS trial. Neurosurgery 2013;72(5):777–95. http://dx.doi.org/10.1227/NEU.0b013e318286fdc8 [discussion: 795].
78. Fiorella D, Derdeyn CP, Lynn MJ, et al. Detailed analysis of periprocedural strokes in patients undergoing intracranial stenting in Stenting and Aggressive Medical Management for Preventing

Recurrent Stroke in Intracranial Stenosis (SAMMPRIS). Stroke 2012;43(10):2682–8. http://dx.doi.org/10.1161/STROKEAHA.112.661173.

79. Chimowitz MI, Fiorella D, Derdeyn CP, et al. Response to critique of the stenting and aggressive medical management for preventing recurrent stroke in intracranial stenosis (SAMMPRIS) Trial by Abou-Chebl and Steinmetz. Stroke 2012;43(10):2806–9. http://dx.doi.org/10.1161/STROKEAHA.112.661041.
80. Failure of extracranial-intracranial arterial bypass to reduce the risk of ischemic stroke. Results of an international randomized trial. The EC/IC Bypass Study Group. N Engl J Med 1985;313(19):1191–200. http://dx.doi.org/10.1056/NEJM198511073131904.
81. Powers WJ, Clarke WR, Grubb RL, et al. Extracranial-intracranial bypass surgery for stroke prevention in hemodynamic cerebral ischemia: the Carotid Occlusion Surgery Study randomized trial. JAMA 2011;306(18):1983–92. http://dx.doi.org/10.1001/jama.2011.1610.
82. Gonzalez NR, Liebeskind DS, Dusick JR, et al. Intracranial arterial stenoses: current viewpoints, novel approaches, and surgical perspectives. Neurosurg Rev 2013;36(2):175–84. http://dx.doi.org/10.1007/s10143-012-0432-z.
83. Mori T, Fukuoka M, Kazita K, et al. Follow-up study after intracranial percutaneous transluminal cerebral balloon angioplasty. AJNR Am J Neuroradiol 1998;19(8):1525–33.

Preoperative Tumor Embolization

CrossMark

Ramsey Ashour, MD[a,*], Ali Aziz-Sultan, MD[b]

KEYWORDS

• Embolization • Onyx • NBCA • Meningioma • Glomus tumor • Juvenile nasal angiofibroma • Carotid body tumor • Spinal tumor

KEY POINTS

- Preoperative endovascular tumor embolization can be used to decrease overall blood loss; to improve visualization at surgery thus facilitating tumor resection; and/or to selectively occlude deep, inaccessible arterial feeders to the tumor.
- Liquid embolic agents (eg, Onyx or NBCA) are the first-line choices for preoperative tumor embolization if distal selective arterial microcatheter access to the tumor is possible; otherwise, particle embolic agents (eg, PVA) can be used.
- Direct tumor puncture with subsequent tumor embolization is an alternative to traditional transarterial embolization for selected tumor types and locations, avoids the need for multiple vessel catheterizations to achieve tumor devascularization, and more reliably achieves intraparenchymal tumor penetration of the liquid embolic agent, which has been suggested but not proven to reduce blood loss at surgery.

INTRODUCTION

Endovascular surgery has emerged as an important tool in the treatment of a variety of hypervascular head, neck, and spinal tumors. Although the concept and first use of tumor embolization date back several decades, recent improvements in catheter design, enhanced angiographic imaging capabilities, and the development of novel embolic agents have all combined to make endovascular intervention safer, easier, and thus more commonly used in the management of selected tumors. However, deciding when and how to use endovascular therapy requires careful consideration of multiple patient- and tumor-related factors to achieve the greatest benefit while minimizing the risk of potentially dangerous complications, which may occur during or after embolization. Embolization can be used in select cases as a primary therapy to reduce tumor-related pain, prevent tumor progression, or stop acute tumor-related hemorrhage. This article focuses on preoperative elective tumor embolization, which is used to decrease blood loss and to facilitate surgical resection.

GENERAL PRINCIPLES

Indications

We are increasingly referred patients with a variety of tumors for consideration of preoperative embolization. In such cases, an *a priori* suspicion exists that the tumor is hypervascular, based on the tumor type, radiographic imaging, or possibly after a biopsy or attempted surgical resection at which time profuse bleeding was encountered. From an anatomic or technical standpoint, if embolization is deemed unfeasible or poses very high risk to a

Dr R. Ashour has no disclosures; Dr A. Aziz-Sultan is a proctor for Covidien, the manufacturer of Onyx.
[a] Department of Neurological Surgery, Lois Pope LIFE Center, University of Miami Miller School of Medicine, 1095 Northwest 14th Terrace, 2nd Floor, (D4-6), Miami, FL 33136–1060, USA; [b] Department of Neurosurgery, Brigham & Women's Hospital, 75 Francis Street, PBB-311, Boston, MA 02115, USA
* Corresponding author.
E-mail address: rashour@med.miami.edu

Neurosurg Clin N Am 25 (2014) 607–617
http://dx.doi.org/10.1016/j.nec.2014.04.015
1042-3680/14/$ – see front matter

patient, it obviously should not be attempted. However, more commonly, the relevant question is not whether embolization is feasible but rather whether it is necessary. It is important to recognize that tumor hypervascularity alone is not a good reason to subject the patient to the added risk of preoperative embolization, particularly if the tumor is small, the major blood supply to the tumor is superficial or readily accessible early at surgery (as in most meningiomas), and/or if the extra blood loss anticipated without embolization is not excessive and would be physiologically well-tolerated by the patient. However, if substantial blood loss is anticipated without embolization beyond what would be medically acceptable in a given patient harboring a sizable tumor in a difficult surgical location with numerous deep, surgically inaccessible arterial feeders, the appeal of embolization becomes readily apparent. Embolization to devascularize a tumor may also decrease procedural time, which certainly increases convenience to the surgeon, decreases anesthesia time for the patient, and may or may not reduce the total cost of treatment. Overall, the combined risks of embolization and surgery should be less than that of surgery alone to benefit the patient. In any given case, several factors may impact the decision to offer preoperative tumor embolization (**Box 1**).

Embolic Agents

Particle embolic agents

A variety of agents have been used for tumor embolization including silk, gelatin sponge, fibrin glue, and gelatin spheres (**Box 2**). Particles, such as polyvinyl alcohol (PVA) or Embospheres (Guerbet Biomedical, Louvres, France), may be used to achieve distal tumor penetration when distal, selective feeding artery catheterization is not possible. Smaller particles penetrate more deeply but carry a greater risk of inadvertent embolization of normal adjacent arterial feeders; choosing the particle diameter that maximizes the effectiveness of tumor embolization while minimizing the risk of nontarget embolization of adjacent vessels is an important step and requires experience with these agents. A major disadvantage of the particle embolic agents in current use is that they are radiolucent; therefore, the extent of tumor embolization must be determined indirectly by contrast injection. Furthermore, they have a tendency to dissipate over time, allowing for vessel recanalization before surgical resection if the embolization is performed too far in advance of the planned surgical procedure.

Box 1
Preoperative tumor embolization: relevant factors

- Lesion size, location, vascularity, edema
- Surgical accessibility of arterial feeders
- Endovascular accessibility of arterial feeders
- Proximity of important vessels at risk during embolization
- Dangerous vascular collaterals and anastomoses
- Flow dynamics within lesion
- Atherosclerosis, great vessel tortuousity
- Medical condition, anesthetic risk
- Open surgical plan and associated risk

Box 2
Embolic agents used for preoperative tumor embolization

Embolic Agent	Indication
Onyx	Intraparenchymal penetration
NBCA	Distal feeding artery occlusion
Particle embolics (PVA, Embospheres)	Flow-directed embolization when unable to achieve distal feeding artery access

Liquid embolic agents

Although particle embolic agents remain widely used at many centers as first-line agents for tumor embolization, the use of liquid embolics, such as *n*-butyl cyanoacrylate (NBCA; Codman, Raynham, MA) and Onyx (Covidien, Mansfield, MA), has increased significantly in recent years. They allow for excellent tumor capillary bed penetration but require selective feeding artery catheterization with distal microcatheter placement. NBCA is a radiopaque liquid adhesive glue that polymerizes rapidly on contact with ionic substances, such as blood, and can be injected to achieve permanent vessel occlusion. NBCA can be mixed with varying amounts of Ethiodol to modify the rate at which it polymerizes and to customize the injection flow rate and depth during embolization, which is truly "more art than science." In general, however NBCA injections must be performed rapidly and continuously and the microcatheter removed in a timely fashion. As injection time increases beyond a relatively short time window, the risk of microcatheter adherence to the glue cast or to the adjacent vessel walls increases, potentially resulting in catheter retention or vessel avulsion.

Onyx, an ethylene vinyl copolymer mixed with dimethyl sulfoxide (DMSO), is a cohesive liquid agent that gradually precipitates in a centripetal fashion after injection as the DMSO diffuses away on contact with blood. Depending on the flow dynamics within the tumor vasculature, lower (Onyx-18) or higher (Onyx-34) viscosity Onyx formulations can be selected for use during embolization. Onyx is less adherent than NBCA, and so a greater degree of reflux around the microcatheter during injection can be tolerated with less risk of catheter retention. Unlike NBCA, Onyx can be injected slowly, and the injection can be interrupted to perform angiographic runs to view the progress of embolization. Because of these properties, a greater degree of embolization can be achieved from a single vessel with Onyx than with NBCA, necessitating fewer vessel catheterizations to achieve the same degree of embolization, as a rule. Despite these advantages, Onyx has been reported to cause DMSO-related angiotoxicity[1] and pulmonary edema[2] and has the potential to create sparks during surgery if contacted by monopolar, or less frequently bipolar, cautery.[3] Furthermore, Onyx has a propensity to penetrate arterial feeders in a retrograde fashion or venous outflow channels, which if not recognized may result in nontarget embolization causing potentially significant ischemic complications.

Embolization Goals

Preoperative endovascular tumor embolization can be used to decrease overall blood loss; to improve visualization at surgery thus facilitating tumor resection; and/or to selectively occlude deep, inaccessible arterial feeders to the tumor. Transarterial embolization has been the traditional method to achieve these goals. Targeted embolization and occlusion of deep, prominent arterial feeders not accessible until late during the course of surgery is particularly useful for selected hypervascular tumors, where delicate microdissection and selective preservation of the normal, nontumor vasculature are necessitated by the site and local anatomy of the lesion. When multiple arterial feeders exist, transarterial occlusion of some may or may not result in significant overall tumor devascularization if others are left patent; however, if the remaining patent vessels are readily accessible at surgery, there may still be a significant benefit to selective embolization of only the deep feeders.

Even when near-complete or complete angiographic devascularization is achieved after preoperative feeding artery occlusion, surgeons may still note that the tumor bleeds significantly at surgery, reflecting collateralization and/or angiographically occult vascularization after embolization. It has been suggested but not substantiated that intraparenchymal tumor penetration of the embolic agent results in less operative blood loss compared with arterial feeding artery occlusion alone.[4] Furthermore, it has been reported that intraparenchymal tumor penetration with Onyx is difficult to achieve by a transarterial route unless the microcatheter is situated within 2 cm of the tumor.[5] In our experience,[6] intraparenchymal tumor penetration of Onyx is best achieved by direct tumor puncture, which is an option in certain types of tumors (**Box 3**), but obviously not all tumors can be accessed directly. Another advantage of embolization by direct puncture is that it offers the opportunity to achieve significant tumor devascularization while avoiding the need to catheterize multiple arterial feeders to the lesion, which may be difficult or dangerous to access transarterially.

TUMOR EMBOLIZATION PROCEDURE DETAILS

Anesthesia

We prefer to perform all tumor embolization procedures with the patient fully anesthetized and intubated. This minimizes patient motion and allows for intermittent suspension of the patient's respirations, which greatly enhances angiographic visualization during embolization. Furthermore, the DMSO in Onyx is angiotoxic and makes injection of this embolic agent quite painful and poorly tolerated in awake patients. For cooperative patients, intravenous sedation and appropriate analgesia without general anesthesia may be considered in selected cases, such as proximal segmental spinal artery occlusions using NBCA.

Angiography

Percutaneous transfemoral artery angiography is performed to delineate the extent of tumor blush, arterial supply, tumor flow dynamics, and venous drainage, and to identify important normal vasculature to be preserved. Using standard endovascular techniques, 5F guide catheters and

Box 3
Hypervascular tumors amenable to embolization by direct puncture

Juvenile nasal angiofibromas
Carotid body tumors
Glomus vagale tumors
Other head and neck tumors

DMSO-compatible microcatheters are generally used to access the target vessels leading to the tumor. Intravenous heparinization is initiated to achieve and maintain an activated clotting time of 200 to 300 seconds. A microangiogram should always be performed before embolization to ascertain tumor vascularity and identify any dangerous anastomoses to the adjacent normal vasculature.

Embolization

Liquid embolic embolization should be performed as close to the lesion as possible to achieve maximal intratumoral penetration of embolic material. Direct tumor puncture can be performed in selected cases using an 18-gauge spinal needle, with subsequent angiography and embolization carried out through the needle, as detailed previously.[6] We typically use NBCA for distal feeding artery occlusion in cases where Onyx embolization is believed to be either too risky or unnecessary. For example, if the local vascular anatomy is such that deep intratumoral penetration of Onyx poses a high risk of nontarget embolization into important adjacent vessels, or if there is not enough of a safe distance proximally on the target vessel to allow for enough Onyx reflux to form an adequate "plug" (which must occur before the Onyx is able to be "pushed" forward), then we favor NBCA to achieve a focal occlusion of the target vessel. In selected tumors with rapid arteriovenous shunting, in which there is concern that an injected liquid embolic agent may inadvertently flow through the lesion and into the venous side, coils may be deployed first to partially devascularize the tumor, making it safer to then use the desired liquid embolic agent.

In those instances where distal selective catheterization is not possible, we prefer to use PVA particles for preoperative tumor embolization. This requires a slightly larger microcatheter than those used for liquid embolic embolization and also demands a careful review of the local vascular anatomy to identify potentially dangerous collaterals and to choose appropriately sized particles.

Postprocedure Care

After embolization, follow-up angiography demonstrates the extent of tumor devascularization and is also necessary to evaluate patency of the important adjacent normal vasculature. Intravenous steroids are often given to mitigate the expected peritumoral edema that occurs as a consequence of embolization. Routine postangiography care includes groin and distal pulse checks and frequent neurologic examinations to detect any clinical deterioration, which may be secondary to ischemia, hemorrhage, or postembolization tumor swelling.

COMPLICATIONS

Complications may occur during or after embolization and are secondary to the inherent risks of anesthesia, angiography, embolization, the embolic agent used, and/or the type and location of the tumor, among other factors. The clinical consequences of embolization-related ischemia, hemorrhage, and/or edema depend highly on the tumor's size and location in addition to the specific details of the embolization procedure that was

Table 1
Tumor embolization complication types and management

Ischemia	Continue heparinization Consider antiplatelet therapy Support blood pressure, fluid status
Hemorrhage	Reverse heparin Lower blood pressure Balloon tamponade or endovascular sacrifice of perforated vessel
Peritumoral edema	Intravenous steroids Resect tumor
Retained microcatheter (stuck to liquid embolic cast)	Pull catheter until it comes out or breaks, if not safe to pull, cut catheter at groin
Allergic reaction to contrast	Antihistamine, steroids, bronchodilators, protect airway, intravenous fluids
Groin hematoma or pseudoaneurysm	Tamponade Ultrasound-guided thrombin injection to obliterate pseudoaneurysm
Retroperitoneal hematoma	Supportive care in most cases Surgical intervention for significant bleeding and hemodynamic instability

performed. **Table 1** summarizes potential complications related to tumor embolization procedures with suggested management options.

SPECIFIC HYPERVASCULAR TUMORS AMENABLE TO EMBOLIZATION

Intracranial Tumors

Meningiomas and hemangiopericytomas

Intracranial meningiomas are often histopathologically benign, dural-based, avidly enhancing lesions arising from arachnoid cap cells; depending on their location, they may present with focal neurologic deficits, seizures, headaches, visual loss, or cognitive dysfunction (**Box 4**, **Fig. 1**). Intracranial hemangiopericytomas are meningeal sarcomatous tumors arising from capillary wall pericytes that often mimic meningiomas but tend to behave more aggressively, are more often hypervascular, and typically are diagnosed postoperatively in cases thought to be meningioma preoperatively. Preoperative embolization has been used to reduce blood loss, decrease operative time, and facilitate more aggressive resection of these hypervascular lesions. In general, because meningiomas are dural-based lesions, their blood supply is often superficial and accessible early at surgery (eg, superficial temporal, occipital, middle meningeal, and posterior meningeal arteries). Therefore, most convexity meningiomas need not be embolized. Meningiomas closely associated with or involving major venous sinuses are riskier to embolize. Deep skull base meningiomas are often difficult and dangerous to embolize, because they may be closely associated with cranial nerves and be supplied by deep internal carotid, vertebrobasilar, ascending pharyngeal, and petrosquamosal middle meningeal branches, all of which are higher-risk vessels to embolize. In our opinion, the type of meningioma that stands to gain most from preoperative embolization is the giant convexity lesion with such exuberant and multidirectional blood supply that simply opening the bone flap can result in catastrophic blood loss. Overall, the role of preoperative meningioma embolization is not well-defined, and there is wide variability across major academic centers in terms of the indications and goals for embolizing these lesions.

Box 4
Hypervascular tumors amenable to preoperative embolization

Intracranial
- Meningioma
- Hemangiopericytoma
- Hemangioblastoma
- Glomus jugulare tumor
- Metastases (renal cell)

Head and neck
- Juvenile nasal angiofibroma
- Carotid body tumor
- Glomus vagale tumor

Spinal
- Hemangioblastoma
- Hemangioma
- Aneurysmal bone cyst
- Giant cell tumor
- Osteoblastoma
- Metastases (renal cell, thyroid)

Hemangioblastomas

Hemangioblastomas are vascular tumors; are composed of endothelial cells, pericytes, and stromal cells; account for less than 2% of central nervous system tumors; and may be sporadic or may occur in association with von Hippel-Lindau disease (**Fig. 2**). They are typically avidly enhancing cerebellar tumors and may be solid or cystic with an associated mural nodule. Hypervascularity by angiography helps to support the diagnosis of hemangioblastoma over other potential tumor types (eg, metastasis) and is also useful to delineate the arterial blood supply in advance of surgical resection.

Cerebellar hemangioblastomas are typically supplied by branches of the posterior-inferior, anterior-inferior, and superior cerebellar arteries. We occasionally perform embolization for these tumors, particularly if the lesion is large, the arterial feeders are deep and inaccessible until late at surgery, and the local vascular anatomy is favorable for microcatheter access. However, because of the presence of important brainstem perforators in this region, the threshold to perform embolization is necessarily higher for these tumors. Furthermore, it must be recognized that after embolization of any posterior fossa tumor, the consequences of postembolization peritumoral edema are significantly increased and potentially life-threatening because of the risk of brainstem compression or herniation.

Glomus jugulare tumors

Glomus jugulare paragangliomas are embryonic neural crest–derived neuroendocrine tumors arising from the adventitia of the jugular bulb. They may present as a middle ear mass with

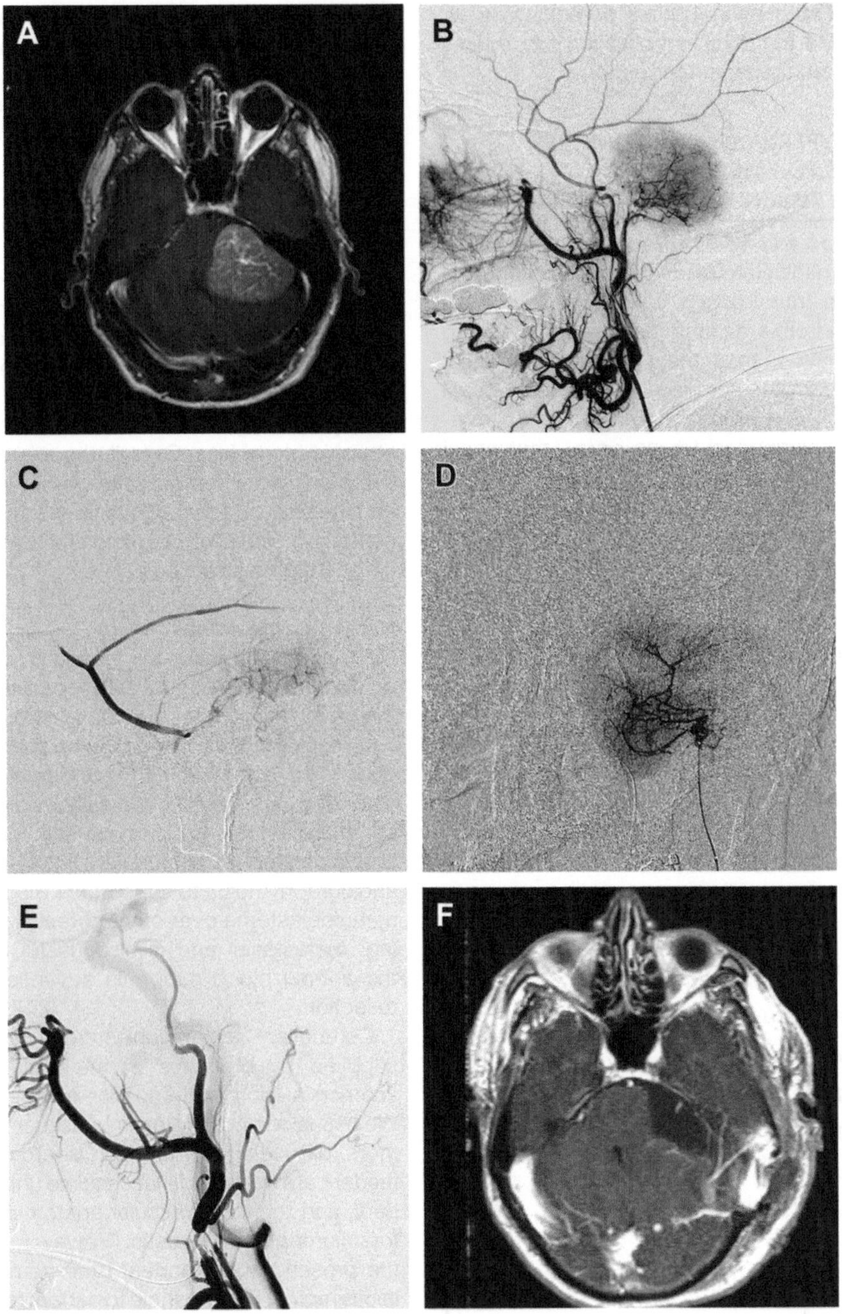

Fig. 1. Large petrous meningioma with prominent intratumoral blood vessels visualized on (*A*) contrast-enhanced magnetic resonance imaging (MRI). (*B*) Left external carotid artery angiogram demonstrating hyper-vascular tumor blush fed by ascending pharyngeal and middle meningeal arteries. (*C*) Left middle meningeal and (*D*) left ascending pharyngeal artery selective catheterization and embolization with Onyx was performed. (*E*) Final left external carotid artery angiogram demonstrates near-complete tumor devascularization. (*F*) Postoperative MRI demonstrates successful resection of the tumor.

tinnitus or hearing loss or may present with lower cranial nerve compressive symptoms including hoarseness, swallowing difficulty, trapezius and sternocleidomastoid muscle weakness, and so forth. Rarely, they may also present with symptoms of catecholamine hypersecretion. They have a classic salt-and-pepper appearance on magnetic resonance imaging and demonstrate

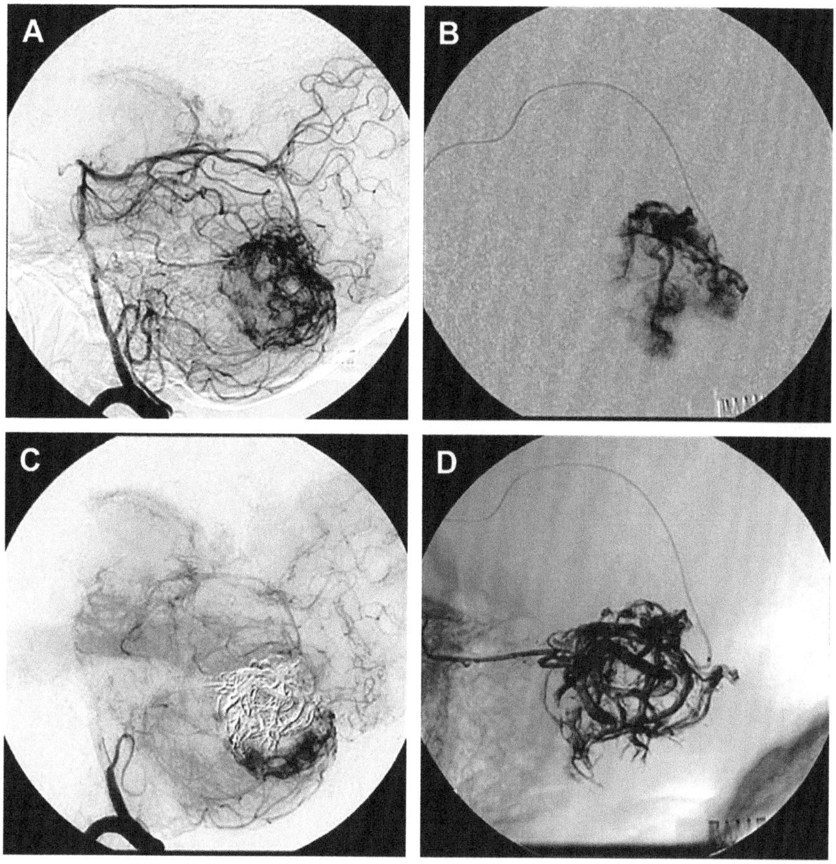

Fig. 2. Cerebellar hemangioblastoma with hypervascular tumor blush demonstrated on (*A*) right vertebral artery angiogram fed by superior cerebellar and posterior inferior cerebellar artery branches. (*B*) Pre-embolization microangiogram after superselective superior cerebellar artery branch catheterization demonstrating the tumor blush. (*C*) Final postembolization angiogram demonstrates significant tumor devascularization. (*D*) Native skull radiographic view demonstrates dense Onyx cast within the parenchyma of the tumor, which was subsequently resected.

uptake of octreotide on single-photon emission tomography scanning because of the presence of somatostatin receptors. Hypervascular tumor blush on angiography helps to support the diagnosis of a glomus tumor and is also useful to delineate the arterial supply to the tumor, the patency of the ipsilateral sigmoid sinus and internal jugular vein, and determine venous sinus dominance, all of which are important surgical considerations. These tumors are typically supplied by the ascending pharyngeal artery, but may also receive supply from the internal carotid, middle meningeal, posterior auricular, occipital, and posterior meningeal arteries, among others. In our recent experience[7] using Onyx by a transarterial route, we were able to achieve excellent preoperative glomus jugulare tumor devascularization (mean, 90.7%) in all 11 cases, but at the expense of permanent cranial nerve neuropathy in two (18%) patients, which has tempered our enthusiasm for embolizing these tumors with Onyx. Others[8,9] have reported success using PVA particles, although the overall number of patients embolized in this manner is small. Currently, the role of embolization in the management of glomus jugulare tumors remains to be defined.

Head and Neck Tumors

Carotid body tumors and glomus vagale tumors

Carotid body tumors are the most common of the head and neck paragangliomas, whereas glomus vagale tumors are relatively rare (**Fig. 3**). Carotid body tumors typically present as a palpable, pulsatile neck mass, which is initially asymptomatic but may later cause pain, hoarseness, dysphagia, Horner syndrome, shoulder drop, tongue weakness, or rarely signs and symptoms of catecholamine hypersecretion. They have a classic angiographic appearance where the tumor can be seen as a hypervascular blush that sits within

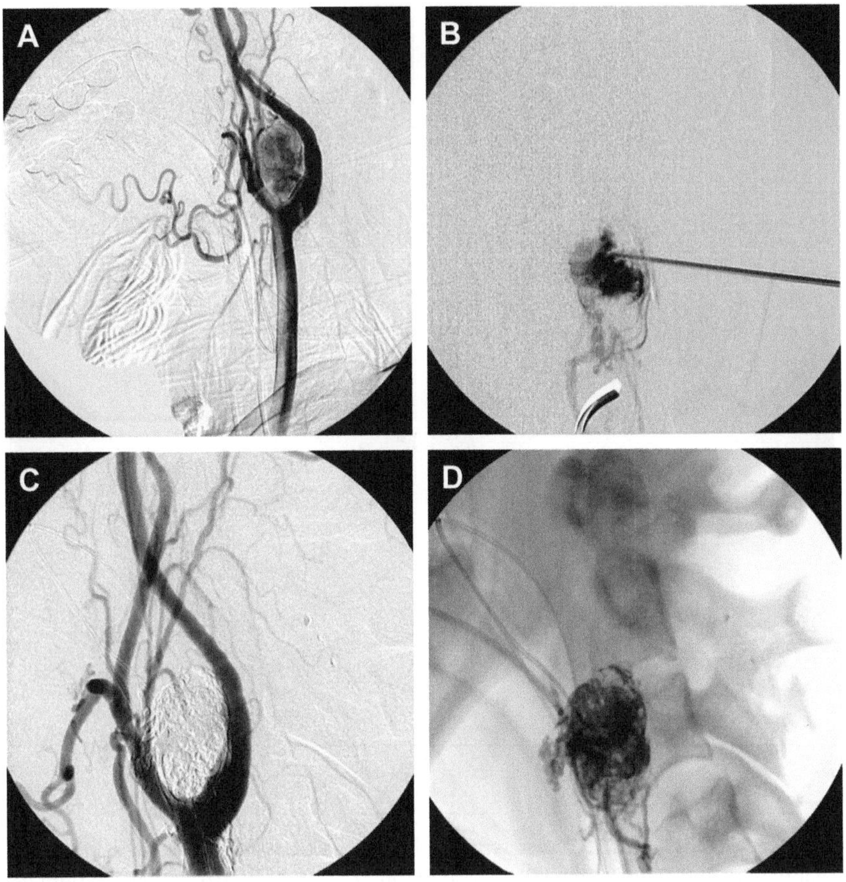

Fig. 3. Carotid body tumor with hypervascular tumor blush splaying the internal and external carotid arteries demonstrated on (*A*) left common carotid artery angiogram. (*B*) Intralesional angiogram performed through a percutaneously inserted 20-gauge spinal needle in advance of Onyx embolization. (*C*) Postembolization left common carotid artery angiogram demonstrates near-complete tumor devascularization. (*D*) Native neck radiographic view demonstrates dense Onyx cast within the parenchyma of the tumor, which was subsequently resected.

the "V" of the carotid bifurcation and "splays out" the internal and external carotid arteries. Furthermore, the ascending pharyngeal artery reliably ascends posteriorly and feeds the tumor from above, although other external carotid branches may also contribute. Glomus vagale tumors occur along the path of the vagus nerve, are situated more rostrally than carotid body tumors, and by virtue of their association with the vagus nerve they tend to push the carotid artery anteriorly rather than splay it while also displacing the internal jugular vein posteriorly. They typically present as a painless pulsatile neck mass near the angle of the mandible, and up to half of patients have evidence of vocal cord dysfunction, secondary to involvement of the vagus nerve. As with carotid body tumors, glomus vagale tumors tend to be supplied by an enlarged ascending pharyngeal artery in addition to other external carotid branches.

Transarterial embolization has traditionally been used to devascularize carotid body and glomus vagale tumors preoperatively, and although this approach is generally safe, direct tumor puncture offers distinct advantages. First, the amount of devascularization achieved transarterially through a single feeding pedicle is often subtotal, and multiple feeders must often be catheterized to achieve near-complete devascularization of the tumor. This translates into an overall increased procedure time and potentially an increased risk associated with multiple vessel catheterizations. Second, small tortuous feeders are potentially difficult to catheterize, which may limit how close to the lesion the microcatheter is placed. This lessens the likelihood of achieving intraparenchymal penetration in some cases when liquid embolic agents are used. Finally, there is a small but real risk of inadvertent embolization into the distal ascending pharyngeal or even into the internal carotid artery when a transarterial approach is used to embolize these tumors. Recently, we have had success using direct puncture for embolization of carotid body and glomus vagale tumors with excellent devascularization achieved and no major complications[6]; this has become our preferred approach to these tumors.

Juvenile nasal angiofibromas

Juvenile nasal angiofibromas are the most common primary tumor of the nasopharynx, tend to occur in adolescent males, and frequently present with nasal obstruction and recurrent epistaxis (**Fig. 4**).[10] They are highly vascular tumors typically supplied by the internal maxillary artery in addition to numerous external and internal carotid artery branches, unilaterally or bilaterally. Preoperative embolization, either transarterially or by direct puncture, is very useful to reduce blood loss and to improve visualization during endoscopic surgical resection of these otherwise bloody tumors. However, although there is little doubt that embolization reduces blood loss, some authors have suggested that embolization may lead to a suboptimal degree of tumor removal at surgery, particularly for those lesions that exhibit deep sphenoid invasion, potentially leading to increased recurrence rates.[11–13] We have evaluated our experience in a limited number of patients prospectively comparing transarterial and direct endoscopically assisted tumor puncture for preoperative juvenile nasal angiofibromas embolization and found no significant difference in blood loss between these two modalities, although there was a trend toward less blood loss and mean devascularization was greater in the direct-puncture group.[14] Care must be taken to avoid embolizing superficial branches feeding the skin of the face, which can lead to discoloration if Onyx is used or lead to ischemic necrosis if the blood supply to

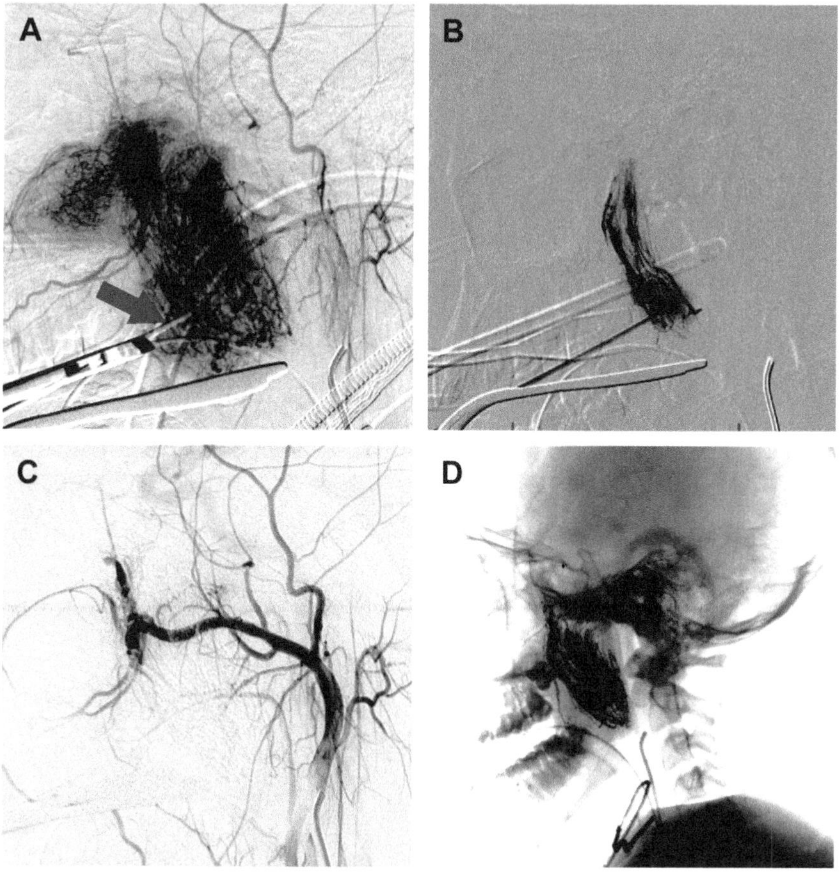

Fig. 4. Juvenile nasal angiofibroma with hypervascular tumor blush demonstrated on (*A*) lateral left external carotid artery angiogram fed by internal maxillary branches. An 18-gauge spinal needle (*arrow*) was inserted directly into the tumor transnasally under endoscopic guidance. (*B*) Intralesional angiogram by contrast injection through the spinal needle in advance of Onyx embolization. (*C*) Postembolization left external carotid artery angiogram demonstrates near-complete tumor devascularization. (*D*) Native skull radiographic view demonstrates dense Onyx cast within the parenchyma of the tumor, which was subsequently resected.

the skin is significantly compromised beyond the compensatory ability of collaterals to the face.[15] Furthermore, care must be taken to visualize and protect the blood supply to the eye, which may arise from the external carotid branches in a small but significant percentage of cases.

Spinal Tumors

Box 4 lists spinal tumors commonly considered for preoperative tumor embolization (**Fig. 5**). When performing spinal angiography to evaluate for preoperative tumor embolization, segmental arteries

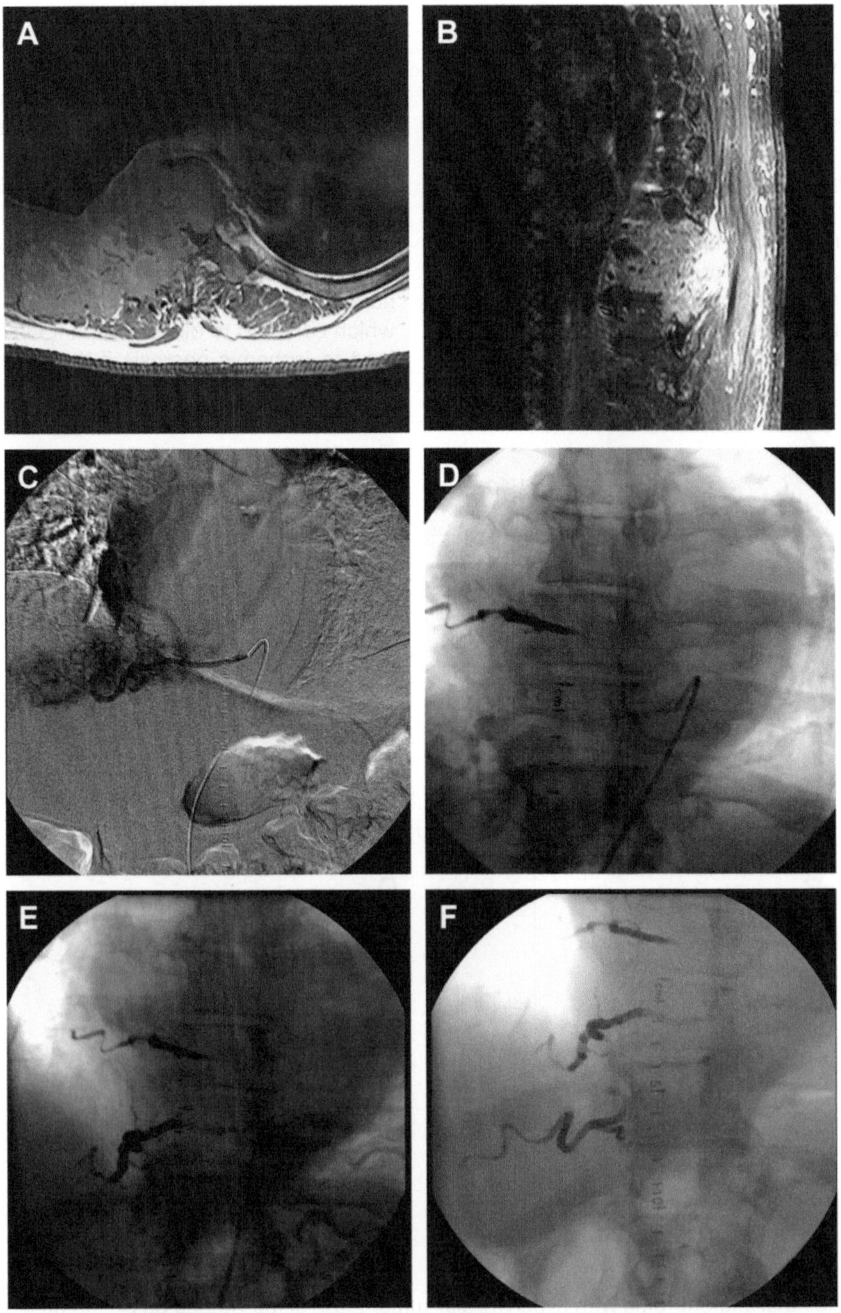

Fig. 5. Metastatic renal cell carcinoma. (*A*) Axial and (*B*) sagittal contrast-enhanced MRI demonstrate a large mass with retroperitoneal, paraspinal, and intraspinal components involving predominantly T8-T9 thoracic levels. Preoperative Onyx embolization of the right T7-T10 segmental feeding vessels was performed. (*C*) T9 segmental artery angiogram demonstrates the hypervascular tumor blush. (*D–F*) Native radiographic views demonstrate Onyx casts within the T8, T9, and T10 segmental vessels (T7 was also embolized but not shown).

must be catheterized at least two levels above and below the level of the tumor to adequately assess its vascular supply and to avoid missing important arterial feeders. The normal blood supply to the spinal cord must also be visualized. For cervical tumors, the vertebral arteries, external carotid arteries, thyrocervical and costocervical trunks, and the supreme intercostal arteries must be injected. For thoracic vertebral body lesions, the right intercostal artery often supplies the anterior vertebral body, whereas the left intercostal artery supplies the posterior vertebral body.[16] In the lumbosacral region, both iliac arteries and the median sacral artery must be injected. The artery of Adamkiewicz and feeding arteries with concomitant medullary supply or *en passage* vessels must be recognized before embolization.

Spinal angiography is performed using anterior-posterior fluoroscopy only with a radiopaque measuring ruler placed on the table to mark the spinal levels during the procedure. Visualization may be improved by suspending respiration during image acquisition, and glucagon can be administered to decrease gastrointestinal mobility. Although the catheters and techniques used for spinal angiography differ somewhat from those used in the head and neck, the same tumor embolization principles discussed for head and neck tumors also apply to spinal tumors. A microangiogram should always be performed before embolization to ascertain tumor vascularity and identify any dangerous anastomoses to the normal spinal cord vasculature. Complications related to ischemia, hemorrhage, and edema may occur after spinal tumor embolization, resulting in neurologic deficits including and below relevant spinal level.

SUMMARY

Endovascular surgery is an important tool in the management of a wide variety of hypervascular head, neck, and spinal tumors, and can be used relatively safely to achieve significant preoperative tumor devascularization to decrease blood loss and facilitate surgical resection. As technology advances forward and further studies are conducted, the indications, techniques, and goals of tumor embolization will continue to evolve in a manner that maximizes the overall benefit to patients.

REFERENCES

1. Chaloupka JC, Vinuela F, Vinters HV, et al. Technical feasibility and histopathologic studies of ethylene vinyl copolymer (EVAL) using a swine endovascular embolization model. AJNR Am J Neuroradiol 1994;15(6):1107–15.
2. Murugesan C, Saravanan S, Rajkumar J, et al. Severe pulmonary oedema following therapeutic embolization with Onyx for cerebral arteriovenous malformation. Neuroradiology 2008;50(5):439–42.
3. Schirmer CM, Zerris V, Malek AM. Electrocautery-induced ignition of spark showers and self-sustained combustion of Onyx ethylene-vinyl alcohol copolymer. Neurosurgery 2006;59(4 Suppl 2):ONS413–8.
4. Elhammady MS, Wolfe SQ, Ashour R, et al. Safety and efficacy of vascular tumor embolization using Onyx: is angiographic devascularization sufficient? J Neurosurg 2010;112(5):1039–45.
5. Gore P, Theodore N, Brasiliense L, et al. The utility of Onyx for preoperative embolization of cranial and spinal tumors. Neurosurgery 2008;62(6):1204–11 [discussion: 1211–2].
6. Elhammady MS, Peterson EC, Johnson JN, et al. Preoperative onyx embolization of vascular head and neck tumors by direct puncture. World Neurosurg 2012;77(5–6):725–30.
7. Gaynor BG, Elhammady MS, Jethanamest D, et al. Incidence of cranial nerve palsy after preoperative embolization of glomus jugulare tumors using Onyx. J Neurosurg 2014;120(2):377–81.
8. Larouere MJ, Zappia JJ, Wilner HI, et al. Selective embolization of glomus jugulare tumors. Skull Base Surg 1994;4(1):21–5.
9. White JB, Link MJ, Cloft HJ. Endovascular embolization of paragangliomas: a safe adjuvant to treatment. J Vasc Interv Neurol 2008;1(2):37–41.
10. Gullane PJ, Davidson J, O'Dwyer T, et al. Juvenile angiofibroma: a review of the literature and a case series report. Laryngoscope 1992;102(8):928–33.
11. Lloyd G, Howard D, Phelps P, et al. Juvenile angiofibroma: the lessons of 20 years of modern imaging. J Laryngol Otol 1999;113(2):127–34.
12. Lloyd G, Howard D, Lund VJ, et al. Imaging for juvenile angiofibroma. J Laryngol Otol 2000;114(9):727–30.
13. Mann WJ, Jecker P, Amedee RG. Juvenile angiofibromas: changing surgical concept over the last 20 years. Laryngoscope 2004;114(2):291–3.
14. Elhammady MS, Johnson JN, Peterson EC, et al. Preoperative embolization of juvenile nasopharyngeal angiofibromas: transarterial versus direct tumoral puncture. World Neurosurg 2011;76(3–4):328–34 [discussion: 263–5].
15. Ashour R, Aziz-Sultan MA, Soltanolkotabi M, et al. Safety and efficacy of Onyx embolization for pediatric cranial and spinal vascular lesions and tumors. Neurosurgery 2012;71(4):773–84.
16. Djindjian RM, Merland J, Djindjian M, et al. Angiography of spinal column and spinal cord tumors. In: Neuroradiologic Atlas. New York: Thieme; 1981.

Index

Note: Page numbers of article titles are in **boldface** type.

Neurosurg Clin N Am 25 (2014) 619–627
http://dx.doi.org/10.1016/S1042-3680(14)00052-7
1042-3680/14/$ – see front matter

D

V

W

X

Y

Printed and bound by CPI Group (UK) Ltd, Croydon, CR0 4YY
03/10/2024
01040377-0003